Effective Practice in Health and Social Care

A PARTNERSHIP APPROACH

Effective Practice in Health and Social Care

A PARTNERSHIP APPROACH

Edited by Ros Carnwell and Julian Buchanan

Open University Press

Open University Press
McGraw-Hill Education
McGraw-Hill House
Shoppenhangers Road
Maidenhead
Berkshire
England
SL6 2QL

email: enquiries@openup.co.uk
world wide web: www.openup.co.uk

and Two Penn Plaza, New York, NY 10121–2289, USA

First published 2005

A catalogue record of this book is available from the British Library

ISBN 0335 21437 1 (pb) 0335 21438 X (hb)

Library of Congress Cataloguing-in-Publication Data
CIP data applied for

Typeset by RefineCatch Ltd, Bungay, Suffolk
Printed in the UK by Bell & Bain Ltd, Glasgow

Contents

Notes on the contributors

Dr Althea Allison is Manager at the Office for Research Ethics Committees (OREC), for Thames Valley, Hampshire and the Isle of Wight and is seconded part-time for one year as Deputy Director of Operations, COREC (Central Office for Research Ethics Committees). Althea is a registered mental health nurse, and previous professional roles have included working as a mental health nurse both in hospitals and as a community mental health nurse. She has also taught and supervised community nurses. She has written for a number of nursing journals, and contributed a chapter on *Ethical Issues in Cognitive Behaviour Therapy* in *Cognitive Behaviour Therapy: An Introduction to Theory and Practice* (1996) edited by Sue Marshall and John Turnbull, Balliere Tindall, London.

John Bates is a qualified social worker and teacher. As a social worker he worked in local authority field social work and in residential work in the voluntary sector. He has been a teacher of social work for many years and is currently head of the Social Welfare and Community Justice Department at North East Wales Institute of Higher Education. His research interests include information technology and social work, men and masculinity, and he has published on both subjects. He is the joint editor of *Protecting Children: Challenges and Change* and is a book reviewer for the British Journal of Social Work. He is also a member of the Institute of Teaching and Learning in Higher Education.

Liz Blyth has worked in health, social care, community development and neighbourhood renewal for the past thirteen years, with experience of work in both the voluntary and statutory sectors. She currently works as Cultural Strategy Manager at Leicester City Council supporting the multi-agency partnership responsible for implementing 'Diverse City: Leicester's Cultural Strategy'. Prior to this she worked for five years for Coventry City Council as Co-ordinator for the Coventry Domestic Violence Partnership, a multi-agency forum developing Coventry's strategic response to domestic abuse. Liz has a diploma in Youth and Community Work and a Masters in Management, Organisation and Change from Loughborough University.

Julian Buchanan is a Reader in Community Justice and member of the Social Inclusion Research Unit at NEWI, Wrexham. Prior to this he worked at the University of Central Lancashire, and University of Liverpool. In the mid-1980s, as a drugs specialist with the Merseyside Probation Service, he pioneered a 'risk reduction' approach, and was instrumental in establishing one of the largest inter-agency community drugs teams in the UK. He has published in a wide range of journals including: *Social Work Education*; *Practice*; *Journal of Social Work in Mental Health*; *Drugs: Education, Prevention, Policy*; *Probation Journal*; *BJCJ*; and *Community Care*. He is currently Deputy Editor of the *Probation Journal*, Series Editor of ICCJ Monographs, and on the British Journal of Community Justice (BJCJ) Editorial Board. His research interests include substance misuse; criminal justice, inequality and social reintegration.

Professor Ros Carnwell worked as a health visitor for eight years, before teaching health visiting and researching in primary care at the University of Keele, Manchester Metropolitan University and the University of Wolverhampton. She is currently Professor and Director of the Centre for Health and Community Research at North East Wales Institute, Wrexham, where she manages funded projects, mainly in primary/community care settings. Her research interests include: developing nursing roles in primary care, evaluation of health and social care provision, and educational research. She is particularly interested in opportunities for collaborative research and creating opportunities to involve users in the research process and to develop research capacity in nursing through involvement of novice researchers in research projects.

Dr Alex Carson is currently a Reader in Nursing Studies at North East Wales Institute. After a number of years as a practitioner in acute surgery, Alex has worked in nurse education for over fifteen years. His main teaching interests have been in health-care ethics. He has a doctorate in sociology from Edinburgh University and has been developing new teaching and research methods, using a narrative-based approach. He has published in nursing and medical journals and is in the process of writing a book about narratives in research, education and practice.

Dr Pat Chambers has been a Lecturer in the School of Social Relations at Keele University since June 2000, working on social work and gerontology programmes. She is Programme Director for the new undergraduate degree in social work. Pat is currently book review editor for the journal *Practice* and a trustee of Age Concern, Cheshire. Recently completed research projects are: 'Lifelong learning in care settings': video and report (Evaluation of a Department of Health funded project carried out by the National Institute of Adult and Continuing Education, NIACE). 'New Horizons – older women and I.T.': report (Working with Age Concern, Cheshire on a project funded by Averil Osborn Fund which seeks to explore the I.T. learning needs of older women). Her most recent publications are: 'Self-indulgence or an essential tool? The use of a field diary in biographical research and narrative analysis' in C. Horrocks, N. Kelly, B. Roberts and D. Robinson (eds) (2004) *Narrative, Memory and Identity* Huddersfield, Huddersfield University Press; Researching 'with' older widows': reflections on the process *Autobiography* (2003).

Dr Michael Clark has been the Research and Development Manager for the last five years for Wolverhampton City Primary Care Trust and its predecessor organizations. Previously, he was a full-time researcher leading to a PhD in quality developments at the University of Wolverhampton. While taking an overview of research across the whole range of activities in the Trust he has developed particular interests in various aspects of mental health and learning disabilities. He is also currently the National Manager for the Mental Health Research and Development Portfolio at the Department of Health.

Professor Brian Corby is at the Social Work Studies Department at the University of Central Lancashire. His research interests are in the field of safeguarding children and child care social work, with particular emphasis on assessment, interprofessional communication and service users' views. He has published widely in these fields and is the author of *Child Abuse – Towards a Knowledge Base* published by Open University Press (2000).

Professor David Jolley is currently Professor of Old Age Psychiatry, University of Wolverhampton; the Director of Dementia Plus, West Midlands and a Consultant Psychiatrist, Wolverhampton City PCT, having previous worked in South Manchester from 1975 to 1995. David moved to Wolverhampton in 1995 where he was Medical Director of the Community Health Trust until retirement in 2003. He continues to work in a clinical role on a part-time basis, and is a member of an expanding team undertaking research, training, education, support and advice at Wolverhampton University and Dementia Plus. David's current research interests are many and varied and include the treatment and outcome in Alzheimer's disease, ethnicity and mental health and spirituality, faith and health in later life.

Thoby Miller is Senior Lecturer in Youth and Community Education at the North East Wales Institute. His research interests include theoretical and practice-based links between informal and formal education and integrating eco-literacy and emotional awareness into formal education settings. Thoby's publications include *The formalisation of education*, a paper delivered to Dilemmas in Professional Practice Conference at the University of Stafford 2000; and Riding the Cusp / Courir deux lièvres à la fois – *European Journal of Social Education* No. 2 – 2002.

Amir Minhas is a probation officer working for the National Probation Service in Merseyside. Amir has worked as a probation officer for seven years, and also has an MA and diploma in Social Work.

Dr Virginia Minogue PhD is Head of Research and Development in the South West Yorkshire Mental Health NHS Trust and Associate Lecturer with the Open University. She has an Honorary Research Fellowship in the School of Medicine, from the Academic Unit of Primary Care, University of Leeds. Virginia's particular areas of interest are mentally-disordered offenders, user and carer involvement in service evaluation, service development and research, and partnership working. She was previously a Senior Lecturer in Community Justice in Sheffield. Prior to this she worked for a number of years in the Probation Service as a manager, research officer, family court welfare officer and probation officer. She is a Director of a voluntary sector mental health organization with specific responsibility for the monitoring and evaluation of services.

Dr Neil Moreland is currently a Research Fellow in Employability at the Open University. His research activities in dementia arose when he took redundancy in 2000 from the University of Wolverhampton, where he was Associate Dean of the School of Education. Neil then became a jobbing researcher, carrying out research projects for Dementia Plus, West Midlands and other organizations involved in rural widening participation activities. Neil obtained his PhD in Applied Social Studies from the University of Warwick.

Lester Parrott is Senior Lecturer in Social Work at North East Wales Institute. He is the author of *Social Work and Social Care*, an introductory text in social policy for social workers. Recent publications include: *Researching the effects of child abuse*, in J. Bates, R. Pugh and N. Thompson (1997) *Protecting Children: Challenges and Change*, Arena, Aldershot; *Social Work and Social Care* (1999), Gildredge Press, Eastbourne; Social Policy (2000), Prospects, Wrexham; *Social Work Values/ Gwerthoedd Gwaith Cymdeithasol* (2000), Welsh Language Development Board/ CCETSW Cymru; *Social Work and Social Care* (2002), Gildredge Series/Routledge, London. 2nd edition.

Professor Judith Phillips is Professor of Social Work at the University of Wales, Swansea. Her research interests are primarily concerned with social gerontology, gender issues, community care social work and social care issues. She has widely researched and published on carers in employment, care management, inter-generational family relationships across Europe and older people living in urban areas.

Dr Richard Pugh is Reader in Social Work at Keele University and has published widely on minority language issues, child care, social work theory, and rural social work. He is currently developing networks of interested practitioners, teachers and researchers and policy makers in rural services. He is a member of the editorial advisory committee for the international journal *Rural Social Work*. Recent publications include: Considering the countryside: is there a case for rural social work? (*British Journal of Social Work*, 2003); Understanding language practice, policy and provision in social work, in J. Kornbeck (ed.) *Language Teaching in the Social Work Curriculum*, Logophon Verlag 2003); Preparing for linguistically sensitive practice, in S. Barrett, C. Komaromy and A. Rogers (eds) *Communication, Relationships and Care: A Reader* (Routledge 2004); Responding to racism: delivering local services, in J. Garland and N. Chakraborti (eds) *Racism, Identity and Community in Rural Britain* (Willan Publishing 2004).

Kate Read took a first degree at Keele University and subsequently a Masters in social work at the University of Kent. More recently she completed a second masters degree in gerontology. She has worked for Wolverhampton Social Services from 1980 firstly as a social worker, approved social worker and team leader. After a period coordinating day services she moved into service development and commissioning, focusing on mental health and, more latterly, older people and older people with mental health needs. In October 2000 Kate became Executive Director of Dementia Plus, the Dementia Services Development Centre for the West Midlands, where she is involved in staff and service development as well as research projects concerning dementia and older people with mental health needs.

Angela Roberts is a qualified nurse and health visitor, currently working as Health Visitor Project Lead for the Welsh Assembly Government-funded Inequalities in Health Initiative: 'Redressing the Balance'. Angela has worked for over 10 years with travellers both locally and nationally, and has presented at various conferences on travellers and health visiting.

Ruth Wilson is the Community Mental Health Nurse Specialist for HIV/AIDS based within the Palliative Care Directorate of Reading Primary Care Trust. She is responsible for the monitoring and care of the mental health of people with HIV in Berkshire and facilitating treatment as necessary, working as part of the multidisciplinary team within the local HIV services. She recently completed her MA in Health and Nursing Studies, researching the lived experience of taking Highly Active Antiretroviral Therapy as the treatment for HIV for her dissertation. Her current research interests are qualitative research into the experience of being diagnosed HIV positive during pregnancy and the ongoing stigma that accompanies HIV and its impact on adherence to treatment.

Ruth Wyner has spent twenty years working in the homelessness sector. She started as a project worker at Norwich Night Shelter in 1979 and a few years later became Deputy Director of the organization running it, St. Martin's Housing Trust. In 1994 she moved to Great Yarmouth where she set up a new hostel with move-on accommodation for the Herring House Trust, and in 1995 she took up post as Director of Wintercomfort for the homeless in Cambridge. Ruth was Chair of the Norfolk Voluntary Hostels Group for five years and was a director of the National Homelessness Alliance. She now works as a group analyst and is co-ordinator of The Dialogue Trust, which convenes dialogue groups for offenders in prisons and in the community. Her book about prison, *From the Inside*, was published by Aurum Press in 2003 and she has published articles in various journals and magazines.

Preface

This book is essentially about effective practice, recognizing that today the needs of a client/patient/service user can rarely be met by one single agency or using one single method of intervention. The book recognizes the realities of practice intervention in the 21st century welfare state where collaboration, working together and partnership between various statutory, voluntary and independent organizations are essential elements of any packages of care.

The book is presented in three parts covering the theory and practice of partnership, with the main emphasis being on effective practice. It draws authors from different disciplines of health, the voluntary sector, probation service, hospitals and social services as well as providing a mix of academics and practitioners. Importantly, the book also includes a service user perspective.

The emphasis on practice is reflected in all three parts of the book, although it is most prominent in Part 2. Hence, the book is not an academic exploration of the meaning of partnership, although the chapters in Part 1 do not duck this issue. The first two chapters explore the theoretical context within which partnership takes place, such as what is meant by partnership, and the political drivers for partnership. The second two chapters, while being theoretical in nature, draw on practical examples to explore the ethical issues raised by partnership, and the challenges of partnership for rural communities. The final chapter in Part 1 is important, as it is a reminder of what the provision of services is all about. In this chapter, Amir Minhas provides a sensitively written personal reflection on his own experience of being dependent upon such services.

Part 2, the main section of the book, examines the role and impact of agencies working together to provide services for a range of key client groups and social issues where a partnership approach is seen as particularly appropriate. The focus of Part 2, however, is not only on providing services for key client groups but also on working in partnership with client groups as well as with other agencies. Client groups covered within Part 2 are: the travelling community; victims of domestic violence; people who are homeless; people who have HIV/AIDS; drug misusing parents; children in need of protection; young people; mentally-disordered offenders; older people and African-Caribbean and Asian elders with dementia. The chapters in Part 2 are written in an accessible style by authors who are able to draw upon considerable expertise, knowledge and skills in their particular field. At the beginning of each chapter is a set of bullet points indicating what the chapter will address. Chapters also include case studies, where possible, to help make the links between theory and practice. At the end of each chapter is a short list of key questions to stimulate further discussion.

The book will be of particular interest to practitioners and students working in settings where partnership work, joined-up thinking and seamless service provision are becoming embedded within mainstream practice due to legislation and policy directive. The book will, therefore, have equal appeal to students, practitioners and managers in health, social and community services, and/or criminal justice settings.

Some of the issues or client groups may not at first appear relevant to some readers who work with a different client group. However, each chapter provides valuable real life examples, expertise and insight into the strengths, struggles and dilemmas of working together with other agencies, as well as with service users, towards establishing a partnership approach to practice. Lessons can be learnt from understanding and reflecting upon the issues others have faced, the ways in which they have overcome them and the models of partnership that have emerged.

In the final section, Part 3, we review the case studies, draw out the lessons of partnership, identify reoccurring themes and issues, and offer 14 principles for best practice. In contrast to the drift towards technocratic and rigidly prescribed practice in accordance with policy practice directives, the drive towards partnership work is much more 'organic' and fluid by nature, and requires different skills that are not easily acquired. However, this book provides the important contextual analysis of partnership, and a thorough examination of the strengths, weaknesses and issues arising from working in partnership with a diverse range of client groups.

Ros Carnwell and Julian Buchanan
June 2004

PART 1

Working in partnership: from theory to practice

1

Understanding partnerships and collaboration

Ros Carnwell and Alex Carson

This chapter will:

- Examine key concepts that will be referred to throughout the book, such as working together, partnership and collaboration.
- Use a concept analysis framework to examine and explore key concepts and outline their distinguishing features.
- Highlight similarities and differences between the concept of collaboration and the concept of partnership, and contextualize these differences within the current health and social policy agenda.
- Discuss the implications of partnership and collaboration for effective working together and how they are understood and operationalized by professionals from different agencies.

Collaboration, partnership and working together: the use of language

Literature in health and social care is replete with synonyms referring to the need for health and social care agencies to 'work together' more effectively in 'partnership' and in 'collaboration'. These words are frequently used interchangeably, often within the same paragraph or even sentence. Much of the use of terminology is policy driven, promoting terms such as 'joined-up thinking' and 'joined-up working', so that services can be delivered 'seamlessly' (NHS Executive 1998).

As a preliminary, we think it worthwhile to distinguish broadly between what something is, that is a partnership, and what one does, that is collaborate or work together. This chapter will initially identify the different models of partnership currently in use, and then look at the way these different partnerships actually operate. One thing that emerges from this discussion is the way that theory (what a partnership is) and practice (what it does) can often drift apart. Sometimes partnership may be little more than rhetoric or an end in itself, with limited evidence that theoretical partners are genuinely working together. Equally, it is possible for different agencies to work collaboratively together without any formal partnerships being in place. It is important, therefore, to tease out the relationships between these concepts so that we can be clear about how effective partnerships are in practice. However, before doing this, it is important to consider the current philosophical and policy context in which these definitions and arrangements have begun to be developed.

Partnerships: philosophy and policy

We live in what many commentators refer to as a post-modern world (Carter 1998). Philosophically and theoretically, post-modernism is a critique of the older 'modern' forms of social health and welfare, the 'one size fits all' policy that characterized the post-war creation of universal health and welfare provision. Lyotard (1992) argues that these huge national schemes or 'grand narratives' have failed to help the people they were created to help. He cites the examples of poor housing and poverty as social problems that have increased rather than diminished in the last fifty years. Lyotard sees these attempts at ameliorating social problems as more about helping the system rather than the people who need the help. This critique of large-scale attempts to solve people's problems has been reinforced by critiques outlining the disempowering effects of professional solutions to social problems. Since the 1980s, both the system and professionals within the system in Britain have largely been seen as disempowering for clients and receivers of services, with the emergence of terms such as 'nanny state' or 'disabling state'. These critiques have in part resulted in an increasing emphasis on client or 'consumer' choice. Health and social care services have been encouraged to allow consumers to become more involved and to have more say in the design and provision of services. Part of the reason for this refocusing on clients as active consumers rather than passive recipients of services may simply be that health and social problems have become more complex and multidimensional and that the older more static models of welfare have outlived their usefulness. In the past, the Department of Health has focused on 'health' issues, while social services have reacted to the rise in 'social' problems. This is increasingly seen as too simplistic a way of tackling more difficult and intractable problems. For example, there is, undoubtedly, a close relationship between illness and poverty.

It is in the context of putting clients at the centre of health and social care that partnerships have become necessary. The complexity of client problems, requiring an input from a number of services, may be more important in designing services than the traditional, centralizing distinctions between, for example, social workers and community nurses. A community may have a need or problem that is peculiar to that particular area or community. For instance, Bournemouth may have greater need of specialized care for older people than other areas. A client with a health problem might need a particular package of care that was previously provided by both the NHS and social services. In the new way of working, both health and social care might join up to provide a seamless 'one-stop shop', which meets clients' needs. People's needs may change over time and place and so partnerships may be formed to meet particular problems.

However, while most people would agree that clients should participate and be involved in the choices that affect their lives, some practical implications need to be considered. The shift is likely to lead to a 'problem-oriented' approach to health and social care and the disappearance of discrete professions such as nursing and social work. With the emphasis of social care and health changing to meet local needs through local solutions, the rationale for generic training might disappear. Moreover, professional 'expertise' is often viewed with suspicion. It is reasonable to suggest that current models of partnership, which are organized around current professional identities, will give way in the long term to 'problem-specific' professions. Within this book there are numerous examples from a range of authors concerning problem-specific partnerships focusing upon areas as diverse as Gypsy Travellers, victims of domestic violence and drug users, to name but a few, but what is evident from their writing is that they can demonstrate explicit examples of partnerships in practice. It is important that this changing political context provides a background for our current ideas of what partnerships are, and what they do. In the next section, we will examine what partnership models are currently in use in health and social care, using Walker and Avant's (1995) concept analysis framework. The process of conducting a concept analysis is useful in that it can clarify the meaning of a single concept (Cahill 1996). Using a concept analysis framework and drawing on examples in the book, this chapter will:

- define partnership and collaboration;
- explore attributes of the concepts;
- identify model, related and contrary cases of the two concepts; and
- discuss the antecedents to and consequences of the concepts.

Partnerships and collaboration: what are they?

The concept of partnership

The concept analysis framework identified by Walker and Avant (1995) requires that definitions of the terms are first sought, including dictionary definitions and those used within the literature. Subjecting the concepts of 'partnership' and 'collaboration' to this process reveals some interesting similarities and differences between them. Dictionary definitions of the term 'partnership' are in Box 1.1 and Table 1.2.

Box 1.1 Definitions of partnership

Collins English Dictionary (1991)

- Equal commitment
- The state of being a partner

The Concise Oxford Dictionary (1992)

- To be one of a pair on the same side in a game
- A person who shares or takes part with another, especially in a business firm with shared risks and profits

The reference to business partnerships is interesting given the recent trends in health and social care towards contracting out service delivery. Use of the term 'partnership' in health and social care settings is profoundly influenced by policy, which is frequently subject to change.

In analysing the concept of partnership as it applies to health and social care, it is useful to consider Rodgers's (2000) concept analysis framework as this takes into account the 'context' of the concept (Gallant *et al.* 2002). Context is important in defining terms like partnership and collaboration, because both terms have changed in use across time and place. This is illustrated by Gallant *et al.* (2002), who points out that 'partnership' has changed over the past five decades, from an emphasis on an equitable, just and free society enshrined within the International Declaration of Human Rights (United Nations 1948), through the need to enable citizens to become more self-reliant and take control over their own health (WHO 1978), to contemporary commentators, such as Frankel (1994), who point out how a better educated and informed public have begun to challenge the quality of services provided and are searching for more meaningful interactions with service providers. This change in policy is poignantly reflected in Minhas's personal account in Chapter 6 of this book, which traces his experiences of accessing health, social and educational services during the past 40 years.

This need for both public involvement and partnerships between service providers is reflected in recent policies, such as the *New NHS Modern Dependable* (DoH 1997), *Modernising Health and Social Services: Developing the Workforce* (DoH 1999a) and the *Health Act* (1999). Indeed, the Health Act demands that health and social services departments must reach planning agreements, and these must identify which services are to be provided by each agency, and how individuals will be assessed. *Modernising Health and Social Services* goes further, in encouraging joint education and employment and deployment of staff, in order to meet the needs of the local population. In addition, The NHS Executive (1998) recommended community development as a means of solving local problems in partnership with statutory agencies. In 2000, *A Health Service of All the Talents: Developing the NHS Workforce* (DoH 2000) also stressed concepts of partnership and collaboration with its emphasis on teamwork across professional boundaries, eliminating boundaries which dictate that only doctors and nurses can provide certain types of care, and developing flexible careers. Although Parrott presents a detailed account of the politics of partnership in Chapter 2, we can conclude here that current policy emphasizes 'three-way partnerships' between health and social care providers and service users, in which there is joint agreement about what services should be provided, and by whom, with joint employment, community development and teamwork seen as means of breaking down existing professional barriers and responding to local needs.

What the above definitions and rhetoric therefore implies is that a partnership is a *shared commitment, where all partners have a right and an obligation to participate and will be affected equally by the benefits and disadvantages arising from the partnership.* What a commitment actually amounts to may vary from one context to another. In the next section, we will trace the limits of what a commitment could amount to. In addition, talk of rights and obligations imply that all parties to a partnership must work to high ethical standards. In effect, this has implications for collaborative working, as this would be substantively defined in ethical terms. Allison takes up this very point in Chapter 3 when she discusses moral obligations placed on professionals when they work together, and the fiduciary relationship, which characterizes the features of a client-professional relationship in which both parties are responsible and their judgements are given consideration.

The concept of collaboration

Dictionary definitions of 'collaboration' are in Box 1.2 and Table 1.2.

Box 1.2 Dictionary definitions of collaboration

The Concise Oxford Dictionary (1992)

- Co-operate traitorously with an enemy
- Work jointly

These two very different definitions perhaps reflect the change of emphasis in health and social care over recent decades. Hence, the need to consider the *context* of the concept (Rodgers 2002) is as important for understanding the concept of collaboration as it is for understanding the concept of partnership. During the 1980s there was considerable suspicion between health and social care professions, to the extent that working together would have been regarded as problematic. However, recent policy reforms illustrated in this book within numerous chapters (see, for example, Wyner Chapter 9 or Minoghue Chapter 14) have encouraged different professional groups to break down barriers and work together collaboratively. It is these changes that have given way to the development of more formal partnerships. It is interesting that a common language of 'working together' and 'breaking down barriers' draws together the two concepts of partnership and collaboration. The close proximity of definitions relating to these two concepts is also reflected in Henneman *et al.*'s (1995: 104) definition of collaboration as being frequently 'equated with a bond, union or partnership, characterised by mutual goals and commitments'.

More recently, the rhetoric around partnership and collaboration is beginning to give way to alternative terms, such as 'working together'. In fact, Burke (2001) cites Service Level Agreements (SLAs) as an example of how agencies have been encouraged to *work together* by the government. Here, it is suggested that both purchasers of health care and the NHS trusts that provide care should draw up SLAs lasting 3–10 years, which should be based on health improvement programmes. Health improvement programmes are also drawn up by different agencies *working together* (Burke 2001).

Defining the attributes of partnership and collaboration

Walker and Avant (1995) propose that once definitions and uses have been identified, the defining attributes of the concept should be explored (see Table 1.2). Derived from the literature, these defining attributes identify specific phenomena and assist in differentiation from other similar concepts. In this case, the process will help to differentiate between the concepts of 'partnership' (who we are) and 'collaboration' (what we do).

Attributes of partnership

Defining attributes that emerged in the literature in relation to partnership are:

- Trust in partners
- Respect for partners
- Joint working
- Teamwork
- Eliminating boundaries
- Being an ally

These attributes illustrate the shared commitment that characterizes partnership and show that it has a substantive ethical content. All partners need to have trust in and respect for other partners. What this amounts to is that partners really need to have a shared identity. As Hudson *et al.*'s (1998) work shows, the key characteristic of partnerships is *integration*, where partners no longer see their separate identities as significant. This means that part of this shared commitment is a shared identity. However, this could lead to a lessening of a long-standing commitment to a previous, separate identity. As has already been indicated, this may mean the gradual erosion of current professional identities in favour of new, more problem-orientated professional partnerships or even, professions. This has led to difficulties with some potential partners feeling that their individual identity is under threat. This may lead to a failure to collaborate as often, as it could be perceived as threatening existing professional boundaries or failing to develop a particular profession (Masterson 2002). Indeed, one could argue that an ideal partnership would be practically impossible, as partnerships need at least two clearly identifiable partners. In the long term, this may happen but at this transitional stage in health and social care provision, partnerships may represent a staging post. Take, for example, trade union reform in recent years, which has seen the amalgamation of many smaller unions who initially formed partnerships with other similarly related unions. While starting off as partners, these reconstituted unions, such as UNISON, took on a new single identity. Over time the sense that this union was a partnership of smaller unions has been forgotten. Therefore, there are limits to what can really be called a partnership. There will inevitably be some tension in partnerships between different partners' identities and all partners' commitment to a shared identity. What determines differences between partnership models is less a shared commitment but more the nature of each partnership's commitment. Types of partnership can be differentiated by the type of commitment they undertake, summarized as:

Project Partnership: These are partnerships that are time-limited for the duration of a particular project. A partnership between the police and other road safety organizations to lower the speed limit may end when their project is successful. Equally, when two companies sign a joint contract to manufacture a particular product, the partnership may end when production ceases. In Chapter 7, Roberts describes a multi-agency 'project partnership' funded by the Welsh Assembly Government, which aims to describe the coronary health status and to redress the inequality of access to health care experienced by the traveller population in North East Wales. Arguably, once the funding ceases and the aims have been achieved, then the partnership could cease to exist.

Problem-oriented Partnerships: These are partnerships that are formed to meet specific problems. Examples of this might include Neighbourhood Watch schemes or Drug and Alcohol Action Teams. These partnerships arise in response to a publicly identified problem and will remain as long as the problem persists. These can be subject to changing definitions of what the 'problem' really is. An example of this can be seen in Minogue's discussion in Chapter 14 of a partnership group established in Leeds to develop a strategic multi-agency approach to provide services for mentally-disordered offenders. It can be defined as a problem-orientated partnership because it arose from a recognition that people with mental health problems who offend were not always dealt with appropriately, and a belief that a partnership response was the most effective way of addressing the issues.

Ideological Partnerships: These types of partnerships arise from a shared outlook or point of view. They are similar in many ways to problem-oriented partnerships but they also possess a certain viewpoint that they are convinced is the correct way of seeing things. A case in point is abortion, in which various organizations, ideologically aligned, form a 'pro-life' or a 'pro-choice' partnership. Another example is the various anti-war and peace partnerships. As with problem-oriented partnerships, ideology can change and develop. For instance, Amnesty International or Christian Aid have evolved into more overt political partnerships as the ideological context has widened. Within this book, this type of partnership is illustrated in Chapter 8, when Blyth describes the Coventry Domestic Violence Partnership, established in the 1980s as a focus group to advise planners and commissioners in health and social care about service gaps and priorities. Although the impetus for the partnership came from the voluntary sector in collaboration with the police and 'safer cities' community safety workers, it has since developed into a strong and dynamic, multi-agency partnership with a wide remit across the spectrum of public and community services. Although, as suggested above, this could be described as a problem-oriented partnership, its long-term dynamic nature is suggestive of an ideological partnership.

Ethical Partnerships: These share a number of features with the above but they also have a sense of 'mission' and have an overtly ethical agenda, which seeks to promote a particular way of life. They tend to be democratic and reflective and are as equally focused on the means as the end. While most partnerships have codes of ethics or ethical procedures, ethical partnerships have a substantive ethical content in their mission and practice.

The above types of partnerships are inclusive; indeed some partnerships might have all of the above types within it. For instance, it would be reasonable to conclude that health and social care partnerships are ethical partnerships since they aim to help people. However, they may also work successfully but be ideologically distinct. Social services may favour a 'social model' approach, while the health care system may favour a more 'medicalized' approach. Project partnerships may take a problem-oriented approach to their work at the behest of one of the partners. Service users may want particular problems solved and demand that service providers address ongoing issues rather than focusing on the big picture.

Gallant *et al.* (2002) also suggest that partnership attributes include *structure* and *process* phenomenon. The *structure* involves partners in the actions of the initiating and working phases within their relationship (Courtney *et al.* 1996). During the initiating phase, they negotiate responsibilities and actions, while during the working phase they evaluate their progress towards the goal of partnership. The structure might also include identification of suitable partners. Most literature relating to partnership identifies partnership arrangements between certain groups, including both service providers and service users. An example of this is Roberts's study (2002), which found that older people welcome advice concerning their discharge from hospital and during the period following discharge, although some preferred decisions to be made for them. Roberts used Arnstein's ladder of citizen participation to analyse the findings, with notions of 'partnership', 'relationship', 'communication' and 'paternalism' being discussed. As will be seen in the chapters of this book, however, involving vulnerable people in partnership can be difficult, when there is still so much work to do in developing multi-agency partnerships. Moreland *et al.* illustrate this point in Chapter 16, when they explain how some community capacity building has been carried out in the 'Twice A Child Projects'. This involves empowering social groups to participate in decision making, which requires skills of involvement and persuasion, as well as the ability to articulate persuasively the needs of the group. They suggest that this limited development of community capacity is due to local political and ideological realities, allied to real issues over current authority policies and practices on service planning, staffing, redundancy and redeployment.

Key to the *process* of partnership is the involvement of partners in power sharing and negotiation (Gallant *et al.* 2002). In partnerships between health and social care agencies, this process might involve considerable negotiation in order to arrive at a shared understanding of roles and responsibilities across multidisciplinary boundaries, as well as the relinquishing of power relationships. Equally in partnerships between clients and professionals, this same process of negotiation and relinquishing of professional power will take place. However, this can be difficult in practice, particularly if professional codes of practice and legal frameworks work against it. In addition, there are safety issues that, while they might help the effective management of a partnership, may restrict the scope of practice. While it might practically be better for a social worker to assess clients' health needs, professionally it might be difficult for a nurse to give care solely on the basis of this assessment. Professional rules may insist on nurses carrying out their own assessments.

Attributes of collaboration

The defining attributes of collaboration include that 'two or more individuals must be involved in a joint venture, typically one of an intellectual nature . . . in which participants willingly participate in planning and decision making' (Henneman *et al.* 1995: 104). Henneman *et al.* further argue that individuals consider themselves to be members of a team working towards a common goal, sharing their expertise and responsibility for the outcome. Fundamentally, the relationship between collaborators is non-hierarchical, and shared power is based on knowledge and expertise, rather than role or title (Henneman *et al.* 1995).

The defining attributes of collaboration can therefore be summarized as follows:

- Intellectual and co-operative endeavour
- Knowledge and expertise more important than role or title
- Joint venture
- Teamworking
- Participation in planning and decision making
- Non-hierarchical relationship
- Sharing of expertise
- Willingness to work together towards an agreed purpose
- Trust and respect in collaborators
- Highly connected network
- Low expectation of reciprocation

As in the concept of partnership, the involvement of the public is central to working collaboratively. Stewart and Reutter (2001) exemplify this, citing evidence from three studies in which peers and professionals collaborated as co-leaders and partners in 21 support groups. The three studies were: survivors of myocardial infarction and their spouses; parents of children with chronic conditions; and older women with disabilities. These three studies, however, are all contextualized around chronic illness, which might not be universally applicable. The current consensus of opinion, for example, is that clients with chronic illnesses have more insight into their conditions than professionals do. Indeed, it is significant that many examples cited in the literature deal with chronic problems such as social care, disabilities and mental health.

Identifying model, related and contrary cases of partnership and collaboration

Having refined the concepts through identifying their defining attributes, the next stage of analysing concepts is to identify a 'model' case, a 'related' case and a 'contrary' case (Walker and Avant 1995). A model case includes all the stated attributes of the concept and is so called because there is no doubt that it represents the concept. Clifford (2003) suggests the model case of 'partnership' between education and service providers would be people (or organizations) willing to join with a partner, together with a shared vision and commitment to making the partnership work. Clifford also remarks that collaborative arrangements should be set up to demonstrate a willingness to share in successes and failures. An example of a model case can also be seen in Chapter 15, when Chambers and Philips refer to the 'Partnerships for Carers in Suffolk'. This could be described as a model case because each partner 'signed up' for the Charter for Carers in Suffolk and, furthermore, each of the partners is committed to implementing an action plan.

In identifying a model case of 'collaboration' it is useful to consider Hudson *et al.*'s (1998) view of a continuum from isolation, through encounter, communication and collaboration, to integration. The characteristics evident within this continuum are identified in Table 1.1.

A model case of collaboration would occur if a Social Services Department joined with a local NHS Trust to identify training needs of their staff and used knowledge and expertise from both partners to produce shared training. In this instance, it seems that collaboration is a means of making 'partnership' work. That is, 'collaboration', the verb, is what we do when we engage successfully in a 'partnership', partnership being the noun. A model case of collaboration would, therefore, comprise the characteristics identified by Hudson *et al.* (1998), such as trust and respect between collaborators, together with joint working, planning and service delivery. This example of a model case would also include all the attributes of collaboration listed in the previous section. There would be few examples of isolation in health and social care agencies, as this would suggest that they never met, contacted or talked to each other. 'Encounters' in health and social care agencies would imply infrequent, ad hoc, interprofessional contact, characterized by rivalry and stereotyping. While it may be assumed that in modern health and social care agencies, such 'encounters' would be rare, Buchanan and Corby's research in Chapter 11 concerning work with drug-using parents would suggest otherwise. The professionals they interviewed about their role in drug misuse felt that although collaboration was important, it was difficult to

Table 1.1 Characteristics of collaboration (Hudson *et al.* 1998)

	Characteristics
Isolation	Absence of joint activity with no communication at all between agencies.
Encounter	Some ad hoc inter-agency contact, but lowly connected networks, divergent organizational goals and perceived rivalry and stereotyping.
Communication	Joint working, but marginal to organizational goals. Frequent interactions and sharing of information as it applies to users whose needs cross boundaries, some joint training, a nominated person is responsible for liaison, expectation of reciprocation.
Collaboration	Joint working is central to mainstream activities. Trust and respect in partners means that they are willing to participate in formal, structured joint working including joint assessments, planning, service delivery and commissioning. There is a highly connected network and low expectation of reciprocation.
Integration	No longer see their separate identify as significant. May be willing to consider creation of unitary organization.

achieve due to other professionals being either ill-informed and ill-trained in relation to illegal drug use, or insufficiently discerning in the way in which they worked with drug-using parents. Stereotyping is also evident in Wyner's discussion of homelessness in Chapter 9. She explains how social services staff are frequently perceived by the voluntary sector as being aloof, unapproachable and not fulfilling their statutory responsibilities. They, in turn, complain that voluntary sector staff do not understand the limits of those responsibilities and fail to appreciate what social services can take on within the parameters of their departments and their scarce resources. Modern health and social care agencies are arguably in transition from communication to collaboration. However, the high degree of trust and low expectation of reciprocation within collaboration might suggest health and social care agencies have considerable progress to make.

Identifying a related case of these terms (Walker and Avant 1995) is a little more difficult, as this requires a similar (but different) instance of partnership or collaboration to be identified. A related case for 'partnership' could be 'associate', as this implies a connection between two organizations or people, but the link would be quite loose and might imply that one of the organizations or people was subordinate to the other. An example of this would be an Associate Director, who would normally act as deputy to the director. At the level of patient-client partnership, Cahill (1996) presents a concept analysis of patient *participation* and suggests that patient *partnership* is a related case for this concept, along with patient *collaboration* and patient *involvement*. She views patient involvement and collaboration as being at the bottom of a pyramid, being precursors to patient participation, which in turn is a precursor to patient partnership. Cahill (1996) goes on to argue that *partnership* is a goal to which all practitioners should aspire. This suggests then that as people become more involved, they begin to collaborate with each other and through this process of collaboration a greater sense of involvement transpires. This sense of involvement can ultimately result in sufficient trust, respect and willingness on the part of different parties for partnership to develop (see Figure 1.1).

A related case of 'collaboration' could be an 'alliance', in which organizations share some understanding, but may lack the joint working arrangements required to be collaborators.

Identifying a 'contrary' case is even more difficult. For the contrary case must have characteristics which illustrate that it is not representative of the concept, although similarities may be present. A contrary case of 'partnership' would be when two organizations or people convey the impression of being partners, when in fact the characteristics they display do not resemble those of a true partnership. We see examples of this with many professional sports personalities. Some professional footballers are accused of not being a 'team player' and some nurses and social workers are accused of the same thing when they do 'their own thing'.

A contrary case of collaboration could be seen in organizations that communicate (Hudson *et al.* 1998) with each other, but only in so far as they need to in order to

Involvement ———▶ Collaboration ———▶ Participation ———▶ Partnership

Figure 1.1 A continuum of involvement

deliver services across organizational boundaries. Frequent liaison may give the impression of collaboration when in fact the expectation of reciprocation may reveal a different state of affairs. This is currently the norm in many areas where services communicate on a case-by-case basis. An example of this can be seen in Chapter 6 when Corby explains how inter-professional training has been variable over the past decade, according to the post-Climbie audit. He goes on to suggest that the child protection system is complex with a bewildering overlap of occupational boundaries and the added complication of disadvantaged and transient families. With such complexity it is not surprising that collaborative working between different professional groups is difficult. Another example is cited by Miller in Chapter 13, in relation to teachers and youth workers. Miller argues that although there is some collaboration between the two, for many teachers and youth workers, there still exists a perceived distance in terms of practice and often a mutually critical attitude towards each other's style of engagement with young people.

Antecedents and consequences

Walker and Avant (1995) also suggest that concepts have antecedents and consequences, some examples of which can be seen in Table 1.2. Antecedents are events that happen prior to the concept occurring, while consequences follow the occurrence of the concept. According to Walker and Avant, exploring antecedents and consequences facilitates further refinement of the defining attributes of the concept. Antecedents for partnerships include local directives, individual initiative and social policy changes. Antecedents can occur at all levels and may spring up in response to individual, local and national perceptions. Doran (2001), for instance, traces the route from policy to practice in the proposed integration of district nursing services with social services to provide a seamless care in the community. Another example of policy antecedents is the recent legislation concerning paedophilia, which arose from a bereaved mother's suffering as a result of her daughter's murder. Partnerships between parents with autistic children and research centres grew out of a 'perceived' increase in cases of autism. In many ways, their antecedents define partnerships. In response to antecedents, for 'partnership' to occur, there must be two sides who are committed to a shared vision about the joint venture and there must be two or more people who are willing to sign up to creating a relationship that will support this (Clifford 2003). Furthermore, partners must value co-operation (Courtney 1995) and respect what other partners bring to the relationship (LaBonte 1994).

According to Henneman *et al.* (1995), antecedents to collaboration include a number of personnel and environmental factors, rather than merely the willingness of one party to work jointly with the other (see Table 1.1). Personnel factors include: sufficient educational preparation, maturity and experience to ensure readiness to engage in collaboration; clear understanding and acceptance of their role and expertise; confidence in ability and recognition of disciplinary boundaries; effective communication; respect for and understanding of other's roles; sharing of knowledge, values, responsibility, visions and outcomes; trust in collaborators. Environmental factors include: a non-hierarchical organization in which individuals can act autonomously and in which reward systems recognize group rather than individual achievements. Furthermore, the parties must be willing to participate in formal, structured, joint working to the extent that they do not rely on reciprocation in order to ensure that each contributes to the shared vision (Hudson *et al.* 1998).

The consequences of 'partnership' can be understood in terms of the benefits and barriers to working in partnership. The main benefits of working in partnership are that multi-faceted problems, such as social exclusion, can be tackled more effectively through multidisciplinary action (Peckham and Exworthy 2003). This would then reduce repetition of service provision from different organizations; the omission of provision of services because each organization believes the other is providing them; unnecessary dilution of activities by agencies as they each try to deliver services; and the possibility of different agencies producing services that are counterproductive to each other. These are what Huxham and MacDonald (1992) refer to as the pitfalls of individualism. However, some see this loss of individualism as a barrier to partnerships. In a recent study, Masterson (2002) saw cross-boundary working as a possible barrier to the development of new professional roles in nursing.

Barriers to working in partnership have also been reported in the literature. One barrier could be the complexity of relationships due to the greater interplay between those involved in the partnership (Gallant *et al.* 2002), an example of this being collaboration to protect children as discussed above in relation to Corby's chapter. Burke (2001) cautions that there is some scepticism about the partnership approach with respect to a number of factors, including how much particular individuals can be representative of the wider public; concern that public participation can lead to both tokenism (as exemplified in Moreland *et al.*'s chapter) and to excessive influence of vocal groups and the possibility that individuals might not wish to be involved in making decisions about their care. Secker and Hill (2001) also report a number of barriers arising from group discussions with 128 participants from 21 organizations working across five service contexts dealing with mental health services. One important barrier was a reluctance to share information about clients due to confidentiality, which, if breached, could result in staff dealing with unanticipated responses from clients with inadequate knowledge and support. This could also be a problem when partnership involves the joint use or joint commissioning of premises in rural areas, where even the simple act of going into a particular building may be witnessed by others and may lead to particular presumptions about what is going on (Pugh, Chapter 5). Wilson supports this view in Chapter 10, when she explains how people who are HIV positive may be reluctant to fill in prescriptions in their home neighbourhood and often hide or relabel medications to maintain secrecy within the home.

Role boundary conflicts and tensions between agencies were also reported as barriers in Secker and Hill's study (2001), such that both learning disability nurses and the police service felt that they were 'dumped on' by mental health services. Such boundary conflicts were reported to arise partly from inadequate resourcing of mental health services, as well as misunderstanding of agency roles, often resulting in unrealistic expectations. Other barriers to partnership included interprofessional differences of perspective (such as those arising from the medical model and the more holistic social model) and differences in approach to risk. As multidisciplinary working becomes more prevalent, blurring of roles may cause some professionals to strive to preserve their own professional identity (Brown *et al.* 2000). Indeed Brown *et al.* argue that boundaries between professions are actively encouraged by the experience of interdisciplinary modes of working. In addition, Gulliver *et al.* (2002) point out some of the legal barriers to closer integration. As well as legal barriers, there may be professional issues of accountability that need to be clearly defined if they are not to become barriers to effective partnerships. In overcoming some of the barriers to collaboration and partnership it may is useful to consider Bates's suggestion in Chapter 4. He proposes four strategies by which health and social care professionals can move forward in a way that embraces diversity: learn from each other; embrace partnership; adopt a value position where anti-discriminatory practice is central; and reflect on practice.

The consequences of collaboration can also be explained in terms of benefits and barriers. The benefits of collaboration include: more effective use of staff as they utilize their skills co-operatively rather than competitively (Henneman *et al.* 1995); demystification of health care with the bridging of gaps between fragmented service provision; sustained energy; cross-pollination of ideas; sharing of effort and, ultimately, sharing of organizational structure (El Ansari and Phillips 2001). There are also a number of barriers to closer collaboration. This may include a fear that individual professions may be threatened as work becomes more problem-focused (Billingsley and Lang 2002). Brown *et al.* (2000) explain how a lack of managerial direction and the encouragement of a more generic way of working can prevent closer collaboration across professional boundaries. In collaboration between service providers and service users, service users may be reluctant to assume an equal role in partnerships. Roberts's study of older people on discharge showed that some preferred service providers to make decisions for them. However, this may reflect older people's perspectives on the relationship between professionals and patients.

A summary of the defining attributes, antecedents and consequences of partnership and collaboration is presented in Table 1.2.

As indicated in Table 1.2, there are a number of similarities between the concepts of partnership and collaboration. Within their defining attributes each share traits of trust and respect for partners, joint working and teamwork. The main shared antecedent is a willingness to participate, while the main shared consequence is increased effectiveness of staff resources. It is interesting that the concept of collaboration has more defining features than does the concept of partnership. This might suggest a more complex concept, which, once achieved, might result in the proliferation of potential partnerships.

The final stage in Walker and Avant's (1995) concept analysis framework is to identify empirical referents to the concept. Empirical referents of partnership and collaboration would be evidenced from behaviour within organizations and people who could be observed. These exemplify the existence of the concept, so that the concept can be measured and validated in order to demonstrate its true existence. A partnership, for example, might be legally binding with a written contract detailing the obligations of each partner. A collaboration could be evidenced by written procedures for joint working. These could then be checked through observation and/or participation to establish the extent of collaboration. Examples of these as they appear in this book are discussed above.

Table 1.2 Attributes, antecedents and consequences of partnership and collaboration

	Partnership	*Collaboration*
Defining attributes	Trust in partners Respect for partners Joint working Teamwork Eliminating boundaries Being an ally	Trust and respect in collaborators Teamworking Intellectual and co-operative endeavour Knowledge and expertise more important than role or title Joint venture Participation in planning and decision making Non-hierarchical relationship Sharing of expertise Willingness to work together towards an agreed purpose Highly connected network Low expectation of reciprocation
Antecedents	Individual, local and national initiatives Commitment to shared vision about joint venture Willingness to sign up to creating a relationship that will support a vision Value co-operation and respect for what other partners bring to the relationship	Educational preparation, maturity and experience to ensure readiness Understanding and acceptance of role and expertise Confidence in ability and recognition of disciplinary boundaries Effective communication, respect for and understanding of other's roles Sharing of knowledge, values, responsibility, visions and outcomes Trust in collaborators Non-hierarchical organization with individual autonomy Willingness to participate in formal, structured joint working to the extent that they do not rely on reciprocation in order to ensure that each contributes to the shared vision

Table 1.2 (*continued*)

	Partnership	*Collaboration*
Consequences	*Benefits* Social exclusion tackled more effectively through multidisciplinary action. Less repetition of service provision from different organizations Less dilution of activities by agencies Less chance of agencies producing services that are counterproductive to each other. *Barriers:* Complexity of relationships Representativeness of wider public Tokenism and excessive influence of vocal groups Desire of individuals not to be involved in making decisions about their care Threat to confidentiality Role boundary conflicts Interprofessional differences of perspective Threats to professional identity	*Benefits* More effective use of staff due to co-operation rather than competition Demystification of health care due to bridging of gaps between fragmented service provision Sustained energy Cross-pollination of ideas Sharing of effort and ultimately sharing of organizational structure

Conclusion

This chapter has set the wider context in which the concept of partnership is located. Partnerships, collaboration and working together need to be seen as new solutions to 'new' problems. It may be the case that the current situation reflects both a negative view of the paternalistic state, with its grand narratives of fairness and equality, and a more positive view that wants to put the client at the centre of things. Whatever the reason, and we suspect that both have played their part, partnerships and collaboration are likely to grow rather than diminish. Evidence discussed above suggests that, despite the potential barriers to partnership and collaboration, they are worthwhile pursuits. Moreover, policy directives are creating the imperative for organizations to work together. However, the evidence for the effectiveness of partnerships and collaborative care arrangements are less clear (El Ansari and Phillips 2001).

This may suggest that partnerships and collaboration are good in themselves, rather than more effective at solving problems. However, there is no doubt that client problems are more complex and require new ways of working. Part of the reason for the paucity of evidence about their effectiveness may be that they need time to be integrated with existing provision. In addition, if partnerships and collaboration are going to be the future ways of working together, old forms of professional education and training will need to be reviewed. The problem with new innovative ways of working may be that they are working within the old context, where professions were discrete entities with their own body of knowledge. So while the policy context is changing to encourage collaboration and partnerships, professional regulation has been slow to catch up. In addition, many clients and potential clients still prefer the old ways of working and may be reluctant to become too involved. What seems clear, however, is that certain problems will, by their nature, be more amenable to a partnership or collaborative approach. As such, more work needs to be done so that the context can keep up with the concept.

Questions for further discussion

1. What attributes of partnership and collaboration have you found in evidence within your own organization?
2. What benefits (if any) of partnership and collaboration have you observed in your organization?
3. How can the barriers to partnership and collaboration be overcome?

References

Billingsley, R. and Lang, L. (2002) The case for interprofessional learning in health and social care, *Building Knowledge for integrated Care*, 10(4): 31–4.

Brown, B., Crawford, P., Darongkamas, J. (2000) Blurred roles and permeable boundaries: the experience of multidisciplinary working in community mental health, *Health and Social Care in the Community*, Nov 8(6): 425–35.

Burke, L. (2001) Social Policy, in D. Sines, E. Appleby and E. Raymond, *Community Health Care Nursing* (2nd edn). Blackwell Science, Oxford.

Cahill, J. (1996) Patient participation: a concept analysis, *Journal of Advanced Nursing*, 24: 561–71.

Carter, J. (ed.) (1998) *Postmodernity and the Fragmentation of Welfare*. Routledge, London.

Clifford, C. (2003) Working in parallel worlds. Key note presentation at Nurse Education Tomorrow Conference, University of Durham, September.

Courtney, R. (1995) Community partnership primary care: a new paradigm for primary care, *Public Health Nursing*, 12(6): 366–73.

Courtney, R., Ballard, E., Fauver, S., Gariota, M. and Holland, L. (1996) The partnership model: working with individuals, families and communities towards a new vision of health, *Public Health*, 13: 177–86.

DoH (1997) *The New NHS Modern Dependable: A National Framework for Assessing Performance*. The Stationery Office, London.

DoH (1999) *Health Act*. The Stationery Office, London.

DoH (1999a) *Modernising Health and Social Services: Developing the Workforce*. The Stationery Office, London.

DoH (2000) *A Health Service of All the Talents: Developing the NHS Workforce*. The Stationery Office, London.

Doran, T. (2001) Policy and practice. Providing seamless community health and social services, *British Journal of Community Nursing*, Aug 6(8): 387, 390–3.

El Ansari, W. and Phillips, C. (2001) Interprofessional collaboration: a stakeholder approach to evaluation of voluntary participation in community partnerships, *Journal of Interprofessional Care*, 15(4): 351–68.

Frankel, B.G. (1994) Patient-physician relationships: changing modes of interaction, in B.B. Singh and H.D. Dickinson (eds) *Health, Illness and Health Care in Canada* (2nd edn), Harcourt Brace, pp. 183–98.

Gallant, M.H., Beaulieu, M.C. and Carnevale, F.A. (2002) Partnership: an analysis of the concept within the nurse–client relationship, *Journal of Advanced Nursing* 40(2): 149–57.

Gulliver, P., Peck, E. and Towell, D. (2002) *Modernising Partnerships: Evaluation of the Implementation of the Mental Health Review in Somerset: Final Report.* Institute for Applied Health and Social Policy, King's College, London.

Henneman, E.A., Lee, J.L. and Cohen J.I. (1995) Collaboration: a concept analysis, *Journal of Advanced Nursing*, 21: 103–9.

Hudson, B., Exworthy, M. and Peckham, S. (1998) *The Integration of Localised and Collaborative Purchasing: a Review of the Literature and Framework for Analysis.* Nuffield Institute for Health, University of Leeds/Institute for Health Policy Studies, University of Southampton.

Huxham, C. and MacDonald, D. (1992) Introducing collaborative advantage, *Management Decision*, 30(3): 50–6.

Labonte, R. (1994) Health promotion and empowerment on professional practice, *Health Education Quarterly*, 253–68.

Lyotard, J. F. (1992) *The Postmodern Condition: A Report on Knowledge.* Manchester University Press, Manchester.

Masterson, A., (2002) Cross-boundary working: a macro-political analysis of the impact on professional roles, *Journal of Clinical Nursing*, May, 11(3): 331–9.

NHS Executive (1998) *In the Public Interest: Developing a Strategy for Public Health Participation in the NHS.* DoH, Wetherby.

Peckham, S. and Exworthy (2003) *Primary Care in the UK: Policy, Organisation and Management.* Palgrave Macmillan, Basingstoke.

Roberts, K. (2002) Exploring participation: older people on discharge from hospital, *Journal of Advanced Nursing*, Nov, 40(4): 413–20.

Rodgers, B.L. (2000) Concept analysis: an evolutionary view in B. L. Rodgers and K. A. Knafl (eds) *Concept Development in Nursing: Foundations, Techniques and Applications* (2nd edn). Saunders, Philadelphia: 77–102.

Secker, J. and Hill, K. (2001) Broadening the partnerships: experiences of working across community agencies, *Journal of Interprofessional Care*, Nov., 15(4): 341–50.

Stewart, M.J. and Reutter, L. (2001) Fostering partnerships between peers and professionals, *Canadian Journal of Nursing Research*, 33(1): 97–116.

United Nations (1948) *Universal Declaration of Human Rights.* http://www.unhchr.ch/udhr (accessed 10 May 2001).

Walker, L.O. and Avant, K.C. (1995) *Strategies of Theory Construction in Nursing* (3rd edn). Appleton and Lange, Norwalk, CT.

WHO/UNICEF (1978) *Primary Health Care.* Report of the International Conference on Primary Care, Alma Ata USSR, 6–12 September, Geneva.

2

The political drivers of working in partnership

Lester Parrott

This chapter will:

- Compare New Labour's discourse of modernizing public services with the previous Conservative governments' approach.
- Introduce a typology of partnership, identifying both a permissive and a directive model.
- Explore the history of partnership culminating in the National Health Service and Community Care Act 1990.
- Explore partnership as an attempt to overcome the boundaries between health and social care, and the adverse effects that a contested responsibility has brought, for example, in relation to residential and community care for older people.

From collaboration to partnership

The development of unified social services departments was promoted in the Seebohm Report (1968) as a necessary reform to overcome the fragmentation between different arms of local government providing personal social services. The post-Second World War legacy showed that while local authorities had responsibility for adults in what were known as welfare departments, there was separate responsibility given to health authorities for community health services, which, in some cases, overlapped with local authorities' welfare departments. This separation resulted in similar services being developed by each separate department with little co-ordination. While the push towards community care remained underdeveloped, these distinctions between departments were problematic but not of sufficient gravitas to provide the impetus for reform. However, as community care began to be seriously considered – particularly in mental health services following the Hospital Plan (1959) – then the rigid distinctions of responsibility between hospital and community began to inhibit the development of care in the community. Ironically, the Seebohm Committee (1968) dedicated as it was to new unified social service departments, did not see the benefits of progressing this integration further. The committee's intention was to reduce the differences between children and adult services by placing them under the umbrella of a unified local authority social service department. The fate of community health services was left in the balance to run separately from local authority social service departments. This was difficult to reconcile when Seebohm saw the need for greater integration in children's services by joining education welfare services to the local authority personal social services, yet was unable to follow through this logic by unifying adult social services and local community health services. Although it was muted by some health pressure groups for more collaboration between the NHS and the PSS (Personal Social Services), the political will and power lay with those who supported a strong PSS, which could become the fifth social service (following health, housing, education and social security) as the final pillar of the welfare state. The idea that local government services were too differentiated and diverse to deliver effective services was an attempt to bring under one universalist roof the welfare functions of local government (Parrott 2002).

As the rundown of institutions holding large populations of people previously considered to be dependent or psychiatric hospitals and special hospitals developed, the Seebohm solution was dead before it had started. Greater collaboration was required between the NHS and the PSS but this was not structurally possible under the Seebohm arrangements with separate spheres of responsibility between the personal social services and the health service. This disjunction between the realities of institutional closure and the abilities of community health and personal social services to work together was cruelly exposed in the 1980s by the pace of hospital closure. Thus much criticism of community care services was encapsulated in the report 'Making a Reality of Community Care' (Audit Commission 1986), in which the existing arrangements for community care were seen to be chaotic.

The push towards community care was made more difficult by the Conservative government's approach in the early 1980s, which took the form of an increased role for the private sector. This policy assumed that subsidizing a growth in private residential care would cope with the increased numbers of older people about to require more intensive forms of care. The intention was that those remaining in the community would be increasingly cared for by a ready and available supply of informal carers, voluntary groups and private providers. This view was repeated at length by successive government reports, yet the policy itself was deemed to be failing (DHSS 1981, DoH 1989). In particular, the chronic lack of co-ordination, failure of joint planning and effective collaboration were all highlighted as major factors that contributed to the problem. Thus after much deliberation the government reluctantly endorsed Caring for People (DoH 1989), which attempted to provide a more coherent solution for care in the community.

In respect to partnership working, the new arrangements hoped to bring greater clarity between the role of the NHS and the PSS. Although some blurring of boundaries was seen as unavoidable, the main hope was that local authorities and the local health authorities would be enabled to work together at the local level (Means et al. 2003). The resulting NHSCCA 1990 gave local authorities the lead role in coordinating community care. The delivery of services was to be developed through a quasi-market in which the provision of services was to be split from the commissioning and purchasing of services, the role then of the PSS as the purchaser of services was crucial in co-ordinating the appropriate mix of services in their particular locality. Partnership at this time was given more attention, as it was encouraged through the development of community care plans, which local authorities were required to produce with the local health service to promote community care. However, given the ideological commitment of the Conservative government to the private and voluntary sectors, new spending on community care would inevitably be directed towards the independent sector. Thus the coordinating role of the PSS was seen as central to the successful outcome of this new policy, which would see a plurality of providers offering individual consumers of community care a service that was (at least in theory) more diverse responsive.

Evaluations of the NHSCCA 1990 have, not surprisingly, been varied. Johnson draws on a number of studies to suggest that, from a positive angle, the new arrangements had:

- A greater degree of accountability
- Greater flexibility and responsiveness
- Greater focus on service users and increased knowledge by them of services available

But on the negative side, a number of problems were identified with:

- Inadequate co-ordination in joint working arrangements
- Difficulties in managing quasi-markets
- Lack of resources
- Rationing and charging
- Poor assessment procedures

(Johnson 1999)

Partnership at this time was less important than the further encouragement of alternative provision through the private and voluntary sectors, so that as long as a mixed economy of care developed, so the local authorities were able to maintain their co-ordinating role. Partnership, therefore, was seen as a necessary aim that could be achieved through a permissive approach to joint working. Thus the NHS and PSS were continually exhorted to collaborate through, for example, more direct guidance from Glendinning (2002). This guidance, as Glendinning (2002) argues, was necessary given the organizational fragmentation brought about by the community care reforms, which had undone much collaborative working through the introduction of the purchaser-provider splits and the development of quasi-markets.

Throughout the 1990s, until the election of New Labour in 1997, there was continual advice and guidance to encourage more collaborative working. Some of these requirements were tied to funding which would promote partnership, for example, the special transitional grant to fund additional community care costs following the NHSCCA (1993) were subject to a precondition that the PSS and NHS develop agreements to work together. In mental health, the Mental Illness Specific

Grant was subject to health agreeing plans with social service for supporting people with mental health problems in the community (see Wyatt 2002). While the PSS and NHS were exhorted and sometimes directed to work together, the reality of partnership working was patchy and still largely dependent upon local authorities and local health authorities to be proactive, with few mechanisms in place from central government to require partnership to happen. The history of partnership arrangements throughout the period under discussion was, as Bridgen (2003) has argued, to be painfully slow with little effective joint working or planning developed on a consistent or national basis.

Following the election of a Labour government, partnership became one of the key strategies for developing public services. The specifics in relation to the PSS and the NHS were not slow to develop. Thus partnership in the early phases of Labour's proposals was seen as a powerful instrument that had the potential for tackling the seemingly intractable policy issues, 'the wicked issues' that challenged local and central government (see Glendinning 2002). To achieve partnership, a raft of initiatives were put in place to stimulate closer working; for example, enabling social service representation on the boards of Primary Care Groups and Trusts. This culminated in this early phase with the Health Act 1999, which introduced more partnership-focused approaches to allow pooled budgets, integrate provider organizations and organize lead commissioning arrangements. Following this legislation, the Health Plan 2000 held out the prospect that in cases of perceived failure of inter-agency working, the threat of introducing mandatory partnership working could be introduced.

The NHS Plan, as Glendinning (2002) observes, proposed the integration of health and social services for specific groups of people in new Care Trusts, which would be responsible for all local health and social care. But, despite the threat of compulsion, by 2000 the Local Government Association revealed that over 75 per cent of local authorities were already actively pursuing partnership arrangements with their health colleagues and had been for many years. Indeed the House of Commons Public Expenditure Committee recognized this in relation to joint working to relieve bed blocking in hospitals where the number of over 75-year-olds delayed in hospital fell from 7,000 in March 1997 to 3,500 in December 2002 (House of Commons 2003). This suggests that the government's threat to compel partnership may have had less substance as local authorities were already voluntarily pursuing this line. These new trusts were given life by the NHS and the Social Care Act 2001, in which the threat of compulsion was removed from local health and social services agencies as the government's powers to compel partnership were removed. Nonetheless although direct compulsion did not materialize, there have been further developments that require de facto partnership working.

The Community Care (Delayed Discharges) Act 2003 places financial penalties on both the NHS and local PSS if they are either keeping individuals unnecessarily in hospital or delaying their rehabilitation into the community. Thus the local PSS will be required to pay a fine to the relevant NHS body in those cases where it has not succeeded in putting together a discharge plan for an individual or where a patient's discharge has been delayed because the local authority has not been ready to provide services. Although government provided £170 million to local authorities in 2002 to develop community-based services to maintain people in their own homes, this has come too late to provide the necessary services. In 2004 local authorities received additional delayed discharge grants of £50 million in order for them to pay the fines that may be incurred under the Delayed Discharges Act 2003. This reflects the relative failure of local authorities and government in developing adequate services if, in effect, the government after instituting the Delayed Discharges Act 2003 has to bale out the local authorities that are unable to meet the legislative requirements placed upon them. Fines for delayed discharges mirrors a similar system in Sweden but this system of fines operates within a context of a more comprehensive infrastructure of community care services compared to the UK (Carvel *et al.* 2004). It is also important to note that the organizational barriers may also be less as in Sweden the local authority is responsible for both health and social care.

Having reviewed the recent history from collaboration to partnership, it is now possible to develop a typology of partnership that reflects the relative ideological positions of the Conservative Party and New Labour to partnership. This is a useful heuristic device to highlight the extent to which New Labour's approach is one which uses partnership as a far more intensive form of governance than that of the previous Conservative administration.

Following Newman's (2001) models of governance some differences can be identified between the previous Conservative governments' approach to partnership and that of New Labour. The Conservative Party reflects a rational goal model, which seeks to disperse power around organizational networks, and relies upon managerial autonomy to use opportunities for partnership. Government is concerned to set incentives to reward partnership behaviour with responsibility for outcomes fixed through contractual relationships with the state and other players in the network. For New Labour we can see that their approach reflects a hybrid rational goal/hierarchical model that uses the previously highlighted strategies over laid by bureaucratic hierarchies that impose rules, guidelines and standards from the top down. This model attempts a 'Third Way' approach by promoting some flexibility at the operational level, while minimizing risk by ensuring accountability to government. Accountability is enforced with the imposition of quality standards to ensure continuity of policy, for example, with the introduction of National Service Frameworks for different service user groups (Department of Health 1999).

In both approaches the nature of state control of the process is not contested, it is the form of control that is significant. This can be highlighted by the respective governments' approach to the quasi-market in community care. For the Conservatives the control of the quasi-market was to be enacted by the local authority as purchaser, whose role was to shape and guide the local market for community care. The local authority could use its role as a consumer of social care to send the appropriate signals to the local providers as to which services would be purchased and those that would not. For New Labour although the quasi-market is retained, its diversity is limited and control of the process moves upwards to government, to ensure that services in the longer term can be planned for and co-operation between providers enforced (see Powell 2003 for an interesting discussion of this process in respect to the NHS).

In broad terms then New Labour's approach can be characterized as a form of entrepreneurial governance (Osborne and Gaebler 1992). In its classic exposition this valorizes competition between service providers, decentralizes authority by embracing participatory management, focuses on measuring performance by outcome and enables public, private and voluntary sectors to come together to solve problems of service delivery.

Governance and modernization

In developing partnership New Labour reflects its intention (which has impacted across all government departments) to modernize British society and the institutions of government. Fairclough (2000) argues that modernization became a key part of New Labour's discourse in order to signify its uniqueness from previous political regimes: from, on the one hand, the Conservative Party and its reliance upon neo-liberalism and, on the other, from those of the 'Old Labour Party' vilified as wedded to the old state bureaucracies. In order to modernize, a new way of governing was deemed necessary to co-ordinate the proliferation of private, voluntary and quasi-public bodies that had mushroomed under the Conservative Party's 18 years of office. Central to this project was the importance given to the concept of partnership in which previously functionally autonomous bodies were encouraged to develop new working relationships, for example, public private partnerships, the Private Finance Initiative (PFI) or through greater co-ordination of government agencies by the Social Exclusion Unit. Thus the previous distinctions between public and private bodies or between operationally independent government departments were to be brought closer together. Such terms as 'joined-up government' or creating 'seamless services' were meant to convey the sense of a new way of organizing and delivering services, for example, the Social Exclusion Unit would target services at groups considered most at risk of permanent exclusion from society. Such groups as young homeless people, care leavers or teenage mothers would receive a package of services that would be delivered together with the intention of integrating these groups into society.

These initiatives all attested to the importance given by New Labour to working across what had previously been considered unhelpful professional and organiza-tional divides, or 'Berlin Walls' as they had been described by various government ministers (Parrott 2002). In *Modernizing Social Services* (Department of Health 1998b), the government argued that the existing configuration of health and social care was contributing to an artificial segregation of services; service users did not present their problems in such functionally delineated ways. In order to deliver its modernization agenda New Labour believed it must break down professional and organizational autonomy when it acted to frustrate the proper delivery of governmental services and the needs of consumers (Malin *et al.* 2002).

In order to reconfigure governmental activity, three related concepts can be identified which became the touchstone of New Labour's policy:

- Governance
- Modernization
- Partnership

Governance

Daly (2002) shows how the idea of governance has emerged over the past 10 years as a dominant concept in framing the academic and political discourse upon government. Although the term has a ubiquitous cloak covering many aspects of academic and policy discourses, it achieves a more solid basis in referring to a form of control of networks within government in which private, state, voluntary and informal sectors are joined together, usually in various forms of partnership. Governance is, therefore, a process by which the state both reflects the existing plurality of relationships and processes between different sectors of society but also reinforces and remakes them to encourage further partnership working. The very process of governance then enjoins participants to be ever more diverse in their working relationships, to look outside their own agencies to make and remake working relationships with other interested stakeholders. Governance is an attempt to encourage and control these newly forged relationships and to further the ways in which the participants can become part of a self-governing network orchestrated by the state (Daly 2002).

Governance can take many forms, for example, as an analysis of the state and the public sphere, or as a focus upon the processes of policy making. For this chapter the focus is on governance as a normative concept, as a set of prescriptions for the way government should manage an increasingly complex society and secondly as a focus on policy implementation through the reorganization of the structure and delivery of services. Governance was the means to achieve this modernizing agenda in which government became an enabler, steering the institutions of government and introducing greater flexibility through the orchestration of the myriad public, private and informal agencies and networks that are a mark of a post-traditional society. The assumption is that power is no longer concentrated in the institutions of government based in nation states but is diffused in global networks, which circulate and shift over space and time. Anthony Giddens, the intellectual guru of New Labour, has argued that a post-traditional society requires a generative politics, which enables individuals and groups to make things happen rather than have things happen to them. Thus a generative politics seeks to reconstitute and regenerate the public domain through an enabling state:

> Generative politics is a defence of the politics of the *public domain,* but does not situate itself in the old opposition between state and market. It works through providing material conditions, and organisational frameworks, for the political life decisions taken by individuals and groups in the wider social order.
>
> (Giddens 1994: 15)

Government must, therefore, respond in more flexible and open-ended ways that seek to orchestrate the new fluid networks of power both nationally and globally. This approach requires networks to be managed through the use of such tools as contracting and collaboration with incentives for co-operation, penalties for non-compliance and the creation of institutional structures with clear principal–agent relationships to effect this change (Brinton Millward and Provan 2003). Governance is the articulation of a new flexibility of control by the state to the new challenges posed by the post-traditional society. The feasibility and desirability of the state's attempt to directly engineer the content of society is replaced by the state's attempt to influence indirectly the content of society through networks which join the state institutions with those of civil society and the economy. The role of the state then is to set the terms and specify the policy aims it wants to achieve, while others carry out the implementation. As Jessop (2000) has argued, it should be regarded as a regime rather than a state in so far as this emphasizes the importance of non-state mechanisms to deliver state sponsored social and economic policies.

The arguments for developing partnership are intimately tied up with new ways of governing society; governance provides the motor for developing new relationships between institutions in society and between professionals. It is through partnerships that, in effect, hybrid organizations are created, joined together to achieve what previous disparate bodies could not do on their own. As Ling (2000) has argued in relation to the NHS: 'In governance, then, partnership enjoys a higher status than in government. Because there is a resource dependency in which state agencies want access to the capacities of other organizations, the relationship becomes less asymmetrical' (p. 88). This suggests that in order for the state to deploy its capacity to govern, it requires its partners to act in a way that does not look only to their self-interest but to the wider social interest as defined by the state. As Ling (2000) argues, this led in the 1980s to the exhaustion of governance, as private partners were unable to relinquish their self-interests for the wider benefit of the state. The new configuration of partnership sought by New Labour seeks to reconcile the particular needs of individual partners with the wider social project of government.

Modernization

Modernization, as the introduction suggested, became a key and unifying concept in the discourse of New Labour. The idea of modernization was aimed at harmonizing two previously opposed and antagonistic forces that had prevented the modernization of British society (at least in New Labour's terms). On the one hand, previous Conservative governments were criticized for an over-reliance on markets which had encouraged a more individualistic culture within public services, fragmenting the nature of public service delivery. On the other, previous Labour administrations were vilified as overly reliant on bureaucratic state machinery that, it was argued, led to rigidities and inflexibility in the delivery of public services. Thus New Labour saw their mission as forging a Third Way, a fusion between what was argued were the strengths of the market, in terms of its so-called dynamism and flexibility, with the capacity of the state and its ability to regulate for social justice to secure a fair and equitable distribution of welfare benefits and services. Both of these characterizations were dualistic and stereotypical. Dualistic in setting up a state or market dichotomy in which New Labour would magically reconcile the two. Stereotypical by exaggerating the differences and simplifying the complexity of previous Labour and Conservative administrations, which had contained elements of both state and market approaches within them. As Newman argues, the Third Way draws 'selectively on fragments and components of the old, and reconfiguring these through the prisms of a modernised economy, a modern public service and a modern people' (Newman 2000: 46). Thus all elements and levels of society were subjected to this modernizing process as a way of redesigning the way New Labour wished to govern society. For the public services, modernization was an essential symbolic element in achieving the goals of New Labour.

In order to achieve these goals, New Labour argued that governments must develop new ways of governing to meet the assumed increasing complexity of a globalized world (Blair 1996). The form that government should take to meet these challenges was one in which government should no longer directly intervene in the complex networks of society but act as an enabler, not by 'government' but through 'governance', to forge a myriad network of partnerships.

Partnership

The active promotion of partnership is seen as the most appropriate way to deal with the problems of the integration of public services as outlined above. Partnership as used by New Labour has a stronger connotation than previously used concepts such as 'inter-agency working' and 'collaboration' in that it means much stronger, permanent and closer relationships at all levels of the organizations involved. In relation to community care it has usually meant joint planning, commissioning and provision of services. In effect, partnership as it is developing now is moving towards integration. For example, in the case of community care with older people, social services are working within local health services to deliver a greater turn around of patients from the hospital into the community or to keep people in their own homes through the development of rapid response teams to prevent emergency admission to hospital. The concept can be seen in the enabling of new forms of service delivery in which management of the process is left to the partners while the service outcomes are set and quality controlled by the state. Professionals within these partnerships are enjoined to work in new ways, to change what may be considered unhelpful working practices and cultures and to reconstruct their professional and practical relationships with one another. Within the field of community care these new ways of working have been vigorously promoted by government. The accepted faith of partnership is one of synergy in which previously separate players whether state, private or voluntary agencies can become more than the sum of their parts by joining in partnership to create collaborative advantage, i.e. in achieving what they could not have done if they had acted separately (Huxham 2003).

Problems of partnership

New working partnerships between the NHS and the PSS have been encouraged by New Labour and have flowed from its critique of existing practice. In relation to community care, the White Paper *Modernising Social Services* (DoH 1998b) was highly critical of the lack of co-operation between the NHS and the PSS. Attention was drawn to the lack of co-ordination between different agencies, leading to the failure to protect both service users and the public from harm. This conceptualization of an aura of failure, as Langan argues (2000), was developed by New Labour to cajole the local authority social service departments in what was argued was their loss of control, for example, in mental health with high profile breakdowns of services to adequately provide for service users and failures to protect the public from violent persons with mental health problems (see Stanley and Manthorpe 2000). As *Modernising Mental Health Services: Safe and Sound* (DoH 1998a) made clear, care in the community had failed to adequately control the small number of people with severe mental health problems who were a danger to themselves and the wider community. These criticisms highlighted the inadequacy of different agencies in their existing arrangements of joint working to prevent these individuals from falling through the net of supervision. These catastrophes were largely identified as problems of the management process rather than inadequate resourcing of community care services.

As part of this modernization process the Personal Social Services (PSS) were to be paid particular attention, in that the existing structure of services was seen as an impediment to the successful implementation of the new government's plans. As *Modernising Social Services* (DoH 1998b) asserts, the focus is on delivery – who provides the service becomes less important than what can be achieved in terms of better quality outcomes. As part of this process, particular attention was given to the lack of integration and collaboration between the PSS and other parts of the welfare state, in particular the NHS. Partnership was the means to overcome these problems and formed a central part of the modernizing process, in which the old structures within local and central government would be reconstructed around partnership. In order to respond effectively to this new agenda, new ways of working within and between the different agencies of central and local government had to be developed. This restructuring of the welfare state was not a voluntary option and New Labour was determined to make new relationships and forge new structures to realize its modernizing agenda.

Partnership as conceptualized by New Labour was not new in the sense that for a number of years successive governments had realized the need for joint working and greater collaboration between the PSS and the NHS. Yet partnership, as argued above, has much stronger connotations and requires of its participants more permanent and co-ordinated actions than those which describe working together or collaboration. As described in the introduction, partnership as it is developing between the PSS and NHS goes beyond any previous conceptualizations and as such (as some argue) may be moving towards integration and even incorporation of personal social services into the health service (Means and Smith 2003). This has increased significance within social care as the creation of Primary Care Trusts meant the movement to these trusts by the majority of social workers working with adults (Baldwin 2002).

The micro politics of partnership

It is too early to assess fully the impact of the new partnership arrangements upon health and the personal social services as they are still in a process of development. However, some evidence is emerging, a report by the King's Fund (2002) shows some encouraging developments for those in favour of partnership – though these are more at the level of ideology. The report suggests that the balance of opinion within health and the personal social services is moving towards partnership, it is no longer questioned by the practitioners surveyed; the focus is not whether partnership should happen but how can it work.

Models of integrated care are beginning to emerge for different service users and a greater concentration of strategic level partnership working is now in place. Yet this report also makes for a more sober assessment in voicing concern that the political agenda of government to solve pressures in the service system for the benefit of acute health services is distorting partnership working. This is problematic then if partnership is seen to solve one of the partner's problems while creating new problems for the other. Partnership working between the PSS and the NHS for the delivery of social care is, therefore, politically contentious, particularly with social workers and local authorities who see in this move a loss of power and control over social care. For social workers in particular, there is a concern that their professional competence and expertise will be compromised within an organization concerned more with the through-put of patients through the health system than the meeting of social need. This concern is supported by a survey carried out by the Local Government Association (2000) that noted the concern over the differential growth in health budgets as opposed to local authority budgets. For local authorities pressures on their budgets acted as a major hindrance to furthering partnership. This anxiety has been further evidenced by the Local Government Association's response to the government's policy towards delayed discharge. Their argument suggests that the government is blaming local authorities for delayed discharges and that the system of fines will be counterproductive in that there is no adequate infrastructure within local authorities to deal with the discharge process from hospital given that responsibility is not wholly with local government but also the NHS (Local Government Association 2003).

Field and Peck (2003) have analysed the potential of the current partnership arrangements from a business merger perspective, which makes rather bleak reading for the supporters of partnership working. They conclude that in the experience of company mergers, partners rarely achieve their strategic objectives leading to an initial loss in productivity and considerable stress and loss of morale on behalf of the workforce. They suggest that for successful mergers to take place then particular attention should be given to the people and their respective organizational and professional cultures, including senior managers and professionals. Field and Peck identify only one study, so far, which has looked at this process within health and the personal social services (Gulliver *et al.* 2001). The findings from this study bring cold comfort, reflecting problems in drawing different organizational and professional cultures together in a form that can ensure positive working relationships.

New Labour has focused understandably upon creating the legislative conditions and mechanisms to achieve partnership but the micro politics of partnership involving the face-to-face practical encounters between different professionals from different organizational cultures and working under different managerial styles has been given less focus. The logic of this approach as Hudson (2002) has noted is that if policies, processes and structures for partnership are established, then partnership at the level of professional collaboration will automatically follow. Yet this logic is flawed. The micro issues at the professional level have received considerable attention identifying many of the problems, which Peck and Field have identified from their broader analysis of mergers. Thus Hudson (2002), although arguing for a more positive approach to partnership, outlines a number of problems at the level of interprofessional working related to professional identity and status, discretion and accountability. Dalley (1996) argues for more scepticism in the promotion of partnership, suggesting that the managerial problems of partnership, for example, in agreeing the control of budgets and line management of staff frequently frustrate the often positive working relationships that front-line staff develop when working together. Rummery (1999), in analysing joint working between health and personal social service professionals, suggests that different models of joint working are crucial in developing or frustrating effective collaboration of front-line staff.

Therefore, different levels of involvement bring with them different benefits – joint working arrangements, which operate at a local area level, bring benefits for managers in developing joint strategies for health and social care services but few benefits for front-line staff. Arrangements that focus on commissioning services for individuals reap benefits for inter-professional working but offer less at the strategic level in terms of service development. The organization of partnership has also been analysed by Carpenter *et al.* (2003), who suggest in their analysis of community mental health services that where mental health and social services are integrated there are significant gains in terms of team functioning. Interestingly the research also highlighted differences in the impact of these arrangements between health service professionals and social workers with social workers experiencing higher levels of role conflict. They argue for more support and supervision for social workers, which may suggest that in the area they researched, this was far from adequate. Glendinning (2003) also supports this view in her research in relation to older people's services. She concludes that structural integration between health and personal social services can transform preoccupation with narrow sectoral responsibilities and boundaries to a 'whole systems' approach to service planning. Yet at lower levels of partnership, barriers to integration remain, including professional domains and identities and differential power relationships between newly integrated services.

Conclusion

This chapter has identified the move towards partnership working between the NHS and the PSS. It has focused on the macro politics of organizational change and has identified the specific approach taken by New Labour to develop new forms of governance that can be separated from the previous Conservative governments' approach. This means that the New Labour approach seeks to maintain consistency in partnership working across different parts of the country, while devolving as much operational power as possible to the partnership organizations themselves.

It has been suggested that much remains to be done in addressing the politics within and between organizations before partnership can be developed further. For example, the government must address the concerns of community health workers that they will not become part of the type of residualized local welfare system characterized by local authority Personal Social Services. Likewise, New Labour must address the concerns of social work and social care staff to not only feel that they will become valued members of the new partnership arrangements but that their distinct-ive professional role and autonomy is not subsumed under a health care orientation. Coleman and Rummery's (2003) research on the experience of social service representatives on Primary Care Group Boards and Trusts (PCGBT) is instructive where despite some encouraging improvements in relationships, social service repre-sentatives still experienced significant levels of non-consultation over services, and the Chief Officers of the PCGBT rated the influence of such representatives to be rela-tively less than other board members. This leads the authors to be very cautious about the assumptions that the new Care Trusts will lead to better integration between health and social services.

At present partnership developments have concentrated on the strategic arrangements between the NHS and PSS, with little reflection upon the politics of organizational and professional change. In addition, as will be argued later, the needs of service users and carers have also been underplayed in relation to the organiza-tional issues. It is clear from the arguments presented above that the macro arguments for the necessity of partnership have been won, however reluctantly in some cases. Nonetheless, having won the ideological argument this should not blind us to requir-ing a further exploration of the implications of governance for the effective organiza-tion and delivery of community care services. A complex network of partnerships may not deliver the requirements of a democratically elected government with an electorate that requires social justice, fairness and equality. The setting of multifaceted partnership networks controlled at arm's length through a system of 'entrepreneurial governance' may militate against those principles and outcomes in terms of equity that citizens require of service delivery. The joining together of the PSS and the NHS at the local level to deliver social care leaves the quasi-market intact. How far the new partnerships will be able to overcome the uneven and fragmenting processes of the previous quasi-market regime is debatable.

The current Minster for Community Care, Stephen Ladyman, has already out-lined in relation to the uneven distribution of residential care homes that it is the local authorities who must resolve the problem, suggesting that if the partnership arrange-ments break down then it could be feasible for the local health authority to commission services (*Community Care Journal* 2003), which in effect would severely compromise partnership arrangements between the PSS and the NHS. What partnership does is to reconfigure the purchaser provider split so that an expanded care trust subverts the local authority as the co-ordinator of community care, something that Margaret Thatcher tried to do prior to the NHSCCA 1990 and which New Labour has finally succeeded in doing. Thus the new care trusts with only a limited representation from the local community will, therefore, find it difficult to be fully accountable. At present there is a fear that a democratic deficit exists within these new arrangements. As Du Gay (2000) argues: 'if the principles of entrepreneurial governance are allowed to set the terms by which the public bureaux are understood and judged, then we should expect the job the bureau has performed and continues to perform for us gradually to disappear' (p. 112).

Glasby and Peck (2004) report on the concerns for accountability and represen-tation on the governing boards of the new partnership arrangements and, in particu-lar, the way in which consultation and the communication of decisions is not spread outwards to the public. This concern is further developed when taking into account the voices of service users and carers who may be acting as representatives on such boards. As Brodie (2003), a service user, suggests there is a conflict of interest that is not easily resolvable: 'I felt torn between the confidential aspects of decision making within the Trust and the needs of users and carers' (p. 67).

The needs of service users and carers has a central place in understanding the politics of partnership but their voices have been given little recognition in the drive to create the new partnership arrangements. Given that the needs of service users are promoted as one of the major justifications for the new arrangements, the failure to include a significant user perspective 'must be seen as a major oversight' (Glasby and Lester 2004, p. 14).

Questions for further discussion

1. To what extent do New Labour's policies result in genuine partnerships in community care?
2. How successful have New Labour's policies been in integrating inter-professional issues in new partnership arrangements?
3. Partnership, governance and modernization are inextricably linked to New Labour's vision of government. How far is this reflected in your organization?

References

Audit Commission (1986) *Making a Reality of Community Care*. London, HMSO.

Audit Commission (1998) *A Fruitful Partnership: Effective Partnership Working*. Audit Commission, London.

Baldwin, M. (2002) New Labour and social care in M. Powell (ed.) *Evaluating New Labour's Welfare Reforms*. Policy Press, Bristol.

Blair, T. (1996) *New Britain: My Vision of a Young Country*. Fourth Estate, London.

Bridgen, P. (2003) Joint planning across the Health/Social Services boundary since 1946, *Local Government Studies*, Autumn 29(3): 17–31.

Brinton Millward, H. and Provan, K.G. (2003) Managing the Hollow State: Collaboration and Contracting, *Public Management Review*, 5(1): 1–18.

Brodie, D. (2003) Partnership working: a service user perspective, in J. Glasby and E. Peck (eds) *Care Trusts: Partnership Working in Action*. Radcliffe Medical Press, Abingdon.

Carpenter, J., Schneider, J., Brandon, T. and Wooff, D. (2003) Working in multidisciplinary community health teams: The impact on social workers and health professionals of integrated mental health care, *British Journal of Social Work*, 3: 1081–103.

Carvel, J., Prasad, R. and Benjamin, A. (2004) Out of Patience, *Guardian* 7 January.

Coleman, A. and Rummery, K. (2003) Social services representation in Primary Care Groups and Trusts, *Journal of Interprofessional Care*, 17(3): 273–9.

Community Care Journal (2003) Interview with Stephen Ladyman, *Community Care Journal*, 24 September.

Daly, M. (2002) Governance and social policy, *Journal of Social Policy*, January, pp. 113–28.

Dalley, G. (1996) *Ideologies of Caring: Rethinking Communities and Collectivism*. Macmillan, Basingstoke.

Department of Health and Social Security (1981) *Growing Older*. Cmnd 8173, HMSO, London.

Department of Health (1989) *Caring for People: Community Care in the Next Decade and Beyond*. Cm 849, HMSO, London.

Department of Health (1998a) *Modernising Mental Health Services: Safe, Sound and Supportive*. HMSO, London.

Department of Health (1998b) *Modernising Social Services: Promoting Independence, Improving Protection and Raising Standards*. The Stationery Office, London.

Department of Health (1999) *National Service Framework*. HMSO, London.

Du Gay, P. (2000) *In Praise of Bureaucracy*. Sage, London.

Fairclough, N. (2000) *New Labour, New Language?*, Routledge, London.

Field, J and Peck, E. (2003) Mergers and acquisitions in the private sector: What are the lessons for Health and Social Services? *Social Policy and Administration*, Vol. 37, No. 7: 742–55.

Giddens, A. (1994) *Beyond Left and Right: The Future of Radical Politics*. Polity, Cambridge.

Glasby, J. and Lester, H. (2004) Cases for change in mental health: partnership working in mental health services, *Journal of Interprofessional Care*, 18(1): 7–17.

Glasby, J. and Peck, E. (2004) *Integrated Working and Governance: A Discussion Paper*. Integrated Care Network, www.integratedcarenetwork.gov.uk.

Glendinning, C. (2002) Partnerships between health and social services: developing a framework for evaluation, *Policy and Politics*, 30(1): 115–27.

Glendinning, C. (2003) Breaking down barriers: integrating health and care services for older people in England, *Health Policy*, 65: 139–51.

Gulliver, P., Peck, E. and Towell, D. (2001) Evaluation of the implementation of the mental Health Review in Somerset: results after thirty months of data collection, *Managing Community Care*, 9, 1: 14–21.

Hudson, B. (2000) Adult Care in M. Hill (ed.) *Local Authority Social Services: An Introduction*. Blackwell, Oxford.

Hudson, B. (2002) Interprofessionality in health and social care: the Achilles' heel of partnership? *Journal of Interprofessional care*, 6(1): 7–15.

Huxham, C. (2003) Theorizing Collaboration Practice, *Public Management Review*, 5(3): 401–23.

Jessop, B. (2000) Restructuring the welfare state, reorienting welfare strategies, revisioning the welfare society in B. Grieve (ed.) *What Constitutes a Good Society?* Macmillan, Basingstoke.

Johnson, N. (1999) The personal social services and community care in M. Powell (ed.) *New Labour New Welfare State?* Policy Press, Bristol.

Langan, M. (2000) Social Services: Managing the Third Way, in J. Clarke, S. Gewirtz and E. Mclaughlin *New Managerialism New Welfare?* Sage/Open University, London.

Ling, T. (2000) Unpacking partnership: Health Care in Local Government in J. Clarke, S. Gewirtz and E. McLaughlin *New Managerialism New Welfare?* Sage/Open University, London.

Local Government Association (2000) *Partnerships with Health: A Survey of Local Authorities*. Local Government Association, London.

Local Government Association (2003) *A Whole in One*. Local Government Association, London.

King's Fund (2002) *Partnerships Under Pressure: A Commentary on Progress in Partnership Working Between the NHS and Local Government*. King's Fund, London.

Malin, N., Wilmot, S. and Manthorpe, J. (2002) *Key Concepts and Debates in Health and Social Policy*. Open University Press, Buckingham.

Means, R., Richards, S. and Smith, R. (2003) *Community Care: Policy and Practice*. Palgrave, Basingstoke.

Newman, J. (2000) Beyond the new public management? Modernizing public services in J. Clarke, S. Gewirtz and E. McLaughlin *New Managerialism New Welfare?* Sage/Open University, London.

Newman, J. (2001) *Modernising Governance: New Labour, Policy and Society*. Sage, London.

Osborne, D. and Gaebler, T. (1992) *Reinventing Government*. Addison-Wesley, Reading, MA.

Parrott, L. (2002) *Social Work and Social Care* (2nd edn). Routledge, London.

Pollitt, C. (2003) *The Essential Public Manager*. Open University Press, Maidenhead.

Powell, M. (2003) Quasi-markets in British Health Policy: A Longue Duree, *Perspective, Social Policy and Administration*, 37(7): 725–41.

Rummery, K. (1999) The way forward for joint working? Involving primary care in the commissioning of social care services, *Journal of Interprofessional Care*, 13(3): 207–17.

Seebohm Report (1968) *Report of the Committee on Local Authority and Allied Personal Social Services*. Cmnd. 3703. HMSO, London.

Stanley, N. and Manthorpe, J. (2000) Reading Mental Health Enquiries, *Journal of Social Work*, 1(1): 77–99.

Timmins, N. (1996) *The Five Giants: A Biography of the Welfare State*. Fontana Press, London.

Wyatt, M. (2002) Partnership in health and social care: the implications of government guidance in the 1990s in England, with particular reference to voluntary organisations, *Policy and Politics*, 30(2): 167–82.

3

Ethical issues of working in partnership

Althea Allison

This chapter will:

- Discuss the ethical and moral issues that may arise in relation to interprofessional working.
- Provide an explanation of ethical frameworks and moral codes, in order that an understanding of these differing frameworks may facilitate the discernment of 'right' decisions.
- Consider the consequences of actions and omissions within the context of professional relationships.
- Consider values and principles specific to practice and to the individual, as well as the theoretical frameworks that need to be applied within the context of practice to have any significance or usefulness for the professional.

Introduction

All professional groups, whether working in isolation or in fully integrated teams, face challenges in the delivery of their particular skills and services. These challenges may be located in many different areas including: increased consumer expectations; evolving cultural boundaries; advances in technology; political and legal norms; government policy initiatives and changes, financial considerations and social mores (Soothill *et al.* 1995). This list is clearly not presented as a definitive catalogue but serves to offer an insight into the complex context of professional practice. An element running through this list which is perhaps more relevant to consideration in this chapter, is that with every item on the list, there are ethical and moral considerations linked to the challenges faced.

Professional groups have a specific remit within society; they meet particular needs within society (Burkhardt and Nathaniel 2002). When one assumes the role of a professional, one takes on certain role-specific duties – in general, those that advance and preserve the special good(s) at which the profession aims. Generally speaking, each professional group has a defined contribution to make that is not shared by others. Bayles (1989) argues that each professional group has its own particular special 'good', its own specific contribution to make. The resulting profession-specific duties impose obligations upon the professional that do not normally apply to everyone else, for example, a doctor is obligated to heal, a lawyer to advance legal justice, a social worker to enhance the well-being of people within their social contexts, a teacher to promote knowledge and facilitate learning, nurses to promote health and care for the sick and dying. It would appear then, that each professional group has some particular service that it provides, some 'good' that others need or want. Arguably, the more professional a job, the greater the responsibilities and obligations that go with it.

An obvious starting point for the individual professional is being clear about the raison d'être or the professional purpose of the group to which they claim membership. While the specific responsibilities may change, influenced by context and development as a professional group, the purpose of the profession does not. This chapter will, therefore, address the following issues:

- Approaches to ethics
- Partnership working and the context of interprofessional practice
- Working together – the fiduciary relationship

Approaches to ethics

Before considering the different approaches to ethics, it is first necessary to distinguish between ethics and morals. There are misapprehensions surrounding the words *ethics* and *morals* embodied in the, sometimes interchangeable, use of the words adopted in various writings in health and social care. 'Ethics' offers a formal process for applying moral philosophy and provides a framework for discerning logical and consistent decisions concerned with questions of how one *ought* to behave in a given situation (Burkhardt and Nathaniel 2002). The word 'morals' has, in a colloquial sense, been narrowed to become synonymous with matters of sexual behaviour, while problems associated with issues other than sexual behaviour are more often referred to using the word *ethics*. In effect then, *ethics* and *morals* can refer to two different areas of ordinary morality (Downie and Telfer 1980). Perhaps the most important issue here is not whether certain acts or judgements are ethical or unethical, but *why* they are deemed to be so. Moral judgement presupposes the moral argument for the case that if something is right or wrong, it will be so for a reason (Fletcher and Holt 1995). Consider the case study in Box 3.1.

Moral philosophy and ethical theories can be useful, therefore, in helping professionals to determine 'right' actions. Moreover, the purpose of moral philosophy and ethics, according to Norman (1983), is an attempt to arrive at an understanding of the nature of human values, of how we ought to live and of what constitutes right conduct. If the pursuit of moral philosophy and ethical theory is to bring greater understanding and insight to practice, a clearer view of the propositions offered by major schools of philosophical thought is required.

Box 3.1 A case study of multidisciplinary ethical care

A GP cares for a family with many health and social care problems. They have five children; the father is a heavy drinker and known to be violent and the mother suffers from a psychotic illness, which is controlled by medication. The mother does not like taking her medication but is visited regularly by the CPN who monitors her care. During her last admission to hospital, the psychiatrist made it clear that if she did not co-operate with taking her oral medication, then he would have to think about prescribing her medication via an intramuscular route. The social worker assigned to the family is most concerned about youngest child, aged two and half, who appears not to be thriving physically and has delayed speech and there is a worry that the child is at risk. She would like to place the child in a day nursery but is faced with a lack of resources. The health visitor to the family has known the mother very well over a great number of years and has developed a very trusting relationship with her. Recently, the mother confided in her that she wanted to stop taking her medication because it made her too lethargic to do anything with her life and was making her fat. She said she wanted to 'be like she used to be' and added that she had been considering telling her husband to go because she was fed up with his behaviour.

   Although it might seem that the psychiatrist was being coercive in making the mother comply with her medication, psychotic illness is devastating for the individual and for those who love and care for them. Hospital admissions can be traumatic for the individual and, in this case, disruptive to the family, particularly the youngest child. The CPN is acting ethically within their professional role in monitoring the medication and progress of the mother but, arguably, there is an element of social control here, which is not primarily in the client's best interest. The health visitor is faced with possibly damaging a trusting relationship, built up over years, if she reports what she knows and is in the unenviable position of considering whether to breech a confidence. The social worker, who sees a way to support the mother and the child, is thwarted by a lack of nursery places. Resource allocation issues are ever present in health and social care. Deciding whose needs are most pressing is both daunting and fraught with ethical considerations. Ultimately, the GP carries the responsibility for the family's health-related needs in the community.

   Is it in the best interest of all concerned to make sure the mother remains well and within the family, or is keeping her on medication, which she is not happy with, using her as a means to an end? Whose frame of reference is being used to decide best interest? What personal qualities within the professional are demanded?

   The main schools of philosophical thought are utilitarianism, deontology and virtue ethics, as discussed below.

Utilitarianism

Utilitarianism, sometimes referred to as Consequentialism, is the moral theory which proposes that right action is that which brings about the greatest utility or usefulness; allowing that no action is, in itself, either good or bad, but rather it is the outcomes that carry moral significance. Central concepts of utilitarianism are 'good' and 'evil' – happiness equating to good and unhappiness equating to evil (Husted and Husted 1991). Although the concept of happiness alone may be criticized as a simplistic notion, utilitarians hold that the only elements that make actions good or bad are the outcomes that can be ascribed to them (Burkardt and Nathaniel 2002).

Deontology

Deontological theories provide a very different framework for assessing ethical questions. Ethical action, within the deontological tradition, is based on 'doing one's duty'. Central concepts within this approach are the notions of 'right' and 'wrong'. The moral agent has a duty to do what is 'right' and to refrain from doing what is 'wrong'. Right action, therefore, consists of doing one's duty, while failing to do one's duty is wrong (Husted and Husted 1991).

The absolute requirement to respect the autonomy and dignity of the person are of utmost importance within this approach, leading to the imperative to treat each individual 'as an end in themselves', not merely as a means for arbitrary use by others. In contrast to the utilitarian school, the rightness or wrongness of an act, then, depends upon the nature of the act, rather than the consequences.

Virtue ethics

The concept of virtue ethics, also referred to as character ethics, presents a challenge to deontological and utilitarian theories. Virtue ethics has experienced a revival in fortune and has re-emerged as an influential framework for examining moral behaviour (Pence 1993). The central tenet of virtue ethics is derived from the view that an individual moral agent will choose particular actions based upon a certain degree of innate moral virtue.

Deontological and utilitarian theories ascribe to the view that ethics provides guidelines to action based on the question, 'what morally ought one to do?' Virtue ethics, however, does not start from this question, but rather starts from the premise that the basic function of morality is the moral character of persons. The question then becomes, not 'what should one *do*?', but rather, 'what should one *be*?' (Burkhardt and Nathaniel 2002).

Behaving ethically and behaving morally are, therefore, different and both terms are frequently used by health and social care professionals when referring to 'professional' behaviour. 'You can't do that, it's immoral' is not an unusual proclamation on the part of caring professionals. Equally, those working in health and social care take pride in their ethical behaviour, which is enshrined in codes of conduct that they are required to follow. However, different codes of behaviour and understanding of ethical and moral rules held by different professional groups have important implications for partnership working.

Partnership working and the context of interprofessional practice

The notion of working in partnership was established into the NHS ideology in the 1997 Department of Health document *The New NHS*. Indeed, inter-agency working and collaboration between professional groups, notably between health and social care, was established as a 'duty of care'. The notion of partnership has continued to gain strength and is now central to NHS ideology and purpose. Indeed, McLaughlin (2004) has argued that partnership provides a 'core theme' within social policy areas as diverse as health and social care, urban regeneration, education, crime and biotechnology (p. 103). While working boundaries between professional groups may become less defined and user perspectives are given greater credence (Biggs 2000), ideological boundaries do not necessarily change by dictat. It remains questionable as to whether different professional groups will be able to make the ideological shift.

The modernization agenda inherent in the policy changes alluded to requires a fundamental culture shift and attitude change by all professional groups at all levels. Fish and Coles (1998) point out that professionals cannot continue to work in isolation from other professional groups. The complexity of contemporary health and social care provision is such that the full range of professional groups must work together as a team. Partnership potentially expands access to resources by virtue of sharing knowledge and expertise. It also promotes cross-fertilization of approaches to intervention. Partnership working also highlights the limitations of single agency working in dealing with complex human problems. Surely this provides an argument for the rationalization of resources, to avoid waste of scarce resources and to maximize the good from resources available. In practice, however, working together as a team is more easily said than done, as Ashwell (2003) has noted in particular relation to health and social care collaborators. Clashes of professional culture, objectives and ways of dealing with the client groups have yet to be fully overcome.

The context of care delivery has been influenced by the changes in the philosophical underpinnings informing political policies: the myriad policy and legislative changes which have emanated as a result; the financial position of the national economy continuing to fuel the quest for cost-effectiveness; continuing technological and scientific advances in health care; the voice and influence of professional bodies; and the demands of stakeholders, including patients and carers. A surfeit of government policies provides an indication of these changes within the NHS, two in particular encapsulating the changing ideology: *The New NHS: Modern, Dependable* (DoH 1997) and *The NHS Plan* (DoH 2000). These policies aim to place consumers at the centre of health care provision and include arrangements for more stringent mechanisms for maintaining accountability in professional practice and for monitoring resources.

Those professionals working in the public service in particular have witnessed unprecedented change in the last 10 years. A fundamental shift in philosophical emphasis is evidenced in the increasing empowerment of consumers of services offered within the public services. Consumers, in response, have become more questioning and articulate in relation to professional expertise and the quality of services offered. Changes in societal expectations have also contributed to an increased emphasis on partnership and respect for individual responsibility in client-professional relationships.

So what does this change mean for the professional in the delivery of their services and expertise? What ethical issues arise in this situation? In the main, professional groups would argue that a central core of the way they work is to make certain that client interests are served as a primary consideration. Professional codes of ethics generally reflect this philosophy, focusing on obligations to individual clients. It is highly likely that individual practitioners from different professional persuasions would believe that they try, in all conscience, to do a good job. To imply otherwise could be considered vaguely insulting. However, health and social care professionals may be faced with very complex situations which call for expertise outside of their normal sphere of practice, resulting in a demand for collaboration and pooling of expertise that locates the client as being central to the exercise rather than being peripheral to it. This inevitably means having sufficient insight to know when one is at the limits of their professional expertise and can be open to working with other professional groups for the good of the client. This can be seen in the case study in Box 3.2.

Box 3.2 A case study of multi-professional working

Sally, a social worker of many years' experience, received a referral following a telephone report from a member of the general public that they thought a child in the street where they lived was being 'neglected'. The child was thought to be under school age, wandered in the street, looked uncared for and asked neighbours for food and drink. There were believed to be three other children of school age but the eldest child, aged about 10, was frequently seen looking after the youngest child.

On visiting the house, the mother, a single parent living on state benefits, appeared to be withdrawn, had difficulty in responding to Sally's questions and the house was dirty, cluttered and cold. When asked about the report that her daughter had been begging for food and drinks from neighbours, the mother just curled up on the couch and closed her eyes.

The potential for many agencies to become involved in this scenario is obvious and, depending on who in the scenario is seen as the client, might include professionals from health, social care and education at the very least. More specialist sections of each of those broad professional groups may also be engaged including, mental health workers, child and family social care workers and educational psychologists. Of course here lies one of the first problems, professional groups may see their primary obligations not only as being of a different nature but also establishing different priorities. One may prioritize the mother, another the child, another the whole family as a unit. One may see it as an emergency, another as a situation that needs intervention but not an immediate threat. Taking the deontological view, then, different professionals will have different views about to whom they should 'do their duty'; while taking the utilitarian stance, it is evident that whatever action the professional takes will have consequences. However, while the individual assesses the possible professional contribution they may make, what remains true for all groups is that they have obligations to their clients emanating from the privileged position they hold.

Obligations to whom?

In the discussion above, it was stated that professional codes of ethics generally focus on obligations to individual clients. Within any client-professional relationship, there are certain moral obligations that are imposed by virtue of the relationship. A professional relationship differs from a social relationship in a number of fundamental ways. In a professional relationship, there is an expectation that the needs of the client will form the focus of the relationship and that the professional will be vigilant to those needs, given that clients will generally become clients because they have a need for which the expertise of the professional is required (Allison 1996). As individuals in our own daily lives, we each will make decisions about our personal circumstances, for example, how we may conduct our relationships, through to a decision about whether we avoid paying the fare on public transport. We have if you like, personal frameworks and *moral* codes by which we live our lives. Within the professional role we inhabit, personal criteria may not be enough. In the context of practice, other considerations fall into the equation, not least the privileged position held by any professional group. Sometimes, the laws and customs of a particular society will determine the scope of moral obligations to be assumed by individuals in that society (Gillon 1986). Possible conflicts between obligations to clients and third parties are also an important consideration in teamworking. Responsibilities of truthfulness, non-maleficence and fairness are implicated here, as indicated in the examples in Box 3.3.

Box 3.3 The ethics of protecting third parties

There is a duty incumbent on professionals to protect third parties from danger. For example, a physician may have good reason to believe that a particular medical condition may present a danger to others, as in the case of a train driver who starts to suffer from unpredictable blackouts. Physicians clearly have a responsibility to provide care and treatment for the client but there is also an obligation to third parties who may be injured. Truthfulness is a basic expectation that a client can expect from a professional, but what about third parties?

There are certainly examples of physicians and nurses being asked by relatives to withhold information about potentially fatal illnesses from a patient and vice versa. However, a terminally ill patient may be denied support and practical help that would support their independence if social service colleagues were not allowed to know the diagnosis. Fairness and truthfulness often combine in forming a dilemma for professionals. Consider the professional who is asked to support an application for rehousing but is expected to exaggerate the circumstances so that a higher priority is assigned.

There are several groups to whom professionals can reasonably be expected to owe an obligation including:

- patients/clients
- patient/client's relatives
- fellow professionals

- employers
- the general public
- themselves and their dependents

Of course it would be exceedingly difficult to serve all these stakeholders in equal measure. When a situation presents itself where conflicting demands are being made, the question is raised of where one's first obligation lies. Arguably, professionals enter a contract with society when they take on a professional mantle. In effect, they agree to provide a specialist service and in return society grants a monopoly around that service. The argument for professional obligations to third parties is located in the role of professions conferred by society (Burkhardt and Nathaniel 2002). The danger in viewing the professional as having a responsibility to society that may outweigh the responsibility to the client is that it relieves the client of responsibility for themselves. This raises the notion of what Bayles (1989) described as the fiduciary relationship.

Working together – the fiduciary relationship

When a client and professional come together, they do so as one human being to another. In essence, they meet as equals, except that a client is generally involved with a professional because the professional has superior knowledge, expertise and gate-keeping abilities that the client does not have. This, therefore, shifts the relationship into more of a dependent one. Bayles (1989) recognized the need for a concept that acknowledged the special contribution of the professional within a client-professional relationship, but also one that allowed the client to retain significant authority and responsibility in the decision making. He utilized the notion of the fiduciary relationship, a concept used in legal relationships to characterize the features of a client-professional relationship. In a fiduciary relationship, both parties are responsible and their judgements are given consideration. However, because the professional is in a more advantageous position because of their special knowledge and expertise, Bayles (1989) emphasizes the special obligation of the professional to be worthy of client trust in a fiduciary relationship. The notion of trust implied in such a relationship is one that accomplishes the outcomes for which the professional has been appointed and which meets the client's needs. Trustworthy professionals, he argues, will demonstrate several virtues within their character. These are listed in Box 3.4.

Box 3.4 Professional virtues as identified by Bayles (1989)
Honesty
Candour
Competence
Diligence
Loyalty
Fairness
Discretion

Although these attributes are offered as a group of virtues that a trustworthy professional can be expected to possess, Bayles (1989) goes further than this, offering that the obligations implied and explicit in these characteristics may be regarded as 'norms of conduct' for the professional practitioner. The possession of these virtues in caring professionals in their relationships with clients might also help to explain the revival of *virtue ethics*.

It would be easy to discard Bayles's list of desirable virtues as only being relevant to the client-professional relationship but what about the other working relationships a professional must engage in? Professional-professional relationships pose particular challenges, especially when considering virtues of candour, loyalty and honesty, as does professional-non-professional relationships with charities and voluntary groups in this time of increasing collaboration. Do the same values and guides to conduct apply? In order to place trust in another person, one must have confidence in them, to be secure that they will act in a particular manner. This is just as true of client-professional relationships as it is of professional-professional relationships. Dalley's (1993) notion of tribalism describes the development of a cultural ideology, which may lead to an inflated notion of superiority about one's own organization, resulting in a lack of respect and trust in another organization with the consequence that there is unlikely to be a willingness to collaborate, even where it is indicated for the good of the client. The sharing of information, expertise and active collaboration in this context is unlikely to be undertaken with confidence. The result of such poor communication between professional groups not only makes us question the possession of ethical virtues discussed above but is also unlikely to promote client-centred care. In considering professional relationships with other professionals think about the example in Box 3.5.

Box 3.5 Behaving ethically in professional life

As a student nurse, I was given a poem to read by a tutor, which was said to have been written by a patient in a long-stay mental hospital. I cannot do justice to the rhyme and language after all these years but the gist of the message was this: Next time you are engaged in a case conference discussing the future of someone else, and you think you are the professional with the most important contribution to make, then think of this image. Imagine a bucket of water filled nearly to the top. Put your hand in and swirl it around until you make a hole in the centre of the water and take note of the impression you have made. Then take your hand out and watch again. The water will subside and eventually it will still, as if no one had ever touched it.

The point of this illustration is that the motivation for 'swirling the water' should not be about self-aggrandizement. Neither should it be short-lived with little to show for it.

It is in the nature of working with other human beings, then, that professionals face ethical and moral challenges in relation to client care. It is not difficult to find issues in any profession that involve the application of general (i.e. non-professional-specific) moral rules and values, such as telling the truth, respecting privacy, keeping promises. Just as in everyday life, many such 'professional' issues are easily resolved without sophisticated analysis, while others are messy and awkward. Some seemingly minor questions do not have unambiguous answers, such as prioritizing where to spend one's professional time and in what proportion. Equally, complex situations may offer more than one alternative strategy for dealing with them, with pros and cons to endorse or eliminate support for competing solutions depending on the gains and losses from a particular perspective.

Client-oriented and professional liaison relationships are not the only trusting relationships in which professionals may engage. A professional is also engaged in a trusting relationship with their employer. Clearly, the obligations imposed in the employer/employee relationship are similar to those contained in the client/professional relationship. Arguably, professionals who are 'self-employed', can be expected to embrace the relevant responsibilities and duties inferred in Bayles's taxonomy of professional virtues listed in Box 3.4. Indeed, one might argue that when one is self-employed, one's client may also become one's employer and as such a greater obligation may be imposed. Certainly, diligence would be a significant requirement in this circumstance. Bayles's (1989) professional virtues are helpful in understanding these wide-ranging responsibilities in the context of interprofessional working.

Honesty

A professional should not be dishonest with a client. This quite obviously includes not telling lies or stealing from a client. There are of course less obvious methods of being dishonest with clients. Stealing time from a client is one example. It could be easy to find a justification to spend time with likeable characters who appear to be appreciative of one's efforts as opposed to spending time with someone who is less responsive or lives in unpleasant surroundings. From an interprofessional perspective, denying a client referral for an assessment by another professional because of personal prejudice or 'baggage' about other professional groups is a theft. In other words, failing to provide access to a service involves dishonesty.

Just as a client can be robbed of respect, lack of respect between professionals can happen too. Where relationships lack respect and value for the expertise possessed by a fellow professional, the client loses out.

Candour

If honesty includes not telling lies, candour carries with it the obligation to offer information. While working in partnership with clients involves sharing information and negotiating aspects of interventions with professional colleagues, this would imply volunteering information in the client's interest. If professional groups are to collaborate in the best interest of their clients, sharing information is arguably a key component. However, professionals often avoid sharing information in order to preserve client confidentiality. Notwithstanding this, the setting of ground rules within a client-professional relationship can make it possible to work in an interprofessional scenario without abusing client privilege (Allison and Ewens 1998).

Competence

There is an ethical obligation on professionals to maintain competence in their area of expertise. Keeping abreast of changes in practice is implicated here. Some professional groups make this requirement explicit, in that evidence of professional development is required for continuous registration on the professional register. Whereas honesty with clients has been cited earlier as a desirable characteristic in a professional relationship, honesty with oneself is also indicated here. Recognizing the limits to one's expertise and competence requires vigilance from all professionals, regardless of how long they may have been doing the job. In interprofessional settings, it is not comfortable to feel ill at ease or unskilled. One might fear losing a professional reputation and be tempted to persevere regardless. Recognizing one's limitations is an essential requirement of the professional in developing self-awareness and determining their own level of competence. It is also the mechanism for developing sufficient confidence to recognize when other professional expertise is required and consequently making it possible to work more closely in interprofessional groups without losing face.

Diligence

Diligence refers to commitment and is closely aligned with competence. To be diligent in one's work implies that the professional attempts to provide competent care complemented with a commitment to the well-being of the client. Irvine *et al.* (2002) notes that the '(re)discovery of the *whole patient*' during the 1970s, provided the forum to reassess the interrelationship between the many new medical specialists, allied technologies and professions (p. 200). This refocusing of how the patient may be viewed established a different way of considering client need. In particular, this included the recognition that patients/clients grapple with difficulties so complex that it would be almost impossible for single agencies acting alone to address them. Increasing credence was also given to recognizing that clients might experience both medical and social needs at one and the same time. Clearly, the implication for all professional groups is that to be a diligent worker, there is a need to pool expertise in the interest of clients.

Loyalty

To display loyalty implies a faithfulness and commitment to duty within the client-professional relationship. However, the client does not have total call on the allegiance of the professional. The professional also has a responsibility to third parties including employers, fellow professionals and themselves. Sometimes, clients may make demands on the professional for a loyalty that would be misplaced. Sharing the burden of difficult and complex cases within an interprofessional setting is an advantage that is likely to be recognized by front-line workers.

Unfair expectations of loyalty may also emanate from employers and/or fellow team members. The potential 'whistleblower', for example, is faced with competing loyalties and responsibilities in a situation where it is inevitable that some individual will suffer harm either by breaking silence or by condemning others to continued harm through lack of action.

Fairness

Fairness relates directly to the principle of justice. It requires the professional to work without discriminating against people on the grounds of race, religion, ethnic origin or gender. Again, these are recognized aspects of conducting oneself in a fair manner. However, there are subtle ways of practising discriminatory behaviour. For all professionals, but especially those working with vulnerable groups, fairness is particularly important. It is important for professionals to be alert to internal obstructions to working in a respectful and egalitarian manner. Such obstructions might include value judgements and attributions about whether a client is 'deserving'.

Discretion

While most professionals feel comfortable with an understanding of what it means to keep confidences, to be discrete may not be so widely grasped. As Bayles (1989) indicates, discretion, perhaps, is not so well recognized. Discretion encapsulates both a broader understanding of the concept of confidentiality and a broad consideration of privacy.

   Clients come from all walks of life. Some may be citizens with very regular lives; others may be very much outside those societal norms. It can be very tempting to comment on the circumstances of the lives of clients. Often, however, encapsulated in those throwaway comments lie value judgements. The two case studies in Box 3.6 illustrate this point.

Box 3.6 Case studies illustrating lack of discretion

Having completed a community assessment following a referral of a person who was believed to be depressed, the professional undertaking the assessment returned to the place of work and announced to the rest of the team that if they lived in a house that resembled the setting of a BBC play, they would not find anything to be depressed about.

   In a very poor area of an inner city, a health professional returned to the health centre following a home visit. The health worker met with the supervisor in supervision. The preliminary part of the feedback from the visit to the client involved the lengthy and graphic description of the poor standard of hygiene in the house. The description was accompanied by strong non-verbal indicators that the poor state of the home environment was experienced as quite shocking to the professional conducting the visit. It was clear that the assessment had included a value judgement about the levels of cleanliness within the house.

   Even if it were feasible to assume that all professionals possess the virtues presented in the section above, given the complexities of practice already referred to, it would not necessarily follow that the obligations inferred would or could be honoured. While the context in which teamworking takes place is important, the individual within a team can seriously affect the ability of the team to function as a team.

An individual practitioner brings with them a personal perspective on teamwork and collaborative working which will profoundly affect the motivation to engage in teamwork, ascribing different values and meaning towards the concept of teamworking. Consequently, this will affect the way in which teamworking may or may not develop. If a member of the team values hierarchy, for example, where leadership is linked to status and power, interactions with others in the team and the respect and value for the perspective brought by other team members may be viewed less favourably.

Conclusion

The ethical implications of working in partnership are complex. This is partly because working within an ethical framework creates personal tensions for individual professionals when attempting to balance potentially competing responsibilities. These tensions are then compounded when working with other professionals either from the same or from other agencies. This chapter has introduced the reader to ethical dilemmas arising in interprofessonal practice and suggested the use of Bayles's (1989) concept of the fiduciary relationship as a guide to practice in reconciling the best way to meet the needs of the client within an interprofessional environment. The increased benefit to the client of combining resources when faced with dealing with complex human problems cannot be ignored and, consequently, brings to bear a clear ethical requirement on the professional to collaborate in the interests of the client.

Questions for further discussion

1. Given that human problems are diverse and complex, what moral arguments can there be for **not** pooling interprofessional expertise in the interest of clients?
2. How far does continuing to engage in 'tribalism' and lack of respect for fellow professionals suggest a lack of virtuous character traits in the individual practitioner?
3. When professional groups fail to work together, to what extent is the duty of care to clients being compromised?

References

Allison, A. (1996) A framework for good practice: ethical issues in cognitive behaviour therapy in S. Marshall, and J. Turnbull (eds) *Cognitive Behaviour Therapy: An Introduction to Theory and Practice*. Balliere Tindall, London.

Allison, A. and Ewens, A. (1998) Tensions in sharing client confidences while respecting autonomy: implications for interprofessional practice, *Nursing Ethics*, 5(5): 441–50.

Ashwell, N. (2003) *Perceptions of Inter-agency Collaboration: Youth and Health*. Unpublished PhD thesis, University of Reading.

Bayles, M.D. (1989) *Professional ethics* (2nd edn). Wadsworth Publishing Co, Belmont CA.

Biggs, S. (2000) User voice, interprofessional and post modernity, in C. Davies, L. Finlay and A. Bullman (eds) *Changing Practice in Health and Social Care*. Open University Press and Sage, London.

Burkhardt, M.A. and Nathaniel, A. K. (2002) *Ethics and Issues in Contemporary Nursing* (2nd edn). Delmar, USA.

Dalley, G. (1993) Professional ideology or organisational tribalism? The health service-social work divide, in J. Walmersley, J. Reynolds, P. Shakespeare and R. Woolfe (eds) *Health, Welfare and Practice.* Sage, London.

Department of Health (1997) *The New NHS: Modern and Dependable.* HMSO, London.

Department of Health (2000) *The NHS Plan.* HMSO, London.

Downie, R. S. and Telfer, E. (1980) *Caring and Curing.* Methuen, London.

Fletcher, N. and Holt, J. (1995) *Ethics, Law and Nursing.* Manchester University Press, Manchester.

Fish, D. and Coles, C. (1998) *Developing Professional Judgement in Health Care.* Butterworth-Heinemann, Oxford.

Gillon, R. (1986) *Philosophical Medical Ethics.* John Wiley and Sons, Chichester.

Husted, G L. and Husted, J.H. (1991) *Ethical Decision Making in Nursing.* Mosby, USA.

Irvine, R., Kerridge, I., McPhee, J. and Freeman, S. (2002) Interprofessionalism and ethics: consensus or clash of cultures? *Journal of Interprofessional Care,* 16(3): 200–10.

McLaughlin, H. (2004) Partnerships: panacea or pretence? *Journal of Interprofessional Care,* 18(2): 103–13.

Norman, R. (1983) *The Moral Philosophers – An Introduction to Ethics.* Clarenden Press, Oxford.

Pence, G. (1993) Virtue theory in P. Singer (ed.) *A Companion to Ethics.* Blackwell, Oxford.

Soothill, K., Mackay, L. and Webb, C. (1995) Troubled times: The context for interprofessional collaboration? in K. Soothill, L. Mackay and C. Webb (eds) *Interprofessional Relations in Health Care.* Edward Arnold, London.

4

Embracing diversity and working in partnership

John Bates

This chapter will:

- Explore whether the pursuit of partnerships marginalizes people from minority groups, or whether it leads to greater opportunities.
- Draw upon research and practice to identify common pitfalls in collaborative practice.
- Highlight theoretical and practical strategies to encourage equal access for all groups when developing collaborative care.

The nature and pursuit of partnerships

A wide range of diverse perspectives needs to be embraced within partnerships if they are to include such groups as ethnic minorities, women, people with disabilities, gay and lesbian people, elders, children, youth, travellers, people living in a rural context, unemployed people, and people with different religious beliefs and cultures. The drive for partnership in terms of service delivery has been a core policy strategy of the current Labour administration. The desire for 'seamless' services has led to an increase in collaborative working in mental health, youth justice, child protection and community care but the reality of delivering such services is in fact complex and fraught with difficulties.

The complex nature of collaborative working has important implications for the delivery of health and social services, which is carried out by an enormous range of providers often to the most vulnerable and marginalized groups in society. Such organizations often create complex and impenetrable bureaucracies, making access to services difficult and the co-ordination of services problematic. The general feeling that services should be arranged around users' needs and not around bureaucratic boundaries and self-interest prompted a number of organizations to experiment with partnership working (Sainsbury Centre 2000). That, coupled with a clear political thrust by the 1997 Labour government, gave partnership working a fresh emphasis. In the Department of Health paper *Partnership in Action* (1998), the government were robust in their condemnation of the fragmented and disjointed provision offered by health and social services agencies:

> All too often when people have complex needs spanning both health and social care good quality services are sacrificed for sterile arguments about boundaries. When this happens people, often the most vulnerable in our society ... and those who care for them find themselves in the no man's land between health and social services. This is not what people want or need. It places the needs of the organisation above the needs of the people they are there to serve. It is poor organisation, poor practice, poor use of taxpayer's money – it is unacceptable.
>
> (Department of Health 1998: 3)

The government's key agenda of social inclusion and community development, although broad, demanded that agencies and service providers work together to facilitate long-term planning and to create a synergy among partner agencies that moves towards the creation of 'one-stop shops' for users and carers. If agencies can work together, then there must be greater efficiency, less bureaucracy and less duplication, which will lead to savings being liberated to be spent on service users' needs. Perhaps most crucially, partnership working is potentially good for service users as they would no longer have to negotiate complex bureaucracies and would find instead a well organized service at the point of contact, which is easy to negotiate and focused on their particular needs. None of this government thrust, however, was statutory and has remained voluntary, leaving local authorities and health authorities to collaborate if they wish. The result was that in 2000 only 20 authorities had engaged with the recommendations in *Partnership in Action* (DoH 1998), which was less than a quarter of the number the government had hoped for. Continued pressure from the government has, however, resulted in some movement since those early days and it is now the case that some form of partnership in the delivery of health and social services would seem a necessity for political, financial and practical reasons although, as the Sainsbury Report points out: 'finding hard evidence that good partnership working actually improves user outcomes is lacking is hardly surprising. Designing and executing a study that could isolate this factor and connect it to user outcomes would be a formidable task' (Sainsbury Centre for Mental Health 2002).

But collaborative working is not only about how complex bureaucracies work together; it is also about how service users, carers and the providers of services work together. What makes for successful collaborative working is, however, complex and not always clearly understood. Simply assuming that various partners share common aims and that conflict is a matter of a failure to align those aims misunderstands the issues. Problems underpinning collaboration may be more deep rooted, relating to values, ideologies, worldviews and other related matters. An example of this is presented in a teaching case study example in Box 4.1.

What the experience in the above case study reflects is that the notions of collaborative working are complex and that simple solutions are likely to be ineffective – in fact they may well make matters worse. Furthermore, as Thompson (2001) argues, the central component to this issue is power. At an individual level it can

---

Box 4.1 A teaching case study of collaboration

My own experience of attempting a joint training project some years ago, although anecdotal, illustrates a number of issues I want to develop later in this chapter. Following the introduction of the Children Act (1989) I was invited by a colleague from the nursing department within the higher education institution in which I was working, to plan a joint training session with my second year diploma in social work students and her district nurse and health visiting students. We designed an involved case study that required knowledge of child health, child protection, mental health and disability issues. The intention was that 'teams' of mixed professionals would work on the case, bringing their different perspectives to a complex and urgent case scenario, thereby encouraging collaborative working and lateral thinking. The resulting session has to go down as one of the worst teaching and learning sessions I have ever managed. What began well enough ended in recriminations and, in one group, students walking out of the room! The case study became the rag doll as 'sides' pulled and fought over it, each one convinced their perspective was correct. As the sides fought, the 'family' became irrelevant as positions became entrenched and defended – illustrating how, even in a simulated classroom event (albeit poorly planned), the family became lost and further marginalized by the self-interest of three separate professional groupings.

---

operate in day-to-day interactions not only among teams, but also across boundaries. Thompson goes on to say:

> At a cultural level, of course, power operates in terms of discourses, and here we have a variety of competing discourses – professional (nurse v. doctor v. social worker; academic (biomedical v. psychological v. sociological); epistemological stance (positivist v. phenomenological v. realist).
>
> (Thompson 2001: 837)

Furthermore, power also operates at a structural level where it relates to social divisions and how people are stratified into class, race, gender or ability. The fact is that professionals working together will *inevitably* hit conflict as their different disciplines rely on different discourses. That is, power and meaning will operate differently within and between groups including, of course, how service users are managed and dealt with – making it necessary for some user groups, for example, to be empowered before they can even begin to play a meaningful role in collaborative provision. Empowering others, however, demands a letting go of power. If statutory bodies like health and social services are not prepared to devolve power to marginalized groups, then 'empowerment' will mean very little (Peterman 2000). The issue is further complicated by the fact that as long as users of services are seen as 'consumers', then little power will be devolved and the most vulnerable will have more responsibilities heaped on them but very little else.

Power is not only a feature of formal organizations, however, but also of informal networks and user groups where relationships are reinforced through familiarity and commonality of interests and indeed can be as exclusive and oppressive as formal bureaucracies (Sullivan and Skelcher 2002). Skelcher *et al.* (1996) suggest a five-point strategy for maximizing the potential of networks to share rather than maintain power:

1. Take positive steps to widen access to potential participants.
2. Ensure that those involved have the opportunity to shape the overall process followed by the collaboration.
3. Codify certain behaviours, that is, that all participants are heard with respect and all decisions are taken through consensus.
4. Ensure that statutory bodies are open to the outcomes of networks and prepared to make changes to accommodate their proposals.
5. Develop networks' ability to learn from their experiences and build their capacity to link with others to form a stronger framework.

The sharing of power then would inevitably enhance collaboration between diverse groups. However, despite the advantages of this sharing of power, a number of pitfalls may occur as a consequence of working in partnership.

The pitfalls of working in partnership

If collaborative working is genuinely to embrace diversity, then clarity is required as to who it is one is trying to reach and why. As Sullivan and Skelcher (2002) point out:

> . . . while collaborations based upon communities of place may experience difficulty in involving their disabled members, collaborations that are focused upon disabled service users may have difficulty in involving young disabled people or black or Asian disabled people.
>
> (Sullivan and Skelcher 2002: 175)

They go on to argue that while groups like young black people and other ethnic minority groups are well targeted the more 'hard to reach' people like travellers, drug users and homeless people remain effectively excluded either because of their very marginalized status or the attitudes of professionals (Keywood *et al.* 1999). In other words, it is not the groups who are hard to reach but the services themselves.

For health and social services projects to seriously embrace diversity it may be profitable to look at current attempts and review their outcomes. Sullivan and Skelcher (2002), in reviewing the impact of the involvement of 'hard to reach' groups in various community initiatives, paint a gloomy picture. They draw on extensive research evidence and conclude that, even when projects have targeted specific people like black and ethnic minority groups, their success has been marginal, with many black groups remaining on the periphery of the action and decision making. Not only were many of the projects, including regeneration activities, marginal in their success in reaching out to the groups they were intended to reach, most took no account of the role women played or were not even asked to monitor their involvement. Even where initiatives were explicitly about community involvement their research showed the dominance of statutory partners on steering groups and management committees. In the same vein, Hague *et al.* (1996) found that, of the survivors of domestic abuse they surveyed, only a small number knew of any initiatives in their area. Although many felt that they would want to make a contribution to any domestic violence initiatives in their area, many felt reluctant to offer themselves because of the power imbalance between the 'professionals' and survivors and even felt that they might be used by the project to give it legitimacy. Sullivan and Skelcher (2002) complete their overview with probably the most startling but relevant research finding. Quoting Lindow's (1996) research, they present a gloomy picture of the involvement of service users in commissioning decisions for the provision of health and social care services. They found that the statutory authorities remained unaware of basic access needs of service users, including wheelchair access and British Sign Language facilities, as well as the religious and cultural observances of specific user groups. Most interesting was Lindow's findings that although training was recommended, many of the professionals did not see this as a necessity.

Barnes (2003) recounts similar histories in relation to disabled people, many of whom have long campaigned for more control over the services on which they are forced to depend. Subsequent developments since the inauguration of the welfare state have compounded the problem as professionally-led provision has become the major problem. He goes on to say

> Whatever the priorities of policy makers, there is a wealth of evidence to suggest that professionals substantially influence the ways in which services are actually delivered. In many ways, disciplinary practices and procedures, professional vested interests and interprofessional rivalries coupled with the control of resources results in the deployment of services for professional convenience rather than user need.
>
> (Barnes 2003: 201)

More worrying is Barnes's later comment that far from improving the lives of disabled people, interprofessional working has made matters worse. He cites extensive research which shows that provision was often unreliable and inflexible. In his own research (2000), he interviewed 26 users, including people who had been labelled 'with learning difficulties' and others who were in the 'mental health system' as users or survivors. His findings confirmed earlier research that often assessment procedures were poor, there was a sense of lack of control, poor reliability of service and inflexible provision.

For users of mental health services the current situation is equally bleak. Projects in which health and social services have been working together are not new, of course. Since 1990 there is evidence that many collaborative ventures have been established, including social workers attached to GP practices and joint mental health risk teams, which have been involved in a case cited by Eaton (1998). According to Eaton, a team of social services, police, probation and psychiatrists shared information on individual cases to bring clarity to the working relationship and to plan and deliver appropriate support. In this particular case, the evidence was positive in that there did seem to be progress and 'team members have a better grasp of what each agency can offer, what the constraints are and what their common concerns are' (Eaton 1998: 215).

However, there is other research which suggests that the co-ordination of services is not so adequate. Leiba (2003) argues that much of the problem lies in the lack of co-ordination of services and that an analytical tool should be applied, which asks some fundamental questions including:

- the degree to which the respective organizations are aligned to the needs of the users, carers and the professionals involved;
- the ability of organizations to address the concepts of users first;
- the ability of organizations to adhere to the corporate goals as well as to work with others.

(Leiba 2003: 215)

It is interesting to note that there are no current policy documents on working with people with mental health problems that fail to mention the importance of working in partnership with all stakeholders, yet the record of working in partnership remains patchy. This may be because the traditional delivery of mental health services has not addressed the concept of inequality in the sense of how mental health has been separated out from other conditions, reflecting the various societal responses that mental 'illness' has evoked over the years. Situating mental 'illness' within an anti-discriminatory framework can help to challenge the historical tradition whereby coercion has often been wrapped up as part of the 'service'. This is a theme I will return to later in this chapter.

Strategies for action

If collaborative provision is to begin to embrace diversity, then health and social services staff need to begin to acknowledge within themselves that a wide range of different perspectives need to be embraced within partnership. Professionals need to move away from the comfortable assumption that there is only one way to see the world and to appreciate that different people operate from different perspectives. For example, when one group believes it 'knows all about' an individual or a condition, a terrible determinism can creep into its dealings with each other and individual service users. This unconscious and often unwitting assumption of a particular type of 'normality' is a persistent feature of inequitable practice. Once an assumption of normality has been made, it is not uncommon for variations away from this assumed norm to be seen, not simply as different, but as abnormal and inferior; thus the norm becomes an ideological one, since it presents one feature as the baseline from which other features are then differentiated. This approach can lead to the devaluation of that which is deemed different, and thus lead to the pathologization of those who possess supposedly 'abnormal' characteristics (Thompson 1998).

In considering the ways in which health and social care professionals can move forward in a way that embraces diversity, four strategies are proposed:

1. Learn from each other.
2. Embrace partnership.

3. Adopt a value position where anti-discriminatory practice is central.
4. Reflect on practice.

Learn from each other

Ideas, actions, interactions and so on do not fall naturally into neat categories – such categories are constructions, sets of representations that help us make sense of the social world (Thompson and Bates 1996). While categorizing things certainly helps us make sense of complex matters, we must recognize that there are problems with sticking too rigidly to such categories. If we are genuinely to reach out to marginalized groups, then discipline boundaries have to become more permeable and we have to become more receptive to learning opportunities that arise from working with other professional groups in the human services. One problem, however, can be that communicating across disciplines can lead to simplification of ideas, as people search for a common understanding. The important challenge is to understand and respect the other discipline without losing the distinctiveness of a disciplinary voice, which can have the effect of acknowledging each other's perspective but also allowing one's own to change and grow.

Social services staff, for example, can learn much from health practitioners' use of reflective practice models and learning from research, while health professionals can learn from colleagues coming from a social work background about the value and importance of embracing an anti-discriminatory framework for practice (Thompson and Bates 1996). Both groups can learn from listening to service users. As Thompson (1998) says, the expert on the client's situation in terms of what 'it feels like' is obviously the client. Fricker (1999) has called this insider knowledge 'epistemic privilege', by which she means that members of an oppressed group have a more immediate, subtle and critical knowledge about the nature of their oppression than people who are non-members. This does not mean that 'non-members' cannot build an awareness of the position oppressed people occupy, but this awareness is not easily realized or directly experienced. I, for example, am never going to experience sexism but I can try to appreciate the subjective reality of a woman, otherwise I might deny the problem and evade any sense of responsibility for its amelioration.

Learning from each other, however, demands hard work and a commitment to learn. This is never easy as people coming together from different professions will inevitably bring with them the perspective of their own organization with its distinct culture, values and procedures. Added to that will be workers' own values, judgements, ideas and uncertainties. Harrison *et al.* (2003) suggest that there are three processes, which are key to creating the foundation for effective partnerships. These require teams to:

- enable the people within the partnership to get to know about each other's organization and to know the people involved both as professionals and as individuals;
- ensure that all partners are involved in ways that enable them to make a full and positive contribution to the work of the partnership;

- develop a consensual way of working, which enables the partnership to develop and implement joint strategies and models of working.

It cannot be assumed that people coming together in a new team will necessarily know how each other's organization works. As Moore (1992) illustrates when talking about child protection matters: 'We . . . take on the values and philosophies of that profession and we take on board the basic concepts and assumptions which form the frame of reference which we use as the set to solve the problems within our own purview. The tools and methods are self evident to us but not to other disciplines' (p. 16).

Embrace partnership

Partnership is a much over-used term but it needs reclaiming in the context of this discussion. Partnership is not so much about simply working alongside people but more about *how* we work alongside others. It is important that teams engage with the concept in its widest context. Within teams effective partnership involves trust, respect, honesty and shared risk taking. Moreover, White and Grove (2000) suggest that true partnership will exist only if there is respect, reciprocity, realism and risk taking. True partnership with service users also involves the same ingredients and will encourage a move towards a more emancipatory practice, which actually involves users in a process and ceases to 'diagnose' the problem and then 'prescribe' the correct 'treatment'. By adopting a more phenomenological approach workers can locate themselves better in the situation in which the service user finds him or herself, thereby becoming better equipped to understand their concerns, their wishes and feelings. Phenomenology in this context is asking us not to take received ideas as if they are tablets of stone but to question them by questioning our culture and our way of looking at the world, so that we may arrive at a more sensitive and insightful view of the experiences of others and our position in the social world. The importance of listening to each other and to service users cannot be overemphasized. By 'allowing' people a voice, especially the marginalized and dispossessed, collaborative provision may begin to have a real impact on the lives of people.

If multidisciplinary health and social services teams want to reach out to marginalized groups, then there are lessons and research evidence to guide them. A common factor that most commentators seem to agree on is that if, for example, a mental health team want to reach out to Asian people, then they will need to involve groups and individuals right at the beginning of the process. The evidence would suggest that unless this involvement is obtained at the start, later attempts will be less than successful as the agenda has become set and no sense of ownership will exist (Brownhill and Darke 1998). Sullivan and Skelcher (2002) suggest that one of the most effective ways of embracing 'hard to reach' groups is by use of skilled outreach workers. They argue that although costly in time and resources, successive projects have identified this factor as one of the most significant. This initiative is more likely to overcome the general mistrust that many marginalized groups have towards statutory services where many individuals may well have had profoundly negative experiences of the 'system'. If outreach workers are not used, they suggest that success has also been obtained by making use of voluntary organizations, such as Women's Aid in the case of domestic violence or 'Mind' in the case of mental health services. These are interesting ideas that teams may want to develop but either way the process of engaging with 'hard to reach' groups needs thoughtful and sometimes creative management. Working with marginalized groups is a time-consuming business and expends a great deal of scarce resources to support individuals to enable participation and it is all too easy to drop back into a culture of 'we know best' but it can be done. Sullivan and Skelcher (2002) present as an interesting illustration, a body called HEAT (Health Equality Action Team), which works as a block to influence events with the Bradford Health Action Zone.

When users are involved in making decisions about their own health needs or community initiatives the results can be spectacular. Sullivan and Potter (2001) describe a number of life-enhancing experiences where service users have worked alongside professionals and developed skills that have enabled them to participate in the true spirit of partnership. All too often, unfortunately, there are as many stories of failure where people have been left feeling exploited and even more marginalized than before (Sullivan and Skelcher 2002).

Adopt a value position where anti-discriminatory practice is central

There is little doubt that one of the most significant changes in UK social work over the last two decades has been a growing understanding of the impact of oppression and discrimination on people and communities. Most social workers now have a much greater understanding of the need to construct a practice that is underpinned by anti-discriminatory measures. This development that began in the 1960s was refined and developed by influential feminist academics like Brownmillar (1977), de Beauvoir (1972) and Oakley (1981), for example, and refined further by a cohort of social work academics in the 1970s and 1980s onwards until it is now mainstream in UK social work programmes. These more radical values gradually had an impact on social work practice and learning, which had traditionally been heavily influenced by psychoanalytical theories. A fresher, sociological analysis led to a more socially and politically aware social work that recognizes the specifics of oppression according to gender, race, class, age, disability and sexual preference. This fresher approach emphasizes the diversity of experience and the validity of each person's experience while seeking to understand both the totality of oppression and its specific manifestations as the preconditions for developing an anti-discriminatory practice (Thompson 1998). The essential building blocks of anti-discriminatory practice are:

- Professionals in the human services need to recognize the socio-political context of the life experience of their clients and of their agency's role and function.
- The dangers of practice not only contributing to but even reinforcing oppression and discrimination must be recognized and guarded against.
- Opportunities to emancipate clients from oppressive and damaging circumstances

should be seized upon as part of the same project, which alerts clients to the social and political basis of their difficulties.

In order to embrace diversity, teams should adopt a position which acknowledges that any intervention in someone's life either compounds their marginalized position or goes some small way to ameliorating it. Examples of this are provided in Box 4.2.

Box 4.2 Examples of how interventions can compound marginalization

- An intervention with a young black person with a mental health problem that fails to recognize both the social construction of 'madness' and the marginalized and oppressed position of black members of the community with all that entails will simply end up providing a disservice.
- An intervention with a young disabled woman that fails to recognize the social construction of both disability and gender and the impact that might have on someone's self-perception will simply add to her oppression.

It is important to remember that oppression is often multiple, which means that teams should work towards adopting a theoretical position that recognizes diversities in patterns of power and inequality, and champion an anti-oppressive alliance. In other words, collaborative teams cannot pay lip service to fighting oppression but it is important to remember that in attempting to gain a better understanding of the life experience of different groups, it is very easy to forget that what is true for the group is not necessarily true for every individual within it. The social locations that individuals find themselves in are not straightforward, influenced as they are by age, class, gender, ethnicity, sexuality and so on. This means that we have to be cautious so that we do not adopt an over-deterministic generalization about people's situations.

As Thompson (1998) argues, workers who impose their own assumptions on other people are denying them their rights as individuals to their own feelings, thoughts and explanations about the world. In practice this can lead to:

- Inappropriate methods
- Inadequate services – this is in itself discriminatory because it imposes beliefs on others and ultimately deprives the service users of services that could enable them to empower themselves
- Inadequate theories, which cannot adequately describe, explain and predict

Reflect on practice

In the monograph entitled *Learning from Other Disciplines* (Thompson and Bates 1996) the authors drew on the extensive experience of nursing and health colleagues in their use of reflective practice as a tool for learning. The conclusions then still hold good today, in that reflective practice is probably one of the most effective tools for developing and understanding practice. Workers in multidisciplinary teams probably more than most need to review constantly their practice in an open and honest fashion. Human services work is often messy, unpredictable and not easy to understand; it is rarely open to off-the-shelf remedies and outcomes are often unpredictable. Nurses' embracing of reflective practice helped them move from seeing their role as a purely technical, functional one to one that emphasized the artistry of practice. Against this, the importance of reflection cannot be over stressed. As Yelloly and Henkel (1995) argue: 'the capacity to draw back in order to reflect on what is happening . . . enables learning to take place in a way which allows thought-less action to become thought-ful' (p. 8).

In addition, critical reflection allows human services workers to identify and question assumptions about content, context, theories and processes. For multidisciplinary teams this is crucial as organizational scripts can dominate a discourse rather than the needs of service users. Reflecting and questioning the frameworks and constructs that are influencing the way practice is being delivered can be an enlightening experience. An example of how teams might work together reflectively is proposed in Box 4.3.

Box 4.3 How teams might work together reflectively

Members of teams might want to share a reflection on a case that demands evaluating practice decisions. Reflection could be guided by the following questions:

1. How have you demonstrated *your* commitment to anti-discriminatory practice?
2. How did you make your decisions in this case?
3. What knowledge and skills did you draw on?
4. How might you do things differently next time?
5. What did you learn from colleagues/service user/supervisor?

The power of this sort of exercise cannot be overemphasized as a learning and developmental tool. As well as developing anti-discriminatory practice by encouraging self-awareness, it provides a forum for critical dialogue allowing the exploration of assumptions about oneself, agency values and, most importantly, it places day-to-day practice in its wider social, economic and political context. Mezirow (1981) describes this process as 'perspective transformation' and defines it as:

> The emancipatory process of becoming critically aware of how and why the structure of psycho-cultural assumptions has come to constrain the way we see ourselves and our relationships, reconstituting this structure to permit a more inclusive and discriminating integration of experience and acting upon these understandings.
>
> (Mezirow 198: 6)

This idea of perspective transformation involves human services workers in challenging the assumptions of our culture and background and starting to unlearn much of the processes of socialization. This is a concept that dovetails with a commitment to anti-discriminatory practice. As Thompson *et al.* (1994) argue:

> Perceptive transformation is a term used by Mezirow (1981) to refer to a funda-
> mental change in how we perceive the world and our relationship to it. It implies
> 'unlearning' many of the restricted patterns of thought to which we have been
> socialised ... This is an important part of anti-discriminatory practice – the
> development of self awareness with regard to the effects of the socialisation pro-
> cess upon us in terms of developing stereotypical and potentially oppressive
> expectations of women, black people, disabled people and so on.
>
> (Thompson *et al.* 1994: 21)

It is clear from this point that reflective practice has to be self-reflective and not simply an exercise in navel gazing. This rigorous approach to reflection allows not only the enhancement of skills and knowledge but develops self-awareness and from that arises a greater opportunity for effective interventions based on the use of self. As Egan (1994) puts it: 'It has been said that self knowledge is the beginning of wisdom. It can also be the beginning of better relationships with others' (p. 20).

Conclusion

The task of collaborating in a way that is inclusive of marginalized groups is not an easy one and it would be naive to pretend otherwise. The government have not helped by being less than confident in the way they have approached the issue. Far from creating ideal conditions for collaborative working they have simply blurred the boundaries, leaving many of the systemic problems well and truly in place. Despite this the challenge for human services workers to reach out to marginalized groups remains. There will be obstacles like misunderstandings, tensions and resource difficulties, but these should not be an excuse to revert to ways of working that may be comfortable but leave the marginalized further away from mainstream provision.

There are clearly problems to overcome and collaborative working which embraces diversity may be able to provide one part of that solution if a new 'profes-sional' emerges who is not allied to individualistic approaches to service delivery and conventional ways of working but is allied to local user groups and committed to a more flexible and holistic way of working. One aim might be to put expertise at the disposal of user groups in order to address and remove the economic, political, cul-tural and professional barriers that have so bedevilled service delivery to marginalized groups of people. This will involve a challenge to established ideologies, practices and policies but conventional approaches are not an option as we make way for models of working that embrace the centrality of partnership and which can overcome the inflexibility created by traditional organizational boundaries. These boundaries have been a factor in so many disadvantaged groups remaining beyond the reach of services and there is no doubt that embracing 'hard to reach' groups will demand solutions to complex problems. There is still much for service users and carers to learn from each other.

Questions for further discussion

1. What strategies could you adopt within your organization to maximize the opportunity to share power with marginalized groups as well as other organizations?
2. What anti-discriminatory practices are most evident in your organization and how are they made explicit within policy and practice?
3. How could anti-discriminatory practices be shared between agencies?

References

Barnes, C. (2003) Disability, user controlled services – partnership or conflict? in A. Leathard (ed.) *Interprofessional Collaboration*. Brunner-Routledge, Hove and New York.

Barnes, C., Mercer, G. and Morgan H. (2000) *Creating Independent Futures: Stage 1 Report*. The Disability Press, Leeds.

Beauvoir, S. de (1972) *The Second Sex*. Penguin, Harmondsworth.

Brownhill, S. and Darke, J. (1998) *Rich Mix: Inclusive Strategies for Urban Regeneration*. Polity Press, Bristol.

Brownmillar, S. (1977) *Against our Will: Men, Women and Rape*. Penguin, Harmondsworth.

Department of Health (1998) *Partnership in Action: New Opportunities for Joint Working between Health and Social Services – a Discussion Document*. Department of Health, London.

DoH (1991a) *Children Act 1989 Guidance and Regulations*, HMSO, London.

Eaton, J. (1998) Arranged Marriages, *Health Service Journal*, 108 (5627): 24–6.

Egan, G. (1994) *The Skilled Helper* (5th edn), Brooks/Cole, Belmont, CA.

Fricker, M. (1999) Epistemic Oppression and Epistemic Priviledge, *Canadian Journal of Philosophy* Supplementary Volume 25, in C. Wilson *Civilization and Oppression*, University of Calgary Press Books, Calgary.

Hague, G., Malos, E. and Dear, W. (1996) *Multi Agency Work and Domestic Violence: A National Study of Inter Agency Initiatives*. Polity Press, Bristol.

Harrison, R., Mann, G, Murphy, M., Taylor, A and Thompson, N. (2003) *Partnership Made Painless*. Russell House Publishing, Lyme Regis.

Keywood, K., Fovargue, A. and Flynn, M. (1999) Best Practice? *Health Care Decision Making by, with and for Adults with Learning Disabilities*. Manchester National Development Team, Manchester.

Leiba, T. (2003) Mental Health in Interprofessional Contexts in A. Leathard (ed.) *Interprofessional Collaboration*. Brunner-Routledge, Hove and New York.

Lindow, V. (1996) *User Involvement: Community Service Users as Consultants and Trainers*. Department of Health, London.

Mezirow, J. (1981) A Critical Theory of Adult Learning and Education, *Adult Education* 32 (1).

Moore, J. (1992) *The ABC of Child Protection*. Ashgate, Aldershot.

Oakley, M. (1981) *From Here to Maternity – Becoming a Mother*. Penguin, Harmondsworth.

Peterman, W. (2000) *Neighbourhood Planning and Community Based Development*. Sage, London.

Sainsbury Centre for Mental Health (2002) *Taking Your Partners: Using Opportunities for Inter Agency Partnership in Mental Health*.

Skelcher, C., McCabe, A., Lowndes, V. and Nanton, P. (1996) *Community Networks in Urban Regeneration*. Policy Press, Bristol.

Sullivan, H. and Skelcher, C. (2002) *Working Across Boundaries*. Palgrave Macmillan, Basingstoke.

Sullivan, H. and Potter, T. (2001) Doing Joined-up Evaluation in Community Based Regeneration, *Local Governance*, 27(1): 19–31.

Thompson, N. and Bates, J. (1996) *Learning From Other Disciplines*. Social Work Monographs. UEA, Norwich.

Thompson, N., Osada, M. and Anderson, B. (1994) *Practice Teaching in Social Work* (2nd edn). Prepar, Birmingham.

Thompson, N. (1998) *Promoting Equality*. Macmillan, Basingstoke.

Thompson, N. (2000) *Theory and Practice in Human Services*. Open University Press, Buckingham.

Thompson, N. (2001) Working Together Across Disciplines, *Nursing Times Research*, 6(5): 837.

White, K. and Grove, M. (2000) *Towards and Understanding of Partnership*. NCVCCO Outlook Issue 7.

Yelloly, M. and Henkel, M. (eds) (1995) *Learning and Teaching in Social Work: Towards Reflective Practice*. Jessica Kingsley, London.

5

Dependent upon outside help: reflections from a service user

Amir Minhas

This chapter will:

- Provide a very personal account from an Asian man in his mid-40s who is physically disabled and uses a wheelchair.
- Share the journey, insights and experiences of being dependent on outside help and support.
- Provide a rich understanding that will be of interest and relevance to any service provider.

Introduction

I am an Asian male born in Pakistan who caught poliomyelitis in early childhood. The impact of 'polio' varies considerably from slight paralysis, in one or other limb to almost total paralysis whereby the individual needs mechanical assistance to breathe and cannot independently move any part of the body apart from the head. In my case, the effect was to paralyse both legs resulting in impaired muscular and skeletal development of both legs. The impact of this impairment is that I am, for the most part, confined to a wheelchair. In a society like Pakistan disabled people have few life chances. There are no developed public sector welfare institutions able to address properly the needs of disabled people. Had I stayed in the country I would probably have been compelled either to beg for a living or to be entirely dependent upon one or other member of my family.

Within this chapter I seek to portray and draw lessons from my life experience with a view to generating a discourse regarding some of the many issues pertaining to the 'human' services and the implications for multi-agency working. In particular, I intend the reader to identify and consider what the issues are, or what they may be. I raise issues for discussion and give personal opinions but am not attempting to provide answers.

Biography

I was born in 1956 in East Pakistan (now known as Bangladesh), the second youngest of six children. I caught poliomyelitis at two years of age and it left me with two paralysed legs. My father died when I was three years old, leaving my widowed mother with six children to raise within the context of an impoverished Muslim society, where women in the late 1950s and early 1960s did not have much opportunity for education, career or social independence. I am informed that, after a fruitless quest by both parents in Pakistan to obtain treatment for the effects of poliomyelitis, my mother and father had planned to send me to England to receive treatment. However, my father's premature death had left the family destitute and, due to the difficult social conditions prevailing in Pakistan, my mother was not able to earn enough to look after my siblings adequately – in terms of providing an education and meeting all our material and emotional needs. Therefore, within this context and being influenced by other relatives, she decided it best to send me to England – telling me that I was going 'on holiday'.

At about five years of age, I was accompanied on an aeroplane by an old friend of my late father who was travelling to England for I know not what reason nor for how long a stay. On arrival in England I understand that my father's friend took me straight to Tite Street Hospital, Chelsea, where he left me in the care of the hospital authorities for several months. I am told that the hospital conducted medical assessments and delivered appropriate treatment to no avail.

After all had been done that could be done, the hospital contacted the local London Mosque, which then took charge of my welfare. It is important to note that the Mosque is not only a building for prayers but is also a tightly knit community under the authority of the Imam. The Imam allocated my care to a young family who took me in as a matter of religious duty rather than with any sense of welcoming acceptance. At some point the local education authority became involved and, in due course, I was sent to a 'boarding school for handicapped children' – Staplefield Place School in Sussex. During the school holidays I returned to the Mosque and to a different family. Some years later an 'uncle' of mine emigrated to England with a view to settling and bringing his own young family to the UK in due course. He had assured my mother that he would locate me and take personal responsibility for my care. The 'uncle' arrived in England and obtained work which necessitated frequent travelling around the country and living in 'digs' at various sites. However, he did locate me at boarding school, assumed guardianship and arranged for me to be looked after by a kind old English lady (who also suffered from poliomyelitis) and her blind and bedridden husband. This lady was only known to me as 'Sister Joan'.

The next year or so was spent at boarding school and with 'Sister Joan' during the school holidays until another friend of my father (Mr Khan) heard about my existence from the Imam at the Mosque. Out of his friendship for my deceased father, Mr Khan sought to take responsibility for my care. He contacted my 'uncle' and arranged for me to live with him and his English wife (Kathleen Khan) and their children during the school holidays. However, Kathleen did not really want to look after me (she had her own three pre-school children to look after) but accepted me out of devotion to her husband. I do not know how for long this arrangement lasted (probably about two years on and off) but it eventually broke down and I returned to live with 'Sister Joan' in the holidays. Staplefield Place School remained for me the only stable environment during my childhood. School holidays had been spent in all sorts of places, including time at a residential children's home in Winchester and being fostered with an Asian family in Farnham, who kept me confined in one room of the house where I spent my days by myself and ate my meals alone.

However, when I was about 10 years old Kathleen Khan contacted the school seeking to look after me during the holidays. It is my understanding that Kathleen's husband had died and that her resolve to look after me as a child was rooted in fulfilling a promise to her late husband. This arrangement lasted for about two years or so when, my 'uncle' and, by then, legal guardian had finally brought his own family over and settled in Liverpool and was keen for me join his family. By this time I had, however, been socialized into Western society culture and values and felt part of Kathleen's family, and although my 'uncle's' family were now settled in Liverpool, he had three pre-school children who had just arrived in the UK from Pakistan and a wife who did not speak English (I had forgotten how to speak in Urdu) and were not integrated into Western society. From the age of twelve, I regularly returned to my 'uncle's' family home in Liverpool during the school holidays and attempted to integrate – notwithstanding the cultural and communication difficulties. By the time I was eighteen I was free from statutory care and dependence and left 'home' in an attempt to lead an independent life.

Initially, I shared a flat with a friend for about two years and then obtained my own independent accommodation. For the next 15 years or so I didn't 'live' life, I didn't try to deal with the difficulties I faced with disability, racism and cultural conflict. Tired of dependence and the stress and traumas it brought me, I simply 'existed'. I claimed all the benefits to which I was entitled, escaped and occupied myself by regularly and excessively taking drugs, watching TV all night and not starting my days until around 2.00 p.m. and ending them in the early hours of the next morning. Not surprisingly, I sank into despair and depression. I formulated a nihilistic view towards life with no purpose or ambition, let alone entertaining thoughts of loving relationships or useful careers. Towards the end of nearly 20 years of purposeless existence, I chanced upon an old drugs misusing friend who had managed to extricate himself from a similar lifestyle. He persuaded me to attend an Access Course (access to higher education for the unemployed). I undertook this course with no particular aim other than it would help fill my days. I successfully completed the course and went on to take a degree course where I established a committed relationship with a fellow student. She 'took charge' of my life. I needed help because by now I was dependent upon heroin. She moved in with me, cleaned up the flat and helped motivate me towards seeking employment. During this period I gained self-esteem and made some significant transitions. I embarked upon a methadone reduction course, achieved a good Bachelor of Arts degree at Christ and Notre Dame/St Kaths College and secured a position as a Community Service Officer with Merseyside Probation Service.

After eighteen months I left my position as a Community Service Officer as I had been sponsored by the Home Office to attend Liverpool University to study a

Diploma in Social Work and Master of Arts (Social Work). Upon successful comple-
tion I was subsequently re-employed as a qualified Probation Officer with Merseyside
Probation Service where I have been employed for seven years.

Analysis/commentary

The reader will note that throughout this brief biography no mention has yet been
made of social work and health-related interventions. During my childhood the
role of the social worker was less formalized and more akin to that of a support
worker cum guardian ad litem or in loco parentis but without stringent, formalized
structures of accountability. Consequently, as well as the potential for more meaningful, organic and 'natural' relationships with clients, the look of accountability
opened the door to the potential for abusive relationships. My knowledge and
experience of the social worker–client relationship is based upon the memories of
the accounts of childhood friends (all of whom seem to have had a social worker).
As far as I am able to recall, no social worker was allocated to my case in the sense
that I, as an individual, had any direct dealings with a social worker. However,
social services must have been involved when I was placed in the children's home
in Winchester and when fostered with the Asian family in Farnham. Essentially,
decisions were made by I know not who, about significant issues without my
involvement at any level, however elementary or basic. Again, this is possibly
nothing out of the ordinary in terms of social work practice during the 1960s and
early 1970s.

It is fair to assume that health, education and social services departments had
been involved to varying degrees in making significant decisions about my physical,
emotional and social welfare at different stages of my childhood development within
the context of an inconsistent and variable 'home/family' setting. Such decisions were
made without even the most basic consultation with me – it may be that as a child
between the ages of five and twelve years it was the prevailing view among the
agencies that consultation would not be appropriate or relevant. Most crucially, and
this is really the main point, perhaps clear explanations (reasons for the decisions)
given in a sensitive and supportive way may have ameliorated some of the sense of
absolute powerlessness I felt when, for example, I was told whether I was to stay with
strangers in Farnham or with Kathleen in Fulham, or whether I was going to the
children's home in Winchester during the summer holidays or to stay with my
'uncle's' family in Liverpool.

On reflection, the main issue for me as a child was not being involved primarily in
actual decision making. Rather it was not having an enduring focal relationship with
one individual who could be both a source of support, information and explanation.
In other words, an allocated social worker with whom a long-term relationship could
have developed. The psychological and emotional need for stability and continuity,
from whatever source, was a paramount need which appeared from my recollections
to be neither recognized nor addressed. However, it is also true to say that the complex and difficult issues of emotional and psychological stability for a child in such
circumstances is a problem which may never have been possible for a statutory
agency to address satisfactorily (social workers come and go). In fairness, my

material, educational and health needs were adequately met in terms of actual provision. The quality of the provision was variable.

The issues of ongoing health care and the provision of aids (wheelchair, crutches, callipers, physiotherapy) were looked after by the residential school authorities directly and so, between the ages of five and sixteen years, I had no direct knowledge of the necessary procedures and processes by which such services and aids could be accessed. The important point here is that, at no time during my school years, was I given information and help to independently access services and aids that I would need to access on a regular basis throughout the rest of my life. The presumption was that the parent(s)/guardian/care-giver would either directly obtain such services and aids on my behalf or would inform me how to facilitate them. Unfortunately, my 'uncle' had no such knowledge or experience and so was not of much use to me in these respects.

On reaching adulthood and independent living all support from my 'uncle' ceased and I was left to my own devices in terms of self-care, obtaining employment, accessing services and aids and expediting daily chores such as cooking, cleaning, shopping, laundry which may be difficult for any eighteen-year-old but are also physically more challenging to a wheelchair user. My early experiences of living independently were fraught with great difficulties and yet I basked in the wonderful sense of freedom from residential care and a home life with my 'uncle', in which the culture, values and communication difficulties had stifled and constricted any sense of joy in being alive. However, that sense of freedom was an important but transitory feeling of elation as the harsh realities of unsupported living encroached upon my consciousness. Loneliness and despair soon became constant companions and my requests for practical support to my 'uncle' came to nothing. Apparently, I had been a difficult child to look after and 'must now live the consequences of my circumstances'. His obligation to fulfil his promise to my mother had been discharged. So, how did I cope?

Well, I coped on an ad hoc basis. I ate as and when I was hungry; I slept as and when I felt like it; I laundered my clothes when the last clean shirt had become so dirty that even I felt the need for a change of clothes. Shopping occurred on a similar basis and cleaning my accommodation was last on the list of chores – except for obtaining employment, which was in all honesty not even on the list! My emotional and psychological circumstances were best characterized as being nihilistic and I very quickly resorted to taking drugs. The drug taking was not exclusively a response to personal despair but was, initially, also a response to my immature understanding of 'the evils of the world'. It was an expression of my rejection of capitalist values, which I held to be the fundamental cause of both global misery as well as my personal misery. It was also a lifestyle choice and recreational activity. As such I socialized with other drug users and constructed an identity that centred on a community of outlaws and misfits – living off the dole, not giving a fig for 'the system' or the norms of society, while inexorably heading towards personal self-destruction without any regard for whether I lived or died.

Paradoxically, it was within this community of misfits and away from formal care, that I formed friendships which became sources of various types of informal support – predominantly emotional and psychological but including practical support by negotiation. For example, in return for food and shelter, one friend would shop and clean the flat or would help to transport the washing to a public laundry. At other times I would provide a taxi service (in the car I got from Motobility) in return for help with the shopping. In other words, my daily needs were being met on the basis of exchange – sometimes direct cash payments for practical help; at other times help was given freely out of friendship. However, any semblance of truly autonomous living was not viable in my particular circumstances without significant support.

With regard to the ongoing need for medical equipment/aids (crutches, wheel-chair), I would approach my GP and he would either make the appropriate referral or supply me with a relevant telephone number and I would then pursue an application to its conclusion. My knowledge of sources of help was sparse in terms of the types of help available. However, I always knew enough to access a starting point. For example, if the need was medically related, then the starting point would be the GP. If it was a benefits issue, then I would approach the Citizens' Advice Bureau. If there was a social issue related to my impairment I would contact the local branch of the British Polio Fellowship or the Liverpool Association for the Disabled. The voluntary organizations were the primary sources of access to information and different forms of help including welfare rights, housing and adult education. Any success I achieved rested upon my ability to communicate and negotiate, with the impetus being generated by personal need and desire. If I did not have enough confidence and ability, then I would not have been able to access such services – and at times I did not do so. There was no single focal point to which I could make an approach and from which the various types of support and help could be accessed. Nevertheless, I did manage to remain housed and fed and eventually undertook relevant educational courses, which led to my becoming more integrated into mainstream society and, ultimately, achieving full-time employment. The desire for integration into mainstream society and wanting to be employed could only have arisen and be sustained once I had been fortunate enough to have established a loving and committed relationship. It was the stability and nurturing aspects of the relationship that helped to heal the emotional and psychological damage sustained by difficult circumstances and a lifestyle that was rooted in a total disregard for personal consequences.

I had always been wary of approaching social services and other statutory agencies since leaving 'home'. After all, I had never had any direct contact with social services and held the same prejudices and forebodings regarding the department's function and role as did all my contemporaries, believing it to be more an agency of control and surveillance rather than a source of help and support. I did once approach social services seeking non-specific help (wishing to discuss my circumstances with a view to changing my self-destructive lifestyle) but the initial assessment interview was such an appalling experience that I was relieved that no further contact was made by the department. The social worker appeared to be absolutely disinterested in my situation and made me feel that I should be grateful for not being even more deprived and oppressed than I actually was!

During my undergraduate days, while seeking to become less reliant upon personal relationships and friendships to meet my everyday needs, I applied to have a home help. At this stage the Home Help Service was provided by the City Council rather than by social services. I received three different home helps over a period of about four years. It was my impression that such people, while being pleasant enough as individuals, were underpaid and, in some cases, not properly trained. Household cleaning was often superficial; shopping would take an inordinately long time; a relationship would strike up in which much of the time was spent chatting and drinking cups of tea (not a bad thing except that it was at the expense of providing a service). Again, the relationship would become characterized in terms of dependency and whether one received a half-way effective service or not depended upon one's social and negotiating skills. It is my personal opinion that home help workers were disincentivized by poor pay, unreasonable work schedules and poor training with little support from management. The priority of the employer would have been 'cost-effectiveness' (as usual). The goal of cost-effectiveness within all public sector service provision too often boils down to doing the job as cheaply as you can get away with and having little or no regard to the consequences for the quality of service delivered or the long-term impact on the client group. It appears to be an abiding governmental principle that is applied to all the public sector services (health, education, criminal justice, social services, police), while 'spin' uses spurious statistics to demonstrate 'successful outcomes'.

It is perhaps significant that my main experience of positive help was not as a client but as an employee during my initial spell of employment with Merseyside Probation Service, then during postgraduate studies at Liverpool University and finally with Merseyside Probation Service again. On first joining the Probation Service as a Community Service Officer, I became aware of the concepts of anti-racism, anti-sexism, anti-oppressive practice and allied 'anti-isms'. In other words, I found myself employed by an organization that expressed anti-oppressive values and sought to promulgate a culture of inclusiveness and a commitment to a fair and just working environment for all its employees. I had very limited previous work experience and this was the first time that I had experienced positive support, understanding and help to facilitate and sustain employment in the context of the employer actively taking into account issues related to disability, with a view to overcoming any difficulties in conjunction and consultation with the disabled employee. For example, any problems or difficulties that did arise were open to discussion with management and with the personnel (sorry . . . human resources) department. I was never made to feel that I was making unreasonable demands upon either a specific individual or the organization as a whole.

In my dealings with colleagues I felt listened to, consulted, taken seriously and involved in the process of finding solutions without being held solely responsible for achieving solutions. In particular, the human resources department responded to issues positively and willingly and continue to so do. A key factor here is that the assistant to the head of human resources (at the time) was available and responsive to me. She was an identified individual whom I could approach with any issues regardless as to which area, section and/or function the issue pertained. A single identified individual with power in the organization developed a working relationship with me, which gave me the confidence to know that whatever difficulties I faced in employment with this organization, together we would seek to resolve issues without my having to take the full responsibility for finding solutions. This was a partnership on equal terms.

One such issue was the physical and emotional toll taken by me in attempting to fulfil my role on a full-time basis. The help initiated by the human resources department is that arrangements were made to involve an organization called the Shaw Trust. In brief, this organization was able to fund one working day. This meant that in recognition of the additional challenges posed by my disability, positive action was taken that enabled me to be allocated 80 per cent of the work of a full-time probation officer, yet continue to receive a full salary and other entitlements of a full-time employee. This was in recognition of the accumulative pressures of working in an environment that demands a high level of personal resources (physical and emotional energy) and, thereby, would not leave me feeling constantly exhausted at the end of every working week. Without this support I would not be able to sustain the role. Eventually, after becoming increasingly dissatisfied with the role of community service officer, I left the probation service and read for a Diploma (Social Work) and Master of Arts (Social Work) at Liverpool University, although this environment too posed additional challenges. Wheelchair access to lecture rooms, seminar rooms, coffee bars, self-service cafeterias, notice boards, pigeon holes, etc., within the university left a lot to be desired. Like the probation service, the university authorities were sympathetic and proactively helpful with achieving solutions. For example, they provided a dedicated parking space (shared) near the entrance to the relevant building, and they relocated the student pigeon hole to a lower height. Wheelchair access is a common issue in both the workplace and public buildings. At university the lecture rooms and tutors' offices were all on the second floor. Access to the only lift (which I think was predominantly designed and used for transporting laboratory equipment) involved convoluted detours down long corridors. However, at least the lift existed – which is not always the case!

While at university I returned to the probation service on my first assessed placement. At this purpose-built probation office all the probation officers were located on the first floor. A lift had been especially installed for a previous wheelchair-bound employee. As a functional object the lift, perhaps better described as a contraption, served its purpose. However, it actually resembled a fork-lift truck with sides (a bit like a veal crate). It didn't look like it was designed for humans. As with so many aids for people with disabilities, the design (style, colour, materials, etc.) of such equipment focused on its functionality with little regard for the ergonomic and/or aesthetic impact upon the individual. If you use a goods lift frequently and are separated from colleagues, you begin to feel like goods.

I have often found that disabled access to places of work or other public buildings is achieved by a side or back entrance, where the entrance is usually locked and the individual first has to locate a member of staff who holds the key, and is invariably difficult to find. The design is invariably functional, crude and the cheapest available. The point here is not just the provision and availability of equipment, services and physical access but where such provision is available it usually serves to separate, humiliate and alienate the individual, while achieving the functional objective (of, in this example, gaining access). Thereby, an accumulation of ad hoc solutions to various problems of disability helps to generate and reinforce an image of people with impairments to the status of childlike dependency at best – at worst a burdensome problem that has reluctantly to be accommodated in order to demonstrate 'inclusiveness' and/or the expression of equal opportunities policies. The missing element is any sense of respect for the dignity or the value of people with impairments for who they are, and what they (intrinsically) have to offer. This is a general point about the expression of social attitudes to disability and the issue of empowering people with impairments to overcome a disabling society.

In my professional role I have become aware how the Criminal Justice System can so often devalue and oppress offenders by increasingly submitting them to processes and interventions without regard to their intrinsic value as a human being and their individual assessment and need. Of course the language of individual assessment and need is a top priority in policy and discourse within the system. However, the actual impact of current policy, dominated by exhaustive bureaucratic form filling and assessments, is to subvert professional judgements in order to fulfil targets, because targets are linked to budgets and are seen as evidence of successful outcomes (if they are achieved) – regardless of the counterproductive impact upon the individual. This obsession with targets pervades public services but when applied to the human services (social work, probation, health and education) the systemic processes oppress those who are subject to them as well as those who are charged with implementing them.

The systems and processes that devalue people with impairments are not consciously formulated and written down as policy, as in the case of the public ser-vices analogy, but are rooted in historic attitudes (as in the case of racism and sexism) and reinforced by both physical and social structures. During my higher education I have been exposed to a variety of sociological and psychological theories from which I have sought to analyse, interpret and elucidate models for understanding the dynam-ics and nature of the oppression of different vulnerable sectors of society, for example, theories regarding racism, sexism, the elderly, children, disabled people and the experiences of immigrants. These theories cover vast areas of psychosocial experi-ences and dynamics, cultural values and belief systems at the personal, familial, communal and societal levels. They seek to explain oppression and disadvantage with a view to informing government policies from which agency policies and procedures are derived which, in turn, inform practice.

The agency policies and procedures are the framework within which the front-line worker is required to implement interventions. However, governmental priority is the delivery of services in a cost-effective manner and so practice guidance and policy frameworks are overlaid with bureaucratic procedures and productivity account-ability systems, which seek to demonstrate successful outcomes in order that politi-cians can evidence so called 'real improvements' in the delivery of public sector services. Inevitably these improvements are measured in terms of achieving targets and targets are linked to budgets. Consequently, the pressure on the public service sector to achieve targets then becomes the agency's top priority. The monumental task of achieving what appear to be arbitrary targets becomes the worker's priority because the achievement of targets is the measure of the worker's, team's, division's and agency's value. If targets are not achieved, financial penalties are imposed which further reduce resource and increase pressure on the worker. If targets are achieved, then they are raised in the next financial year. The point here is that the *quality* of service delivery is undermined and subverted by such imperatives. In my own life experience I often received the services I needed, but it was the way the services were delivered that undermined the benefit of them to me, and at times it possibly created additional difficulties. This is a subtle but crucial point.

Conclusion

In conclusion I would make the following points. First, during my childhood and schoolboy years I did receive help and support from education, social services and the health departments. However, none of it, at any time and as best as I can recall, actively involved me as an individual in any of the assessment and decision-making processes. I received a number of different interventions, some of which should have involved my active participation at various stages. Statutory obligations were discharged by the relevant agencies, but I was often left feeling powerless like a 'straw in the wind', for example, the school holidays spent with the Asian family in Farnham. This foster placement appears to have been arranged on the reductionist assumption that, because I was Asian, I would be best placed with an Asian family, as if Asian people are a homogenous group. This was despite the fact that I was no longer able to speak Urdu and had never met the family prior to being placed with them. No account of my Western socialization, developing identity or personal preferences had been taken into account.

Secondly, when I did leave the residential school and my 'uncle's' home in Liverpool, there arose a tension between continuing to seek support from various agencies from which I had often felt powerless and patronized, and the freedom of living autonomously and independently. I opted for autonomous living with all its difficulties problems and dilemmas – most of which I did not foresee. For those I did foresee I did not have ready-made solutions but attempted to resolve problems on an ad hoc basis. The solution depended upon the nature of the problem, the resources available at the time and my own inner resources. The point is that the lack of information, coupled with previous difficult experiences when I did receive help, reinforced an aversion to availing myself of necessary support from the relevant statutory agency.

Thirdly, during my 'non-productive' adult years obtaining appropriate help and support was often a case of trial and error. Myriad organizations existed, both statutory and voluntary, yet I could only access assistance if I was capable and skilled enough to negotiate the bureaucracy and conduct myself in a manner that attracted a sympathetic understanding. There was no single, focal access point (as in the contemporary City Council initiative of one-stop shops).

Fourthly, significant support was made available when I obtained full-time employment with Merseyside Probation Service. The support given has enabled me to sustain a demanding job and to develop both in my practice as a probation officer as well as in other personal areas as a human being – notwithstanding managerial imperatives to fulfil targets set by Home Office officials. Of course, the rhetoric of impacting upon offending behaviour is prevalent throughout the Criminal Justice System and the intention in so doing is sincere and appropriate. However, it is the mechanistic application of the business model (in the interests of being cost-effective) to all the human services that I believe will ultimately prove to be counterproductive to the main purposes of any given agency. It is not the basic analyses and ideas in their entirety which are at fault, it is the inflexibility of target-driven initiatives that damage both the client group and the workers who have to implement them.

Fifthly, we live in an increasingly complicated and difficult world in which, as workers, we have to take into account various issues, many of which are only partly understood, sometimes contradictory, sometimes irreconcilable and which present dilemmas in practice, in order to practise our professions. With the increasing momentum towards multi-agency practice (involving different agency protocols, agendas and priorities) there arises the danger of compounding the complexities of delivering services and interventions. While we become preoccupied with negotiating the dynamics of multi-agency working, the prospect of losing sight of the purpose of all this work becomes a real possibility, and the client group risks becoming increasingly peripheral to the purposes of multi-agency partnerships and projects. Meetings will be held, e-mails exchanged, minutes circulated, documents sent out for consultation, faxes sent and received, working parties attended, and the telephone never stops ringing – in the midst of all this you might find 10 minutes to talk with the client!

Finally, I think what I am seeking to impart to the reader is that, from personal experience as a recipient of services as well as a professional seeking to deliver services, you cannot underestimate the importance of engaging with whatever client group you work – in a spirit of truth, honesty, justice, care and respect. These attributes are harder to measure, they will probably not find their way into the mechanistic detail of targets, outcomes or deliverables. It is quite feasible for a partnership to demonstrate how successful it is 'on paper', yet fail to deliver on these crucial values. From my experience, the single most important issue is not increasing the range of services we deliver, but it's the manner in which we deliver them that counts. It's not so much what we do but the way we do it that matters most to clients.

Questions for further discussion

1. How far does the account presented here reflect the experience of clients with whom you have had contact?
2. In your experience, has there been an improvement in user involvement since the 1950s and 1960s? If yes, what has been the nature of this improvement?
3. To what extent is the way in which a service is provided more important than the actual service itself?

6

Working in partnership in rural areas

Richard Pugh

This chapter will:

- Explore the rural context of health and social care provision.
- Look at the challenges to providing services in rural areas.
- Investigate why agencies and workers need to work in partnership in rural settings.

Introduction

The British countryside is home to substantial numbers of people, but rural life is often subject to idealization and oversimplification. The reality is that there is no simple picture of an ideal community, there are many different experiences of rural life. The interplay of location and different dimensions of demographic difference, such as class, gender, age and ethnicity, result in a complex and variable set of social circumstances in which agencies have to establish and provide services. Unfortunately, few courses of professional training in health and social services offer any preparation for rural work and existing research into rural practice provides limited guidance as to what might be considered best practice (Craig and Manthorpe 2000). This chapter draws upon previously published material in which a fuller account of the complexity of rural settings and the professional neglect of rural work can be found (Pugh 2000).

Rural areas are disadvantaged by two factors: the urbanist nature of the assumptions that are often made about needs and services; and the continued under-funding of rural services. However, we contend that collaborative practice between agencies should not simply be a pragmatic response to scarce resources, but is a desirable feature of service planning and delivery in settings where the relationship between those who require services and those who provide them is often distinctively different to that in urban districts. Nevertheless, effective joint work is not easily achieved. There are potential risks for both public sector and independent and voluntary agencies in any collaborative enterprise, and without support in the local community there may be resistance to any new partnership developments.

The rural context

The question of what is rural is a surprisingly complex one and raises issues that go beyond the scope of this chapter. Barnes (1993) in a useful review identified four different ways to define 'rural':

1. to define urban areas first and then classify the rest as rural;
2. to define villages and settlements below a certain population size as being rural;
3. to identify particular characteristics that are thought to indicate rurality, such as population density, distance from a larger urban centre, or types of economic activity, and then apply these to existing administrative divisions such as electoral wards, parishes, local authority districts or postal districts;
4. to ask people and organizations to define themselves.

Different ways of defining rural emphasize some features or perceptions rather than others, and may have important consequences when decisions are being made about priorities and resources. For example, when the size of the community is used as the defining feature in decisions about the provision of public services, then other aspects, such as the degree of geographical isolation may be ignored. Thus, the question of defining 'rural' should not be naively viewed merely as a technical question, it is one that may have some resounding consequences, as some ideas and needs may come to predominate to the exclusion of others. A useful review of the definitions used by health researchers can be found in the Institute of Rural Health's study (1998) and further information on the definitions used by the Office of National Statistics can be found on the web (www.statistics.gov.uk/geography/urban_rural.asp).

Regardless of which definitions are used, a significant number of people live in the British countryside. For example, one estimate provided by Age Concern (1998) suggested that there were 11.5 million people in rural areas in the UK, including Northern Ireland. However, the work of the Office of National Statistics suggests that the figures are much higher. At the time of writing, a full analysis of the 2001 census is not available, but the first analysis that provides figures for England alone indicates that the proportion of people living in the countryside rose from 27.6 per cent in 1991 to 28.5 per cent in 2001, and that the rate of population increase is much higher in rural areas at 5.5 per cent compared to 0.7 per cent in urban areas (DEFRA 2002). Most of this increase in numbers is due to migration. In the most rural districts of Scotland and Wales – the Western isles, Orkney, Shetland and Powys – the proportion of the population living in rural areas is significantly higher with 50–70 per cent living in the countryside. In total, there are 24 local authority areas in the UK where more than 20 per cent of the population lives in the countryside (Denham and White 1998).

In general, the rural population reflects broad trends evident throughout the rest of the UK – increased divorce rates, smaller families with fewer children – but there are some points of difference. The proportion of young children up to four years of age is smaller than in urban areas, and there is a smaller proportion of young adults between 18 and 29 years of age. While this latter group constitute 18.7 per cent of the population in English urban areas, they comprise only 14.6 per cent in rural areas. For those aged over 75 years, the typical pattern is of a slightly higher proportion of older men in rural areas compared to urban areas (Denham and White 1998). Of course, these overall figures mask more marked variations in particular localities, such as those with declining employment opportunities, or those rural areas that have become popular destinations for retirement.

While the degree of ethnic diversity in rural areas is generally lower than in most urban areas, every area of the UK has some minority ethnic population within it. For example, the 1991 census indicated that for just one group, i.e. those describing themselves as 'Afro-Caribbean', there were over 33,000 people living in small villages and the wider countryside (OPCS 1992), and Jay (1992) estimated that there were between 26,200 and 36,600 people who might be perceived as black living in south-west England, that is, Cornwall, Devon, Dorset and Somerset. The most recent census shows that the proportion of residents born outside of the UK including those from the EU and Eire, range from:

- 1.03 per cent in Blaenau Gwent
- 2.28 per cent in Cumbria
- 4.16 per cent in Devon
- 8.74 per cent in Herefordshire
- 8.79 per cent in Cambridgeshire

(ONS 2003)

Changes in the structure of the rural population – evident in the changing social composition of many villages as new residents move into them – have led to conflict. For example, in some Welsh-speaking communities, the influx of English monoglots has raised fears of cultural dilution. Elsewhere, incomers may oppose any further development and resist proposals for new housing, new business and new roads. This can prevent villages from changing or growing, and may have other far-reaching effects upon local communities. For example, planning restrictions upon new building can lead to localized housing shortages, resulting in house prices and rents rising beyond the means of other local people. This in turn can lead to an increasing polarization of the socio-economic structure of the community, as the proportion of relatively wealthy incomers increases (Murdoch and Marsden 1994). The growing numbers living in the countryside, who commute to work in urban areas where they also conduct their personal business and do their shopping, have begun to reshape the rural context by diluting demand for local services such as bus transport, doctors, schools and post offices.

A recurring feature of social problems in rural areas is that they are often unnoticed by policy makers and service providers. In part, the 'invisibility' of rural problems stems from the uncritical acceptance of rather idealized conceptions of what rural life is like. Thus it is assumed, rather than based upon fact, that poverty is not an issue, that there are no drug problems, and that loneliness and isolation cannot be a problem in rural communities. This oversight is often underpinned by the assumption that rural communities are self-sufficient, homogenous entities which lack both the diversity of urban areas and the sorts of problems associated with urban life. Thus, racism or homophobia are not seen to be an issue because these forms of difference upon which discrimination may be based are presumed not to exist in the countryside. Consequently, one of the most fundamental problems facing rural dwellers is getting public services to recognize their particular needs and the diversity of problems in the first place. In the absence of service, many potential service users struggle because they lack other financial or social resources which they could mobilize to meet their needs. Thus, poverty, sexism and racism, along with other types of discrimination, can lead to disadvantages which are not unique to the countryside, but are reinforced by the rural context. Furthermore, such individuals who are perceived as 'different' or not 'belonging' may not have the support of any wider community of similar people, and can be further exposed to significant risks arising from intolerance and hostility (Chakraborti and Garland 2001; Dhalech 1999; Garland and Charaborti 2004; Henderson and Kaur 1999; Jay 1992).

Service planners and providers need to look beyond stereotypical notions and gather accurate information about the communities they are supposed to serve. Although the diversity of rural areas may seem insignificant in comparison to the obvious diversity of many urban areas, every rural community will contain some social minorities. However, in recognizing this more complex picture of the rural context, we should be wary of assuming that the experience of health and social problems in the countryside is universally shared. For:

> people living in the same place, with access to similar levels of housing, service and employment opportunities, and with similar levels of wealth and income, may experience rural life differently. Their needs may be different; their expectations may be different; their willingness to cope with problems as part of everyday life may be different; their cultural view of what rural life should be like may be different; their strategies for coping with rural life may be different, and so on. Rural problems are thus experiential as well as material, and seemingly similar material conditions obscure important differences in the way that rural people feel marginalized by a lack of power, choice and opportunity, or in the way that they cope with the strong relative differences in rural life which are accentuated as the affluent live cheek by jowl with the less affluent . . .
>
> (Cloke *et al.* 1997: 165)

The point is that we should not make deterministic assumptions about what people's lives are like until we have learned from them how they perceive and experience their particular situations. Therefore, we cannot assume that every gay man or lesbian woman, or every person from an ethnic minority will necessarily be subject to homophobia, bigotry or racism. Indeed there is some anecdotal evidence which suggests that some people have been able to find a place for themselves in a small community, where they have become known and accepted for who they are rather than being perceived as a stereotypical member of some larger grouping (Pugh

2004a, 2004b). Nevertheless, even such acceptance, if present, cannot be assumed to be a continuing feature of a person's life. For some people, their apparently secure position is always fraught with the threat of discrimination and exclusion (Williams 1997).

Rural service provision

Craig and Manthorpe have noted that an explicit rural dimension is lacking from many reports into policy and practice development in rural areas (2000). This is indicative of the wider problem facing rural services, which is that, in the absence of any specific consideration of rurality, urban models are the de facto norm. Frequently, central government requirements, advice and guidance to public services are given with the presumption that their activities are based in urban areas, and if rurality is acknowledged, it is often done so in a way that ignores the diversity among different rural areas (Hill and Fraser 1995). The provision of health and social services in rural areas poses particular challenges for such agencies. Many of these arise from distance, poor transport and dispersed and sparse populations, which offer few possibilities for economies of scale and result in relatively high per capita service costs. For example, in 1999 Wiltshire Social Services calculated the unit cost of providing residential care for older people in the largest homes to be £232 per week, while the cost in their smallest home was £365. More recently, the Scottish Executive reported that the unit cost for residential care on the islands served by the local authority of Argyll and Bute was £640, compared to £377 on the mainland (Wilson 2001). Studies into the use of health services show that their utilization by some groups in rural areas diminishes the further away that people are from the services (Deaville 2001; Higgs 1999). As well as the obvious geographical isolation that accompanies residence in a remote location, such as the Highlands and Islands of Scotland, even people living comparatively close to local services may have difficulty in accessing them. A person may live only a few miles from a doctor's surgery or a day centre, but because of features such as hilly terrain, estuaries, open moor land, a consequent lack of roads and poor public transport, they may find that their journey to obtain such services is disproportionately lengthy. In the most extreme examples, a return visit to some of the remoter Scottish Isles can take up to three days (Wilson 2001).

Among rural dwellers, women, older people and the rural working class are less likely to seek medical care, and when they do seek it, their illnesses are often at a more serious or chronic stage and, consequently, they have poorer outcomes. The uneven geographical distribution of health services (Benzeval and Judge 1994) is compounded for some people by increasing difficulties in accessing GP services because of the closure of branch surgeries (Watt 1999), inconvenient surgery hours and unsatisfactory appointment schemes. Unsurprisingly, difficulties in transport are a major factor too. Furthermore, there is a complex relationship between access to services and other aspects of the rural environment. For example, the absence of alternative child care services, dial-a-ride and community care schemes, as well as fewer opportunities to 'piggyback' services upon existing services/centres, may also impede both the provision and take-up of services. Aside of transport difficulties, the main differences in the nature of general practice in health care between urban and rural areas are:

- increased emergency and minor casualty work;
- specific rural diseases and illnesses (especially those arising from farming and contact with animals);
- difficulties in cover for absences and out-of-hours work.

(Institute of Rural Health 1998)

The 'post code lottery' which is evident in rural health services (White 2001) – that is, where a person's chances of receiving a satisfactory service vary according to where they live – is also apparent in social services. Numerous reports into rural social services have demonstrated that rural dwellers are much less likely to receive a service that is comparable with their urban counterparts (Department of Health 1996; Gregoire and Thornicroft 1998; Hayle 1996; Spilsbury and Lloyd 1998). For example, a study of unmet mental health needs in Wensleydale found 1,360 elderly people with mental health problems, two thirds of whom were suffering from depression or anxiety-related conditions sufficient to warrant support, yet most 'were receiving little or no help, and isolation and loneliness were identified as major influences on their mental health' (Rickford 1996: 26). A similar picture prevails for many aspects of children's services, with Mullins *et al.* (2001) finding that those who cared for children with disabilities were under considerable strain.

Higher costs

Dispersed populations and transport difficulties generally result in rural services costing more to access and more to provide than in urban areas. For example, a study by the University of York (1998) indicated that the additional cost element for the provision of domiciliary care services in rural areas was around 20 per cent, and some preliminary research undertaken for Shropshire Social Services found that the travel times of home care staff as a percentage of the contact hours varied from 11 per cent in the least rural areas to 19 per cent in the most rural ones (Shropshire County Council 2000). Wiltshire Social Services have calculated that their rural social workers average an additional 3,777 miles per year than their workers based in urban areas (Craig and Manthorpe 2000). Because service users are often scattered and some distance from other service users, there may be few opportunities for economies of scale in such services as meals on wheels. This may be compounded by the absence of other public services, which could otherwise be used as points of access or distribution, such as schools and health care centres. Similarly, the more limited involvement of voluntary organizations, such as Age Concern, the Children's Society, MIND, NCH, SCOPE, Shelter and so on, means that there are often no alternative sources of help available.

Higher costs may also be incurred when agencies seeking to develop new services simply assume that what has worked in urban areas will work in rural ones (Gibson *et al.* 1995). For example, Mason and Taylor, in a report to the Gulbenkian Foundation, found that it could take much longer to establish voluntary sector initiatives in rural areas (1990) and Pickering in a more recent review of good practice (2003) has made the same point. It is likely that this is also true of the statutory sector as well. This longer setting-up period can arise from a number of factors, including poorer infra-structure, local resistance to new developments, and the more personalized basis of formal relationships in small communities where professionals often live within the communities they serve, and where the credence afforded to a new initiative may be closely related to personal perceptions of competence held about workers (Pugh 2003).

Lower funding

Despite the higher costs associated with rural service delivery, national government funding for rural social services has not generally included any premium to offset these additional costs (Hayle 1996; Rural Development Commission 1998a). For example, the County Councils Network found that the Standard Spending Assess-ment (SSA), the government's measure for resource allocation to local authorities, for shire counties was consistently lower than the average of all English authorities, that is

- the SSA for a child at risk in Cumbria was 77 per cent of the average for England;
- the SSA for domiciliary care in Dorset was 82 per cent of the average for England;
- the SSA for elderly residential care [sic] in North Yorkshire was 77 per cent of the average for England.

(Shropshire County Council 2000: 3)

Such inadequacies in service funding largely derive from the formulae that are used to calculate the funding allocation to local authorities, and while population sparsity is included as a relevant factor, insufficient weight is given to it. However, there are indications that central government is beginning to recognize some of the difficulties, as the Social Services Inspectorate noted: '. . . services, information and facilities are more expensive and/or difficult to access than in urban areas. This means that they are much less likely to be used, leading to a breakdown in provision' (Social Services Inspectorate 1999: 2). Furthermore, local authorities vary in the extent to which they internally formalize rurality as a factor in distributing resources. Thus, while one department may provide additional funds for rural teams, another may not (Social Services Inspectorate 1998a). Variation in local decision making about services and priorities also contributes to the differential chances of receiving services. For example, Foley (2001) in his research into support services for children with special needs in East Sussex by health and social care agencies found that not only were there marked disparities in the provision of respite care between urban and rural districts, but that there were also significant variations between different rural districts. While Pizey and Lyons contend that:

Less money is made available for older people who live in rural areas . . . because it is assumed (rather than based on fact) that . . . [they] are less likely to need help, and that the amount needed for their care will be lower. Smaller proportions of older people are expected to need social services help in rural areas than elsewhere; and local authorities in rural areas are expected to spend significantly less on social services for older people than other types of authority.

(Pizey and Lyons 1998: 12)

Similar problems are evident in primary care. The much criticized General Practitioners' Deprivation Payment Scheme, which operated from 1990 until recently, was a scheme for providing additional funding to reflect the workload of GPs in deprived areas. Unfortunately, this scheme was developed using an index based solely upon urban settings. Thus, the particular problems of transport and travel time in rural practices were not even considered (Deaville 2001). Following lobbying by the Royal College of General Practitioners Rural Group the new contract for GP services does include some recognition of the additional travel costs of delivering primary care in rural areas, but does not include any uplift for the diseconomies of scale in small practices (www.bma.org.uk/ap.nsf/Content).

An additional problem for many aspects of public service is that population 'thresholds', which are widely used in the distribution of public funds, tend to discriminate against areas with small populations. Thus, class sizes, levels of need and so on, may not reach the levels that ensure the continuance of existing services, or trigger new funding. Whatever the reason, there is no doubt that many people in rural areas do not have equal access to services, and even when they do get them, they may not match the levels found elsewhere.

Lack of knowledge, lowered expectations and resistance

As in urban areas, many potential users of services lack knowledge of how particular services may be able to help them. In rural areas, this is compounded by the reduced opportunities for the dissemination of information. The Social Services Inspectorate noted that 'innovations such as databases in libraries and advice centres tended to be located in towns' (1999: 9), and the distribution of other sources of information, such as that found in many local free advertising papers, is often very limited. Nonetheless, some services are becoming more proactive in this respect. For example, some have provided mobile information centres that go out to villages and schools, while others have developed farmers' health initiatives where nurses attend auctions, farms and WI meetings to provide advice and minor treatments (Deaville 2001).

Although expectations of public services may vary considerably, especially in areas where there are a substantial number of middle-class incomers, there is some evidence that rural dwellers generally have lower expectations of services. It is likely that these arise in part from traditional notions of independence and stoicism, and partly from the realization that health and social services are scarce anyway. Indeed, the Social Services Inspectorate have noted that 'people in rural communities have lower expectations regarding quality of services and this obliges them to be more self-sufficient, particularly in terms of self help' (1999: 2). It is also likely that a lack of anonymity, and fears of stigmatization, especially in regard to mental health issues, some physical illnesses and some types of family problems, may also contribute to this situation. For example, MacKay in her report on Women's Aid services in rural Scotland noted that women in rural areas were reluctant to seek help if the mere act of using public transport or entering a particular building or office would make them visible to other people who might know them (2000). Lambert and Hartley similarly note a reluctance to seek mental health care because 'stigma may be more strongly experienced in rural areas where people know whose car is parked by the mental health centre' (1998: 957).

Attempts to localize services may not always have the desired effect of increasing take-up. While attempts to meet local needs and reduce transport costs by recruiting local workers may appear to be an effective way of improving services in rural areas, there may be objections. As the Social Services Inspectorate have noted, local workers may 'not always be acceptable to service users who . . . [will be] concerned about confidentiality or . . . reluctant to have service, especially intimate service, from neighbours whom they . . . [have] known for many years' (1999: 10).

The situation of members of ethnic minorities is likely to be worse. Comparatively little research has been done into service provision and take-up for ethnic minorities in rural areas, but what there is shows patchy or non-existent provision allied to very low expectations of service from minorities (Social Services Inspectorate 1998c). For example, while the low take-up of child care among parents and carers from ethnic minorities is partly due to financial constraints and lack of information, it is also due to their perceptions that existing provision is 'a white service to a white clientele' (Stephens 2001: 9). Although further information will become available as one of the requirements of *Best Value* (HMSO 1999), it is up to local authorities to monitor the ethnicity of people who are assessed for service and those who receive them, and even so the immediate prospects of improvement are not promising. The relatively small numbers of ethnic minorities in rural areas means that there is less pressure for culturally appropriate services in the first place, and fewer knowledgeable people and organizations who are available to advise or directly provide them (Patel 1999).

The impetus to better services and joint working

It was noted earlier that national government is becoming more attuned to rural needs and problems, and since the *Care in the Country* report (Social Services Inspectorate 1999), there have been a number of significant developments. In 2000 the rural white paper, *Our Countryside, The Future*, established a Rural Services Standard at the same time as the government sought to ensure that all of its polices were 'rural proofed', meaning that they had been considered and developed not solely from an urban perspective. The Standard sought to: '. . . give people in the countryside a better understanding of access to services they could expect . . . [and] update and refine the Standard over time as the modernisation of public services proceeded and rural access was improved' (The Countryside Agency 2003b: 2).

Although much of the Standard relates to schools, the police, employment services and access to benefits, there are a number of elements that bear upon health and social services. These include:

- collecting evidence to be used to develop rural standards and targets, for example, mapping rural public and private child care provision, and mapping distance travelled to dentists and GPs;
- efforts to improve access to information about available services, especially through the use of IT technology;
- efforts to improve access to services themselves, for example, by improving public transport in rural areas, and improving GP appointment systems;
- establishing clear lines of responsibility for rural issues across government departments;
- a presumption against further closures of schools and rural post offices.

Progress in regard to health and social care has so far been limited, and as the Department of Health themselves have noted, 'there is scope for improvement' (Countryside Agency 2003b: 12). It is also expected that the newly established Commission for Health Care Audit and Inspection, and the Commission for Social Care Inspection will consider the extent to which health and social care services meet the needs of rural populations and will be developing further performance indicators to measure progress.

It remains to be seen whether these efforts at developing more responsive services will be successful. Hopefully, these moves to improve and develop access for potential users of services should increase the impetus towards co-operation between agencies, especially where resources are scarce. However, one should not forget, that these imperatives are but the latest in a long series of policy initiatives aimed at improving co-operation and joint working in child care, mental health services and community care, such as *Working Together, Sure Start, Framework* plans, *Building Bridges* and *Better Government for Older People*, initiatives whose very existence unfortunately testifies to the limited impact of previous efforts.

Working together

The widespread acceptance of the need for partnership approaches to practice owes much to the failings revealed by inquiries into numerous child protection cases where children's safety has been compromised by inadequate co-operation and communication between agencies, and also to the failure of earlier community care initiatives prior to the National Health Services and Community Care Act 1990. Partnership may also be driven by:

- statutory requirement or policy directive from central government;
- economic necessity, where no single agency can afford to fund a project alone;
- common commitment to a project to which no agency alone bears sole responsibility;
- the need to broaden the base of support by enlisting other people and other agencies to help carry an existing initiative forward, or to extend its field of operation;

- common recognition that a multi-agency approach is a necessity to meet the needs of service users;
- desire to seek acceptance and to legitimate an initiative that might otherwise be controversial or be resisted by a particular community or potential service users.

Nevertheless, research into joint working has revealed a number of difficulties. Hague (1999) in a review of multi-agency initiatives indicated some of the more general problems which were:

- the tendency of some agencies to 'defend their own turf';
- potential confusion about roles and responsibilities;
- a tendency to marginalize equality issues such as gender and ethnicity;
- using multi-agency initiatives as a face-saving strategy to avoid confronting shortages of resources;
- the consumption and wastage of scarce resources, especially of smaller agencies, in unproductive discussion;
- the futility of attempts to co-ordinate systems that are already inadequate or disorganized;
- the difficulties in resolving differences of power, resources and philosophy between agencies;
- a tendency for larger agencies to take over the work and marginalize the smaller agencies, or alternatively, to leave too much of the work to smaller ones;
- a tendency to marginalize service users and prospective clients.

These difficulties are neither inevitable nor intrinsic aspects of joint working, and it is sensible to consider them as potential risks which, with foresight, commitment, clear aims and explicit strategy, can be avoided or mitigated. There are three aspects of partnership working where the rural context is likely to have a particular bearing upon how this may be undertaken:

1. Enlisting community support and enhancing user input
2. Service development
3. Staff training and support

Enlisting community support and enhancing user input

The use of partnerships to enlist local support and to avoid potential opposition can be a crucial element in rural initiatives because there is often resistance to agencies coming in from outside and imposing their 'solutions'. This resistance is frequently interpreted as political conservatism, and indeed in some instances it may be so, but often the reasons for it are structural. Small communities may engender solidarity by avoiding overt dissent and will often work hard to establish the appearance of consensus, especially on contentious issues. Thus, resistance may have complex foundations. Sometimes it may arise from a desire not to 'rock the boat' or to avoid social division or conflict, while at other times it may be focused upon the specifics of a proposal which are felt to be inappropriate or unnecessary. For example, Dhalech in reporting the development of anti-racist initiatives in south-west England noted that some:

> Black agencies come into the area wanting to undertake development work but they typically lack an understanding of rural issues . . . An officer from a national agency offered support for developing a telephone help line modelled on a London borough. The several meetings between the officer and representatives of local Black agencies proved to be remarkably unconstructive because there was no recognition of rural issues. As soon as the local agencies started discussing the idea between themselves an immediate consensus was reached and the ideas were developed.
>
> (Dhalech 1999: 29)

This illustrates a very important point, which is that success is most likely when a community or a group takes on board the need for change itself and determines its own direction, its own priorities, and commits itself to the development and implementation of the proposal (Francis and Henderson 1992). As the following case study illustrates, this principle of trying to understand the social context and work with it, also extends to efforts to encourage and enhance service user input into service planning.

Service development

Despite the risk of joint working being used as a 'face-saving' initiative when resources are scarce, it can be a legitimate response to scarcity providing that the shortage is explicitly acknowledged and that care is taken to avoid the unwitting exploitation of the scarce resources of smaller agencies in rural areas. In fact, in rural areas where higher service delivery costs are often unavoidable, in the medium term at least, it is often the most practical way of improving user access and choice. Probably the most common form of partnership involves the joint use or joint commissioning of premises in rural areas, but caution is needed as client confidentiality can easily be compromised in small communities where even the simple act of going into a particular building may be witnessed by others and may lead to particular presumptions about what is going on. A study that looked at innovative methods of service delivery in rural areas and examined a range of different approaches, including shared premises, concluded that there was no 'first best solution [and that] good practice could be identified as linking community transport initiatives with outreach services' (page 1, www.scotland.gov.uk/library5/rural/gprd-08.asp). Poor public transport networks and lack of access to a private vehicle remain prime barriers to service for many people. However, for agencies with a statutory duty to provide transport for clients, the Countryside Agency notes that 'joint contracting arrangements with voluntary or private transport providers can reduce the overall cost to each agency. By working in partnership to assess requirement, service planners can gain an overview of demand

Case Study

Powys is a large rural area but until Powys Mental Health Alliance, a voluntary organization, started its work, mental health service users and their families were often isolated, having little input into service development. In addition to the typical rural problems of poor transport networks and scattered populations, there were few places for
service users to meet and they were often unprepared or uncertain about participating
in service planning through such bodies as Patients' Councils. The Alliance organized a
series of day workshops at eight different locations to bring users into contact with
each other and promote their input into service development. Each event was facilitated by service users who had received training using discussion and role plays to
develop skills and confidence in facilitating meetings and recording discussion.

The workshops were held in comfortable locations, such as hotels or inns, and
transport and child care was organized for those participants who needed them. Particular attention was paid to publicizing the events by local voluntary groups, home care
workers and mental health workers. In total 130 people attended and the groups varied
from 8–21 people. From the morning discussions a list of common concerns was
established. These ranged from concerns about informed choice of treatment and
medication, hospitalization, stigma and public attitudes, information and so on. In the
afternoon, the groups were asked to consider their preferences in terms of formal and
informal support. These included: a desire for some half-way house provision to avoid
admittance to hospital; a 24-hour helpline, the availability of counselling; temporary
foster care places for children and someone to mind pets during hospitalization, drop-in
centres, befriending schemes and self-help groups.

The project helped service users to share their concerns, and encouraged them to
elucidate and express these to service providers. Indeed, many agencies were sur-
prised to learn that service users felt that professionals, such as social workers, doctors and nurses, lacked empathy, were unresponsive and did not really understand their
situation, and in particular, did not seem to appreciate their social isolation. Following
the events, service users made a greater input into service plans and were able to
influence service priorities. Most significantly, they were able to do this knowing that
they had some 'constituency', i.e. that other users shared their views.

(Pugh and Richards 1996)

in a particular area and tailor services accordingly' (2003a: 25). Furthermore, a
study into the joint provision of services that examined many successful initiatives,
including 'tandem services' (that is, where two or more services share premises or
facilities), found no firm evidence about the scale of cost savings from these ventures
(Rural Development Commission 1998b).

Obviously, some areas of service require joint commissioning, particularly when
people's problems do not fall exclusively within the realm of one service, for example,
where people with learning disabilities or frail elderly people also have mental health
problems. One difficulty that faces smaller voluntary organizations in rural areas is
that because many funding initiatives are short term, they often create pressure to bid

quickly for funds and if successful, to spend money within a relatively short period of time. This can lead to inappropriate attempts to apply models of service delivery which have been developed in an urban context into a rural one, and thus, fail to take sufficient account of differences in geography, demography and attitudes to services (Gibson *et al.* 1995). The importance of adequate 'lead-in' time was noted in a study of community-based partnership in rural areas (Edwards *et al.* 1999), which found that:

> The lead-in time for preparing bids to programmes, and partnership initiation, is frequently too short to enable appropriate structures and sustainable relationships to be constructed. ... This 'establishment phase' is particularly crucial as partnerships tend to be very stable once set up.
>
> (1999: 2)

Similarly, a review of partnership working in rural regeneration projects (Edwards *et al.* 1999) concluded that partnerships in rural areas need sufficient time to allow effective partnerships to be established and that these may typically take much longer to get established than in urban areas. Indeed, one person commented, 'I don't think that three or four years is a very long time. All the literature says seven or ten years' (Edwards *et al.* 1999: 3).

Staff training and support

With the exception of the commendable efforts of the Institute for Rural Health, most health and social welfare professionals receive no specific education or training focusing upon rural issues. Yet there are five aspects of rural practice that are likely to make particular demands upon those who deliver public services and where there is much to be gained by developing services and training together. These arise from the:

- increased visibility of professional workers in small rural communities;
- lack of separation of personal and public roles;
- difficulties in maintaining client confidentiality;
- relative professional isolation from support networks and training opportunities and the impact these may have upon professional advancement;
- shortage of resources and the lack of alternative services.

Furthermore, there are some indications that recruitment and retention of public sector professionals in rural areas is becoming more problematic. Clearly, professionals moving into rural practice do so for a number of reasons including their expectations regarding their quality of life, but it is also likely that the lack of preparation for rural practice may have some influence upon their decisions.

Conclusion

We have tried in this short account to give readers some idea of the variability and complexity of rural contexts, and in particular, have warned against any simplistic assumptions about what rural life is like. Indeed, the social context of any community requires particular attention. Good local knowledge and careful study will lessen any tendency to simply apply 'what works' elsewhere. While many of the advantages and disadvantages of joint working in rural areas are similar to those pertaining to urban areas, the rural context may have other features that impact upon the necessity and the feasibility of partnership practice. Some of these, such as increased costs, the lack of alternative provision and the generally poorer infrastructure, can be a stimulus to joint working as agencies seek to maximize scarce resources and address the marked disparities in service provision that occur between different areas. Other features, such as those that arise from the social context, may make it difficult to get new developments established and accepted, and may also militate against what might otherwise seem to be efficient solutions to the disparities and difficulties of rural service provision. As noted earlier, concerns about confidentiality, a desire to keep one's business one's own, and fears of stigmatization, may not only inhibit potential users from seeking service, but should also give those who are planning multi-agency initiatives cause for thought. The fact that an initiative appears practical and effective to those who provide services, does not mean that rural dwellers will necessarily use it.

We should remember that the rural context is not 'out there', agencies and their workers are a part of it. Living and working in the same place may bring many advantages in terms of workers having local knowledge and awareness of local sensibilities. In many instances this will make it easier to gain acceptance and build personal credibility. In communities where as an elderly man said 'you are a long time living with your mistakes', prospective service users may be initially wary of engaging with services. Service users may often attempt to 'place' the worker; that is, to discover something about the worker's background, family and personal networks, and above all, their professional capability, before committing themselves. Consequently, when workers make mistakes or fail to deliver what they promise, credibility may be under-mined and a poor reputation, as with a good one, may often precede the worker's engagement with potential users. The personal credibility of workers is more likely to be based upon a wider consideration of their behaviour and social comportment within the rural community. For many workers this is a positive experience, they value the sense of belonging, recognition and achievement, but for others it can be a more isolated experience as they struggle to establish themselves and their service without the support of a larger team of colleagues, and without other professional support networks.

Finally, we would encourage readers to conceptualize multi-agency practice in a much broader fashion than it is typically conceived, that is beyond simply envisaging cooperative efforts at direct service provision, to include research and development, community capacity building, social inclusion strategies, and anti-discriminatory initiatives. As we indicated earlier, working with the grain of a rural community, that is with local people and organizations, is not simply desirable, it is often a practical and professional necessity. Service providers have much to gain from a broader range of partnerships. For example, Action with Rural Communities in England (ACRE) developed a poverty mapping project in Dorset in partnership with the county council and Oxford University. Mixed partnerships often facilitate access to sources of funding, such as charitable organizations and research bodies, which would not otherwise be available to one or other of the partners. Such initiatives sit well with the developing rural guidance and policy emanating from national and local government (DEFRA 2002; Haskins Review 2003; LGA 2001). Creative and thoughtful approaches to multi-agency work in rural communities can develop more effective provision, which can ultimately deliver more equitable services to rural communities.

Questions for further discussion

1. If the local social context is so important in rural work, why is social context not considered more in urban settings?
2. How can isolated professionals in rural areas support one another?
3. To what extent do people in rural communities have a right to expect to receive a service comparable to that available in large cities?

Note

The author would like to record his thanks for the supporting research undertaken by Debbie Williams, formerly of North East Wales Institute of Higher Education.

References

Age Concern (1998) *Developing Rural Services to Older People.* Age Concern, London.

Barnes, L. (1993) *Getting Closer to Rural Communities.* NCVO, London.

Benzeval, M. and Judge, K. (1994) The determinants of hospital utilisation: Implications for resources allocation in England, *Health Economics*, 3: 105–16.

Chakraborti, N. and Garland, J. (2001) An invisible problem? Uncovering the nature of racist victimisation in rural Suffolk, *International Review of Victimology*, 10(1): 1–17.

Cloke, P., Goodwin, M. and Milbourne, P. (1997) *Rural Wales: Community and Marginalisation.* University of Wales Press, Cardiff.

Countryside Agency (2003a) *Local Transport Plans.* Countryside Agency, Wetherby.

Countryside Agency (2003b) *The Rural Services Standard: Second Progress Report 2002/03.* Countryside Agency, Wetherby, and is also available at www.countryside.gov.uk.

DEFRA (2002) *The Way Ahead for Rural Services: A Guide to Good Practice in Locating Rural Services.* Department for Environment, Food and Rural Affairs, London.

Craig, G. and Manthorpe, J. (2000) *Social Care in Rural Areas: Developing an Agenda for Research, Policy and Practice.* Rowntree Research Findings, 5110, http:dRwww.jrf.org.uk.

Craig, G. and Manthorpe, J. (2000) *Fresh Fields: Rural Social Care: Research, Policy and Practice Agendas.* Joseph Rowntree Foundation/York Publishing Services, York.

J. Deaville (2001) *The Nature of Rural General Practice in the UK – Preliminary Research.* Institute of Rural Health, Gregynog.

DEFRA (2002) *Population Trends in Rural Areas of England.* Rural Statistics Unit, Department for Environment, Food and Rural Affairs, London.

Denham, C. and White, I. (1998) Differences in Urban and Rural Britain, *Population Trends.* Office for National Statistics, London.

Department of Health (1996) *Developing Health and Social Care in Rural England.* The Stationery Office, London.

Department of Health (1997) *Taking Care – Taking Control*. Social Services Inspectorate, The Stationery Office, London.

Dhalech, M. (1999) *Challenging Racism in the Rural Idyll*. The Rural Race Equality Project, Exeter.

Eaton, S. (1995) *Multi-agency Work with Young People in Difficulty*. Rowntree Research Findings, Social Care Research 68, http://www.jrf.org.uk.

Edwards, B., Goodwin, M., Pemberton, S. and Woods, M. (1999) *Partnership Working in Rural Regeneration*. Rowntree Research Findings, 039, http://www.jrf.org.uk.

Foley, R. (2001) *The Role of GIS in Health and Social Care Planning*, unpublished paper presented at Keele geography seminar, Keele University, 6 February.

Francis, D. and Henderson, P. (1992) *Working with Rural Communities*. Macmillan, London.

Garland, J. and Chakraborti, N. (2004) *Racism, Identity and Community in Rural Britain*. Willan Publishing, Collumpton.

Gibson, F., Whittington, D., Pattenden, A., Rahmin, L. and James, D. (1995) *Day Care in Rural Areas*. Rowntree Research Findings, Social Care Research 72, http://www.jrf.org.uk.

Gregoire, A. and Thornicroft, G. (1998) Rural mental health, *Psychiatric Bulletin*, 22(5): 273–7.

Hague, G. (1999) Smoke screen or leap forward: inter-agency initiatives as a response to domestic violence, *Critical Social Policy*, 53: 93–109.

Haskins, C. (2003) *Rural Delivery Review – A Report on the Delivery of Government Policies in Rural England*. www.defra.gov.uk/rural/ruraldelivery/default.htm.

Hayle, R. (1996) *Fair Shares for Rural Areas? An Assessment of Public Resource Allocation Systems*. Rural Development Commission, London.

Henderson, P. and Kaur, R. (1999) *Rural Racism in the UK*. The Community Development Foundation, London.

Higgs, G. (1999) Investigating trends in rural health outcomes: a research agenda, *Geoforum*, 30: 203–21.

Hill, C.E. and Fraser, G.J. (1995) Local knowledge and rural mental health reform, *Community Mental Health Journal*, 31(6): 553–68.

HMSO (1999) *Explanatory Notes to the Local Government Act*, http://www.hmso.gov.uk.

Institute of Rural Health (1998) *A Study to Obtain a Definition of Rurality and to Investigate the Problems Encountered by Practitioners who Work in Rural Health Settings*. Institute of Rural Health, Gregynog.

Jay, E. (1992) *Keep Them in Birmingham: Challenging Racism in the South West*. Commission for Racial Equality, London.

Lambert, D. and Hartley, D. (1998) Linking primary care and rural psychiatry: where have we been and where are we going?, *Psychiatric Services*, 49(7): 965–6.

LGA (2001) *All Together Now? – Social Inclusion in Rural Communities*. Local Government Association www.lga.gov.uk.

MacKay, A (2000) *Reaching Out: Women's Aid in a Rural Area*. East Fife Women's Aid, St Andrews.

Mason, S. and Taylor, R. (1990) *Tackling Deprivation in Rural Areas: Effective Use of Charity Funding*. ACRE, Cirencester, Gloucestershire.

Mullins, A., McCluskey, J. and Taylor-Browne, J. (2001) *Challenging the Rural Idyll*. The Countryside Agency, Wetherby.

Murdoch, J. and Marsden, T. (1994) *Reconstituting Rurality*. UCL Press, London.

ONS (2003) *Census 2001: Key Statistics for Local Authorities in England and Wales*. Office for National Statistics, The Stationery Office, London.

OPCS (1992) *Census 1991*. Office of Population Censuses and Surveys, HMSO, London.

Patel, N. (1999) *Community Care Services For Black and Ethnic Minority Elders*, unpublished paper presented at CCETSW/University of Wales seminar at the North East Wales Institute, Wrexham, 19 February.

Pickering, J. (2003) Innovative methods of service delivery in rural Scotland: A good practice guide, *Good Practice in Rural Development, 8.* The Scottish Executive, www.scotland.gov.uk/library/rural/gprd-08.asp.

Pizey, N. and Lyons, R. (1998) *Developing Rural Services to Older People.* Age Concern, London.

Pugh, R. (2000) *Rural Social Work.* Russell House, Lyme Regis.

Pugh, R. (2003) Considering the countryside: is there a case for rural social work?, *British Journal of Social Work*, 33: 67–85.

Pugh, R. (2004a) Responding to racism: delivering local services, in J. Garland and N. Chakraborti, (eds) *Racism, Identity and Community in Rural Britain.* Willan Publishing, Collumpton.

Pugh, R. (2004b) Difference and discrimination in rural areas, *Rural Social Work*, 9(2).

Pugh, R. and Richards, M (1996) Speaking out: a practical approach to empowerment, *Practice*, 8(2): 35–44.

Rickford, F. (1996) Country myths, *Community Care*, 25–31 July: 26.

Rural Development Commission (1998a) *Local Authority Social Services in Rural Areas.* Rural Development Commission, London.

Rural Development Commission (1998b) *The Joint Provision of Services.* Rural Development Commission, London.

Shropshire County Council (2000) *Reflecting Rural Issues: Implications for Performance Management.* Discussion Paper.

Shropshire Regeneration Partnership (1998) *Fairer Funding for Shropshire Public Services.* Shropshire County Council.

Social Services Inspectorate (1998a) *Inspection of Community Care Services in Rural Areas – Dorset County Council.* Department of Health, Bristol.

Social Services Inspectorate (1998b) *Inspection of Community Care Services in Rural Areas – Wiltshire County Council.* Department of Health, Bristol.

Social Services Inspectorate (1998c) *Inspection of Community Care Services for Black and Ethnic Minority Older People.* Department of Health, Bristol.

Social Services Inspectorate (1999) *Care in the Country – Inspection of Community Care Services in Rural Areas.* Department of Health, London.

Spilsbury, M. and Lloyd, N. (1998) *1997 Survey of Rural Services – A Report to the Rural Development Commission.* Rural Development Commission, London.

Stephens, S. (2001) *Challenging Inclusion – Childcare: The Way Forward.* Suffolk ACRE, Ipswich.

University of York (1998) *Population Distribution and Sparsity: Effects on Personal Social Services.* Centre for Health Economics, York.

Watt, I. (1999) Access to care in J. Cox and I. Mungall (eds) *Rural Health Care*, Radcliffe Medical Press, Oxon, pp. 105–15.

White, C. (2001) *Who Gets What, Where and Why?* Institute of Rural Health, Gregynog.

Williams, C. (1997) 'Colour in the pictures': a Welsh Guyanese childhood, *Planet*, 125: 25–30.

Wilson, M (2001) *Changing for the Future – Social Work Services for the 21st Century.* www.scotland.gov.uk/library3/social/tlr-05.asp.

PART 2

Partnership in action: examples from practice

7
Working with Gypsy Travellers: a partnership approach

Angela Roberts

This chapter will:

- Explore the origins of Gypsy Travellers.
- Assess the impact of the legal system upon Gypsy Travellers.
- Discuss the cultural identity of this community.
- Identify one project and its multi-agency approach to addressing the health needs and problems of access to services for this socially excluded group.

Throughout this chapter I will identify the theories of origin purported by the many gypsiologists who have studied groups of Gypsies and Travellers throughout the centuries and across the nations. In order to explicate the problems faced by these much-maligned groups of people, I will look at some of the attitudes and stereotypes underpinning the legal reform used to assimilate or exclude Gypsy Travellers. Readers will begin to understand the impact of history, prejudice and politics on their culture, social well-being and health.

A multi-agency approach to assisting this group to access appropriate primary and secondary health care will be described and proposed as one model which may create good partnership working and good practice.

The origins of Gypsy Travellers

Wibberley (1986) defined travellers as a nomadic people who sold the products of seasonal work. Other contemporary definitions allude to the ethnicity of those descendants of Irish Travellers and Romanies who continue to live by the cultural norms of that society (Okely 1983). Many generalizations are available about the origins of Gypsy Travellers; some lead from a need to romanticize this group and this is exemplified in songs about 'raggle-taggle' gypsies and the freedom of roaming. Additionally, there are stories about those who can cast curses, read the future from crystal balls and predict life chances and happenings from a palm reading or with tarot cards, and it is true that many Gypsies previously made their living from such pursuits. In order to hold such abilities there is a need to look the part, hence the image conjured up is one of a man with swarthy good looks, slick black hair and a brightly-coloured neckerchief. The women in this myth are good-looking, slim, flamboyant, dark-skinned and surrounded by children. For many Gypsy Travellers this is only the stuff of legend and story telling, since a good number of Gypsies and Travellers are fair skinned and fair or red haired. In my working life with Gypsy Travellers I have only seen one highly-coloured neckerchief amongst the denim jeans.

There are many groups who refer to themselves as Gypsy Travellers and these include Eastern European and Mediterranean Gypsies and Roma, English Gypsies said to be of Roma origin, Scottish, Welsh and Irish Travellers; and New Age Travellers. For the purpose of this chapter, I will not address the issues surrounding New Age Travellers as these differ vastly to the other groups.

It is said that Gypsies living in Britain can be traced back to the sixteenth century. There are historical accounts of these first recordings of Gypsies being mistaken for and named as Egyptians. Okely (1983) gives a good account of the many and varied categories and representations that she found in her social anthropological study of 'The Traveller Gypsies'. In the study she describes the plethora of explanations of the component groups, their ascendancy, their Romanic and secret languages and the differences and similarities between the hundred or so groups of nomadic peoples across the world. Theories include one of Indian descent, which was first postulated in the nineteenth century (Smith 1880, as cited by Okely 1983). There is evidence to suggest that many Indian entertainers and craftsmen moved continents to escape slavery and became the first recorded nomads to be known as Gypsies, or more correctly Roma, initially inhabiting what is now modern Greece and Turkey (Kenrick 1998).

There are nomadic groups of 'Gypsies' found across Europe and these are categorized according to ethnic grouping in Table 7.1. These groups, while retaining their own identities and having distinctly different histories and life experiences, nevertheless share similar values, culture and traditional lifestyles including that of nomadism (either throughout their lives or at intervals until old age makes travelling prohibitive).

Table 7.1 Ethnic groupings of gypsies across Europe – reproduced from Citizens Information Base 24 September 1999

England, Ireland, Scotland, Norway, Sweden	Spain	France	Portugal	Italy	Netherlands	Eastern Europe, European Union	Germany
Gypsies Travellers	Gitanos	Manush and Tsignes	Ciganos	Zingari	Woonwagenbewoners	Roma	Sinti

The actual number of Gypsy Travellers in the UK is unknown. Estimates have been made of the broader definition of amounts of travelling peoples including English, Welsh and Scottish Gypsies, Irish travellers, new/new age travellers, Roma, fairground travellers and boat dwellers (bargees). These estimates vary, around 2–300,000 (Morris 1996). In some rural parts of the UK, Gypsies and Travellers make up the largest ethnic minority in the region.

Historically there has been legislation dating back to the sixteenth century that outlawed gypsies and travellers. Initially much confusion arose from the descriptions given of early nomadic peoples in this country and it was generally thought that their dark skin was due to them originating from Egypt. Early laws passed referred to them as 'outlandish people calling themselves Egyptians', and during the reign of Philip and Mary (1553–58) the law made it a felony punishable by death to reside in this country as an Egyptian, unless you agreed to enter into service and give up the travelling lifestyle (Morris 1996). Effectively many of these laws aimed to make the travelling lifestyle illegal. An example of this type of legislation is the Housing of the Working Classes Act 1885, which placed controls on 'nuisances in tents and vans' (Hawes and Perez 1996).

Romany (Gypsy) history

It is thought that the origins of the Romany Gypsy lie in India where as nomads they were entertainers and craftsmen and there is historical evidence to suggest that as early as AD 855 persecutions began in Syria. Movement of Roma probably began around the thirteenth century when recordings took place of Romany shoemakers residing in Greece. Roma arrived in Europe in 1445. Twelve thousand people who 'looked like Egyptians', were transported from Bulgaria for slave labour and in 1471 the first anti-Gypsy law was passed in Lucerne Switzerland (Patrin Timeline, Kenrick 1998).

Kenrick (1998) states that throughout the sixteenth century further anti-Gypsy laws were passed across Europe including in Germany, Spain and Italy. Throughout medieval times Roma Gypsies were thought to be traitors to Christianity and were accused of witchcraft, child kidnapping and banditry. The first recordings of Gypsies in the UK are in Scotland in 1505 – this group are thought to have travelled from Spain – the first recording of Gypsies in Wales is in 1579. During the sixteenth century there are numerous recordings of Gypsies being banished and deported from many European states and countries. Assisting with transportation into England was punishable by a severe fine for the transporters, usually a ship's owner or captain, and death by hanging for the Gypsy passenger. In 1541 Scotland passed its first anti-Gypsy law. Around the same time Edward VI of England introduced branding and enslavement for Gypsies. In 1560 the Swedish Lutheran Church issued an edict to its priests forbidding the christening of Gypsy children or Christian burial of their dead. Later that century, Spain forbade the wearing of distinctive Gitanos dress, punished those who travelled in groups of more than two, condemning them to a period of up to 18 years in the galleys and later altered legislation to death for all nomads. Similar legislation existed in England at the same time. In the early seventeenth century, Spanish Gitanos were forbidden to trade in horses and vigilante groups were permitted by law to pursue Gitanos. Sweden introduced harsh anti-Gypsy laws in 1637 and any Gypsy men not complying with expulsion orders were to hang (Kenrick 1998).

Throughout Europe, between 1600 and 1800, anti-Gypsy laws were beginning to take a hold. Indeed punishment for pursuing a nomadic lifestyle and speaking Romany included: flogging, branding, banishment, deportation, shooting, mutilation, forced labour, whipping and hanging. In Germany, Gypsy children under the age of ten could even be forcibly removed from their families to be brought up by Christian families. During the eighteenth century authorities throughout Europe made further attempts to deal with Gypsies. These included forced public work, incarceration in poor houses, being pressed into service or into factory work, sentencing to the galleys and many other attempts at banishment, reform or assimilation.

It is apparent that Gypsy history is one of constant prejudice, hatred and harass-ment. Hunted down like animals, prohibited from speaking their own language, con-stantly moved on or incarcerated, Gypsies have a historical right to be wary of Gajos or Georgios (the name given to non-Gypsies) who clearly do not believe that being a nomadic Gypsy is a legitimate way of life.

Effects of recent legislation

In 1960 the Caravan Site and Control of Development Act effectively disbarred willing private landowners from providing temporary or permanent sites. This was followed by the 1968 Caravan Sites Act, which placed a duty on local authorities in England and Wales to provide static sites for Gypsies. This law was often not enacted and faced enormous opposition from the general public. The main impact of these laws is twofold; firstly, they send clear messages that a nomadic lifestyle is not accept-able in the UK and, secondly, they attempt to assimilate nomadic peoples into the settled population by making travelling illegal and enforcing a working life.

In addition, legislation further establishes static sites provision, sending messages to local authorities that Gypsy Travellers should be contained. Latest legislation, under the jurisdiction of the Criminal Public Order Act in 1994 initiated by a con-servative government, seemingly exorcised by the need to contain 'raves' and large groupings of New Age travellers, had the effect of removing the duty to provide sites and gave police forces increased powers of eviction. Despite the fact that this law was unpopular and contested by both the Country Landowners Association and the Association of Chief Police Officers it has been used repeatedly to prevent unauthor-ized camping by Gypsy Travellers. We can see from the aforementioned examples that the law has been used to assimilate this minority group and curtail the nomadic lifestyle.

Local authorities have responded to legal requirements by closing off many traditional stopping places and green lane camping areas and providing legal encampments on council owned and managed sites instead. In doing so, they have incited local prejudice. Those country landowners who would willingly have allowed small Gypsy Traveller encampments on their land have been prohibited from doing so, and since Gypsies were first recorded in Britain, they have been moved on without stopping rights or provision.

More recently the Race Relations Amendment Act 2000 gave Gypsies and Irish Travellers ethnic status. This means that they have the entitlements of nomenclature as shown in capitalization of the first letters of Gypsy and Traveller and are afforded the protection of the law, in the same way as other ethnic minorities. This law is often broken. How many times have you seen signs saying 'Travelling people are not welcome here'? Are we shocked by those words and how would it be if the same signs read 'Blacks not welcome here' or 'Jews not welcome here'? *The Traveller Times* recently (2004) reported an incident where a well-known motorway fast food chain refused entry to their restaurant for a small family of Travellers. A public apology was forthcoming but is this enough to stop this overt racial discrimination?

How does the Human Rights Act 1998 impact upon Gypsy Travellers? The two articles of the European Convention on Human Rights, enacted in the UK in 2000, which relate to the plight of Gypsy Travellers, are Article 8 and 14 (see Table 7.2).

The latter requirements of Article 8, referred to in Table 7.2 are limitations to Article 8.1 seen in Article 8.2. In respect of planning application from Gypsy Travellers wishing to reside on their own land this set of laws clearly expects that Town Councils should take the view that unless Article 8.2 is applicable then the requirements of Article 8.1 are clearly enactable. In respect of Article 14, there have been occasions when the democratic suppositions of the Article which particularly relate to Gypsies and Travellers have worked both for and against those people it was designed to assist. The main benefits derived have been that it has at least shown that the court is willing to consider complaints on an individual basis and, furthermore, each case heard has included comment relating to the UK governments' failure to deliver an international commitment towards minority groups.

In relation to the Criminal Justice and Public Order Act 1994, Cemlyn (1997) found that attitudes to Travellers and Gypsies varied across local authority and social services interfaces. Regarding the eviction of Gypsies and Travellers, her sample suggested that only 8.8 per cent of social service departments had corporate policies

Table 7.2 The European Human Rights Act 1998 as it applies to Gypsy Travellers

Article	Application to Gypsy Travellers
Article 8 refers to the right to respect for private and family life, home and correspondence.	Article 8 should, therefore, enable Gypsy Travellers to determine their own family way of life, in so far as it does not cause a problem of national security, public safety, economic well-being or disorder and crime to others.
Article 14 prohibits discrimination on any ground such as sex, race, colour, language, religion, opinion, national or social origin, association with a national minority, property, birth or other status.	Article 14 has limitations in that it does not apply to indirect discrimination and where discrimination occurs between private individuals and organizations. In such cases, the complainants must seek redress through pre-existing Acts of Parliament, such as the British Race Relation Act 1976.

wherein the police limited their use of the Act. Cemlyn was attempting to explore the interaction between the Children Act and the Criminal Justice and Public Order Act (CJPOA) and determined that the CJPOA had a low profile in the documents she analysed. The laws that continue to criminalize a Traveller lifestyle are in the majority and Acton (2000) notes that there has been no move to repeal the anti-Gypsy sections of the 1994 Criminal Justices Act. He further contends that while successive governments have promised to give administrative guidance to avoid the unnecessary evictions carried out under the auspices of this Act, this is no substitute for human rights.

This section has examined the laws relating to and acting to criminalize a Gypsy Traveller traditional way of life. The consequences of the enactment of these laws can be seen to impact on the life chances of Gypsy Travellers. Laws of this nature criminalize innocent children and their families. The impact on health and social inclusion can be devastating as Gypsy Travellers are either assimilated into the dominant culture or forced to travel continuously. This will impact on literacy and education, development and behaviour and disable Gypsy Travellers from obtaining continuous and appropriate health and social care. Demonizing this section of society increases the prejudice and harassment suffered by many Gypsy Travellers on a daily basis. Perhaps more fundamentally a review of service provision for Gypsies and Travellers undertaken by the National Assembly for Wales in 2003 drew attention to the impact of policy in its failure to provide adequate stopping places. This review quotes from the advisory committee of the European Union's Framework Convention for the Protection of National Minorities and states that, 'The Advisory Committee notes with concern the lack of adequate stopping sites for Roma/Gypsies and Travellers . . . and the effect this has on their ability to preserve the essential elements of their identity, of which travelling is an important element' (p. 50).

The cultural identity of the Gypsy Traveller communities

Gypsy Travellers are not a homogenous sector of society, however, despite their diverse origins they do all have similarities in culture, many of which are defined by the nature of living a nomadic lifestyle. There are still a small number of Gypsies living in the UK who have their roots in their Romany origins. These include: the Kale in Wales, the Romanicals in England, the Minceirs of Ireland, and the Nawkens of Scotland. In recent times these numbers have increased as Gypsies have migrated from Eastern Europe (Acton 2000). Okely (1983), among others, defines their culture as one based on economic need and its evolution. Traditionally, Gypsy Travellers were horse traders, musicians, sellers of homemade crafts and seasonal labourers who followed seasonal agricultural work around defined routes across the UK. More commonly these days, scrap metal dealing, tarmacking, roofing, domestic service trading, tree felling and landscape gardening have filled the gap left by the decline of seasonal picking and agricultural work. Travellers of Irish origin more commonly were tinsmiths, as were their Scottish counterparts, and were known as Tinkers or Tinklers. A small number of Gypsies follow a more settled life, which has included full time long-term education and a work life similar to others. Often these Travellers do not admit to their origins and roots for fear of prejudice.

My daughter works in a good position in the bank, but she dare not ever own up to being a Gypsy. Some days she comes home to me and says, 'They're at it again, calling us fit to burn.'

Scottish Traveller (as related to the author)

Gypsy Travellers are adept at modernizing their traditional pursuits while retaining a self-employed independence (Okely 1983). Many Gypsy Travellers remain illiterate, dismissing formal schooling as irrelevant to their way of life. This, however, does not make them ignorant of the world or their local community. Attempts to assimilate Gypsy Travellers into the dominant society continue to fail and I list a number of reasons for this:

- Gypsy Travellers do not wish to live in a house all their lives. Those who do may continue to treat the house as though it were a caravan, spending a good deal of time out visiting kin on legal or transient sites.
- Formal education has little to offer a traditional nomadic lifestyle.
- All housing has internal bathrooms and toilets and for those Gypsy Travellers who continue to observe the notions of 'mochadi' or cleanliness it is an anathema to them to have these indoor facilities integral to living, cooking and sleeping areas.

It is impossible to do justice to an explanation of the cultural difference in this chapter. However, I will attempt to illustrate some cultural differences, which colour the way that many (but not all) groups of Gypsy Travellers view the world. Gypsy culture is largely governed by superstition. Some typical superstitions held by Gypsies are listed in Box 7.1.

Box 7.1 Some examples of Gypsy superstitions

- To speak of the Devil will make him appear.
- If a daddy long legs walks over you, you will have new clothes.
- A baby born at full moon will be lucky but if born at midnight before the Sabbath, it will be under a curse.
- An itching of the right eye means sadness.

(Superstitions, Jarman and Jarman 1991)

I asked a number of Irish Travellers if these sayings had any meaning for them and they agreed that, while not identical, some of these myths exist in similar forms in their culture as well as in the Welsh Romany. However, it is important to note that most Irish Travellers whether living in Ireland or Britain are Catholic (Kenrick 1998).

Cultural beliefs, whether they arise from superstition or religion, determine much of the Gypsy way of life. Marime or Makadi (Mochadi), for example, is the Romany Gypsy hygiene code requiring that different wash-bowls are used for clothes, dishes, the body, and for cleaning the home. The more common observance in the Irish Traveller community is two bowls, one for the dishes and one for cleaning. Even in a modern caravan with toilet facilities these remain unused and outside facilities are required. There is debate about the extent to which Mochadi is understood or practised by modern-day British Gypsies and whether this continues to further extend to traditional beliefs about being unclean around menstruation and childbirth.

Additionally, beliefs about death and the ghost of the deceased have resulted in the burning of all belongings including the caravan of a Gypsy elder. While still clearly understood by the descendants, this seems to have varying degrees of observance. Some workers with Travellers report that following a death it is likely that Gypsy Travellers will move on, as they do not constantly wish to be reminded of the deceased (Derbyshire Gypsy Liaison Group 2004). This may be due to a fear of coming into contact with a spirit of a dead person. Traditionally two or three people kept vigil with the body of the deceased, for fear of a possible confrontation with the spirit (Jarman and Jarman 1991). This ritual may be further extended to include abstinence from a dead relative's favourite food or drink for many years as the belief was held that this might be perceived by the spirit as an invitation to join in.

Romany and Irish travellers will travel across the width and breadth of the country to visit a sick relative or good friend. This is seen as a mark of respect, and a large number of visitors in the vicinity of a very ill person will be the measure of the esteem in which the person is held. This is carried through to the funeral, which is inevitably a huge affair with a large following and which lasts many days and nights.

Traditionally, Romany Gypsies and Irish and Scottish Travellers are bashful of sex education, sexuality, pregnancy and childbirth and the needs of young children are the concern of the women only. Indeed fathers do not usually stay with their wives during childbirth – it is more likely that the maternal grandmother will attend the birth or possibly an older sister who herself has had children (Derby Gypsy Liaison Group 2003).

What remains apparent is that the majority of Gypsy Travellers' caravans gleam and sparkle and Gypsy Traveller women are taught to clean relentlessly from a very early age. These hygiene practices do not always translate into a clean external environment and again the extent of cleanliness varies from the caravan, its facilities and the defined pitch. Many sites have immaculate well hosed down pitches smelling strongly of bleach and disinfectant but the boundaries may be littered with rubbish. Many Gypsy Travellers believe in the concepts of purity and impurity and Vernon (1994) relates these to notions of good and bad fortune. This tends to impact upon health and illness behaviour, as can be seen by the following transcript from a conversation I had with a female Irish Traveller:

Me: How is your grandson? I believe he had a serious accident in Ireland.
Traveller: It is a miracle, he was run down by a lorry on the road by the site and they thought he was dead. He was spared and it's thanks be to God.

A multi-agency approach to addressing the health needs and problems of access

A recent survey of Travellers' views was undertaken in Scotland and this identified five key areas of concern raised by Travellers with various organizations. These are:

1. Access to housing and sites
2. Access to education
3. Legal advice and its charges
4. Access on health care
5. Advice on benefit and debts

The Wrexham Multi-agency Forum has existed in Wrexham in North Wales for some years. Its membership has functioned and changed and for a period of time its existence was contentious resulting in it being temporarily disbanded. Since 1999, however, the Multi-agency Forum has gained in representation, membership, strength and purpose and currently meets at two monthly intervals with representation from:

- Social Services (a Senior Manager acts as Chair)
- Health Services
- Midwifery Services
- Domestic Violence Officer (Police Force)
- Commission for Racial Equality
- Police Diversity Officer
- Site Management Team
- Housing Officer
- Voluntary Services including Home Care Services
- Traveller Education Service
- Youth Offending Team
- Youth Work Service
- Community Housing Association
- General Practice
- Catholic Traveller Education Forum
- Roman Catholic Church
- Traveller representatives

In the early stages of the development of this team the emphasis was on 'how best can we work together', developing terms of reference for the group, and identifying the skills, knowledge and expertise held within this diverse gathering of professionals and lay interested parties. As the group grew there was a recognition that individuals were working independently of each other, attempting to address many of the same themes that were identified by Scottish Travellers as important issues in their lives. The Wrexham Forum continued the attempt to address the needs of the local Traveller population through an inter-agency model with varying degrees of success until 2001.

It should be noted that a number of areas across the UK have operated inter-agency groups with the aim of targeting this socially excluded sector of society, most notably Pavee Point Northern Ireland. In addition, Streetly (1987) gives a good account of equal access for health care for Travellers, with services supported by representation from the Department of Education, Health and Social Services and other interested parties in Kent.

In 2001 the Welsh Assembly Government announced the availability of funding to redress inequalities in health in the Gypsy population. Some of this funding was targeted at reducing chronic disease and increasing access to health care. For some years, readdressing these inequalities in health has been a priority for health policy development across Wales. A number of strategic and policy documents, including 'Better Health Better Wales' (Welsh Assembly Government 1998) and 'Better Wales/ Plan for Wales' (Welsh Assembly Government 2001) have paved the way for the development of the Inequalities in Health Funded Projects. Particular attention was given in those documents to raising awareness of how cultural issues impact upon service delivery. In 2002 the Chief Medical Officer for Wales noted in his report the disproportionate impact of inequality in health on marginalized groups including Travellers. Similarly, England, Scotland and Northern Ireland documents have high-lighted the plight of Gypsies and Travellers in the UK. A successful bid to the Inequal-ities in Health Fund in Wales resulted in refocusing the ability to deliver an effective multi-agency service, in addition to providing an on-site health service to the Traveller community (Roberts *et al.* 2004).

The project: coronary heart disease and Gypsy/Travellers

The Wales Inequalities in Health Fund was designed in part to implement the National Assembly for Wales Service Framework, 'Tackling Coronary Heart Disease in Wales: Implementing through Evidence' (DoH 2001). One evidence-based standard from the plan states that:

> Health Authorities through their local groups and with local authorities in partner-ship through local health alliances should develop and monitor evidence based programmes to address tobacco use, diet and physical activity targeted at the most disadvantaged communities in Wales.
>
> (p. 23)

One of the requirements of the fund was that the responses made should be multi-agency in origin. A project steering group was formed from the existing Multi-agency Traveller Forum. Initial membership of the steering group has changed and now includes a Project Health Worker, a full-time researcher to evaluate the impact of the project, a Professor of General Practice in North Wales who is the research supervisor, myself as Project Lead and the Chair of the Multi-Agency Traveller Forum. This group steers the direction of the project ensuring that it will deliver upon its stated aims and objectives.

The major aims of the project are to describe the coronary health status and to redress the inequality of access to health care experienced by the traveller population locally. At the present time the project is well underway and Figure 7.1 identifies the process as a continuous cycle.

As indicated in Figure 7.1, at all stages of development, the project has needed to take account of new challenges, changing needs, differing perspectives and overlapping areas of responsibility. The funding allowed for the purchase of a refitted motorized caravan, which enabled service delivery on site. Additionally, the Traveller community perceive the mobile caravan to be a private space, within which discussions concerning culturally difficult issues can be raised. These have included sexual

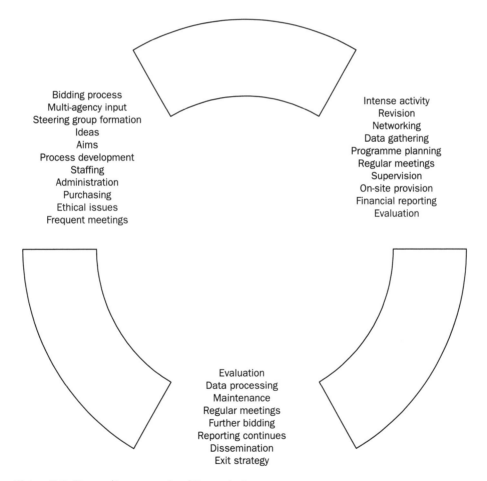

Bidding process
Multi-agency input
Steering group formation
Ideas
Aims
Process development
Staffing
Administration
Purchasing
Ethical issues
Frequent meetings

Intense activity
Revision
Networking
Data gathering
Programme planning
Regular meetings
Supervision
On-site provision
Financial reporting
Evaluation

Evaluation
Data processing
Maintenance
Regular meetings
Further bidding
Reporting continues
Dissemination
Exit strategy

Figure 7.1 The continuous cycle of the project

health topics, pregnancy, informal counselling, domestic violence and mental health worries.

The mobile unit has provided a focus for delivery of health and social welfare information and advice. The members of the Multi-agency Forum can deliver their own service, if required, from this vehicle by a collaboration partnership with the Project Health Worker. Appropriate triage for medication advice, referral, liaison and treatment is available from the mobile unit, which visits the site three days a week. Settled Travellers can also access this facility or arrange home or clinic visits via this facility. The Multi-agency Forum is the inner core and building block of this project and this partnership way of working is illustrated in Figure 7.2.

The project views the Multi-agency Forum as an enabling, physically and emotionally supportive agency, which hosts a number of developments and approaches to the delivery of health and social care services. This form of inter-agency liaison is said to be vital and is highlighted in the work of Lawrie (1983) and Rose (1993). It enables service delivery and this project would echo those authors' conclusions. To date, the project's early findings have indicated value found in shared alliances between agencies, dissemination of good practice between organizations and provision of an outreach service, which provides for the cultural differences of Gypsy Travellers and respects their right to adopt a nomadic or semi-nomadic lifestyle while retaining the ability to access services. In common with Cemlyn (1995), we take the view that best practice is illustrated through service development, which includes mainstream development, encouraging 'flexible agendas; creative working areas across geographical departmental, professional and agency boundaries' (p. 288).

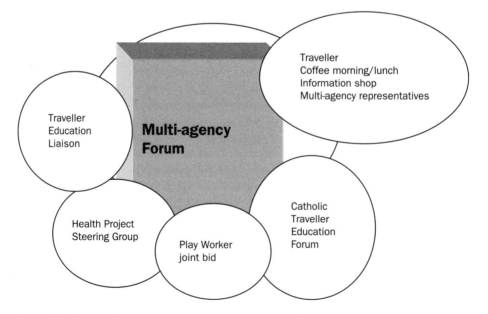

Figure 7.2 Partnership way of working, with multi-agency forum at the central core

Underpinning a good deal of the social exclusion that characterizes the life of Gypsy Travellers is the problem of discrimination. Across the UK there is documented evidence that Gypsy Travellers are subjected to widespread prejudice and discrimination (Cleemput 2000). Anecdotal accounts are regularly reported in the *Traveller Times*, a magazine for travellers edited by the Rural Media Company, and there are examples of widespread and vehement local opposition to the establishment of sites and stopping places (DoE 1982). Some authors take the view that conflict exists between travellers and the settled society because of a lack of recognition of the nomadic way of life (Friends, Families and Travellers 2000). Ethnocentrism in the service delivery population is described by Smaje (1995) as resulting from an assumption formed on the basis of the majority example, which displays attitudes of prejudice and bias towards the minority needs of these groups. Further anecdotal evidence of discrimination is illustrated in the Scottish Survey of Travellers' Views (Lomax *et al.* 2000) and includes from a school child an account of bullying and children advising each other 'not to talk to the tink' (6.2). Further evidence from the report suggests that medical staff 'expected travellers to be dirty and treated them differently' (6.9).

The Multi-agency Forum creates opportunities for joint training aimed at dispelling stereotypes and encouraging cultural understanding. Good practice can be disseminated through the agencies' representatives to their fellow workers and the wider community. A recent report (Review of Service Provision for Gypsies and Travellers, National Assembly for Wales 2003) suggests that stereotypes around what is a 'real Gypsy' are misleading and used as an excuse to follow up with discriminatory comments. Multi-agency groups need to include representation from the Commission for Racial Equality to ensure that their membership challenges discrimination and prejudice at every level in the organization they represent. Groups should also include representation from the Gypsy Traveller community to offer guidance when developing service provision.

An English survey by Hussey (1989) demonstrated a lack of inter-service collaboration in health care, while Cemlyn (1995) comments upon the lack of specific policies and practices in social services departments reacting to Travellers at times when they become more vulnerable through eviction. Morris and Clements (2001) conclude that the extent of unmet need for services provided by social services departments (children's or community care services) is unknown. Multi-agency partnerships, therefore, need to include representation from these services.

Conclusion

In this chapter I have illustrated the background tensions, cultural differences, legal interpretations and nomadic lifestyle influences that impact upon the ability of Gypsy Travellers to access health and social care services. Legislative changes are explained to demonstrate the interface issues which surround and compound the difficulties faced by this disadvantaged and hard to reach group. Cultural examples are also offered which have implications for the delivery of services, and the need to gain the trust of individual Gypsies and Travellers becomes apparent.

An example of a multi-agency approach is offered with an emphasis on the collective experience, expertise and partnership working capability. Shared experience, including that of service users themselves, is essential to prevent discriminatory practice. Anti-discriminatory training is crucial for service providers in these partnerships. I am aware of many other good models across the UK and would point the reader towards national associations, which seek to share good practice throughout their membership. The National Association for Health Workers for Travellers is a good starting point as is Pavee Point in Dublin.

Questions for further discussion

1. What problems might a worker face when advocating on behalf of Gypsy Travellers and how might these be addressed?
2. What considerations might your organization need to make before planning or carrying out care for Gypsy Travellers?
3. Prior to engaging in the care of a Gypsy or Traveller who is in need of your service, what should you learn about that individual and what skills will be required?

References

Acton, T.A. (2000) *Patrin, The Revival of Romani Lobbying in Great Britain.* The Patrin Web Journal. www.geocities.com/Paris/5121/lobbying-gb-htm.

Cemlyn, S. (1995) Traveller Children and the State: Welfare or Neglect? *Child Abuse Review* 4: 278–90.

Cemlyn, S. (1997) *Policy and Provision by Social Services for Traveller Children and Families.* A Research Study. Nuffield Foundation.

Cleemput, C. (2000) Health care needs of Travellers, *Archives of Disease in Childhood*, 82(1).

Commission for Racial Equality (2000) *Strengthening the Race Relations Act.* CRE, London.

Criminal Justice and Public Order Act (1994) Home Office, London.

Department of the Environment (1982) Management of Local Authority Gypsy sites: DOE/Welsh Office.

Derby Gypsy Liaison Group (2004) Ernest Bailey Community Centre, Matlock, DE4 3FE.

Derbyshire Gypsy Liaison Group (2003) A Better Road, Ernest Bailey Community Centre, New St, Matlock, DEA 3FE.

DoH (2001) Coronary Heart Disease National Service Framework Implementation Plan For Wales: Tackling Coronary Heart Disease in Wales: Implementing through Evidence. National Assembly, Wales.

Friends, Families and Travellers (2000) Community Base, 113 Queens Road, Brighton, BN1 3XG.

Hawes, D. and Perez, B. (1996) *The Gypsy and the State: The Ethnic Cleansing of British Society.* The Policy Press, Bristol.

Hussey, R. (1989) Equal opportunities for Gypsies, *Public Health*, 103: 79.

Jarman, A.O.H. and Jarman, E. (1991) *The Welsh Gypsies; Children of Abram Wood.* Cardiff University Press, Cardiff.

Kenrick, D. (1998) *Patrin Web Journal*, Timeline of Romani (Gypsy) History. www.geocities.com/Paris/timeline.htm.

Lawrie, B (1983) Travelling families in East London – adapting health visiting methods to a minority group, *Health Visitor*, 56: 26–8.

Lomax, D., Lancaster, S. and Gray, P. (2000) Moving on: A survey of Travellers' views. The Scottish Executive Central Research Unit. http://www.scotland.gov.uk/cru/kd01/blue/moving-01.pdf.

Morris, R. (1996) *Factsheet: Travelling People in the United Kingdom*. Traveller Law Research Unit, Cardiff Law School.

Morris, R. and Clements, L. (2001) *Disability, Social Care, Health and Travelling People*. Traveller Law Research Unit, Cardiff Law School (not cited in text).

National Assembly for Wales (2003) *Review of Service Provision for Gypsy Travellers*.

Okely, J. (1983) *The Traveller-Gypsies*. Cambridge University Press, Cambridge.

Pavee Point Travellers Centre. Dublin: Pavee Point.

Rose, V. (1993) On the Road, *Nursing Times*, 89: 33–1.

Roberts, A., Lewis, H., Degale, J. and Wilkinon, C. (2003–4) *Coronary Heart Disease and Gypsy/Travellers Redressing the balance*. Annual Report 2003–2004 Welsh Assembly Government IIH Fund.

Smaje, C. (1995) *Health, Race and Ethnicity*. King's Fund Institute, London.

Streetly, A. (1987) Health care for Travellers: one year's experience. *British Medical Journal*, 294: 492–4.

The Travellers Times (2004) Issue 20, Summer. The Rural Media Company, Hereford.

Vernon, D. (1994) The Health of Traveller-Gypsies. *British Journal of Nursing*, 3(18): 969–72.

Welsh Assembly Government (1998) Better Health Better Wales.

Welsh Assembly Government (2001) Better Wales/Plan for Wales.

Wibberley, G. (1986) *A Report on the Analysis of Response to Consultation on the Operation of The Caravan Sites Act* (1968) London: DoE www scotland.gov.uk/kd01/blue/moving-10.htm-30k.

8

Not behind closed doors: working in partnership against domestic violence

Liz Blyth

This chapter will:

- Discuss the nature and extent of domestic violence and the implications for service providers.
- Explore the context of multi-agency work on domestic violence and explain why effective collaboration and co-ordination is important.
- Examine some of the challenges, obstacles and opportunities created by working in partnership across the boundaries of statutory, voluntary and community organizations.
- Draw on research and experience of multi-agency partnership work on domestic violence to provide examples of good practice.

This chapter examines some of the issues, obstacles and opportunities created by working in partnership to challenge domestic violence. It is based on research carried out for a Master's dissertation, as well as practical experience of working in a multi-agency context. Until recently the author worked as Domestic Violence Co-ordinator in Coventry, a post based in the local authority and working with a multi-agency partnership of 20 organizations to improve responses to domestic violence in the city. The Coventry experience underlined the importance of working in partnership when seeking to challenge complex societal problems such as abuse. Domestic violence is a complex issue, which creates complex problems for individuals, service providers and communities. No single agency is able to successfully respond to this complexity alone and therefore real 'joined-up' working between the statutory, voluntary and community sectors is essential. The chapter explores some of the key issues for partnership work on domestic violence, using practical examples from the Coventry Domestic Violence Partnership to illustrate that analysis.

Domestic violence: the social context

In Britain, over the last decade, there has been a significant societal shift in the public perception of domestic violence as a private, family matter to be excused, ignored, dismissed or even ridiculed. The view that what goes on behind closed doors is somehow outside the usual boundaries of acceptable behaviour, and indeed beyond the scope of legal jurisdiction, is finally being challenged. Domestic violence is the subject of increasing public concern and condemnation and there is a much greater understanding of the nature of abuse and its serious, long-lasting consequences.

This increased level of awareness is largely due to the determined efforts of refuges (safe houses) and other women's organizations that have forced the issue of domestic violence from the margins to the mainstream. Since the first refuges were set up in the 1970s, the Women's Aid Federation of England (WAFE) has developed a network of over 300 projects providing helpline, drop-in and outreach services as well as 500 refuge houses across England (WAFE, 2004). Working alongside academics and practitioners, Women's Aid has been the key driver in ensuring increased co-ordination through multi-agency fora, as well as successfully lobbying for a number of significant changes to legislation in order to protect women and children and bring perpetrators to justice. Public awareness has also increased as women have found the courage to tell their stories, celebrities have spoken out about their personal experiences, and cinema, TV 'soaps' and awareness campaigns have explored the issue of domestic violence and the impact on family lives.

The increased profile has, in turn, led to policy responses at local and national levels. During the 1990s, statutory bodies, particularly the police and local authorities, showed a marked improvement in their response to domestic violence with new guidance and legislation. This included inter-agency guidance from the Home Office in 1995 and 2000, new legislation in the 1996 Family Law Act, and 'Living Without Fear', a cross-departmental strategy document from government (Women's Unit 1999). In 2003 the new Domestic Violence, Crime and Victims Bill was announced and is intended to improve the protection given to those experiencing domestic violence (UK Parliament 2003). There has finally been a recognition that the responsibility for supporting women and children experiencing domestic violence cannot be left to the voluntary sector alone. However, the current position remains one of inconsistent and under-resourced responses, depending much on the profile of domestic violence in a particular local authority area and on the awareness and commitment of individuals. Many refuges and voluntary sector projects struggle to access mainstream funding despite increased awareness by statutory agencies of the nature and extent of domestic violence and its impact on core statutory duties, such as child protection or mental health service provision.

Domestic violence: the nature and extent of abuse

Domestic violence is the everyday life experience of many thousands of women and children. According to the British Crime Survey domestic violence accounts for one quarter of all violent crime (Women's Unit 1999). Research by Professor Betsy Stanko in October 2000 found that in the UK the police received a call for help every

60 seconds and that an incident of domestic violence took place every six to twenty seconds (Stanko 2000). According to the Home Office, over half of all female homicide victims in England and Wales are killed by a current or former partner and approximately one woman dies every three days as a result of domestic violence (Home Office 2000). In 2001/02 Women's Aid supported over 140,000 women and 114,000 children with more than 40,000 staying in their refuges (WAFE 2004).

Research and practical experience have shown that domestic violence can affect anyone, regardless of gender, ethnicity, race, sexuality, age, marital status, disability or lifestyle. However, the majority of abuse is perpetrated by men against women, usually by a partner or ex-partner. Although men do experience abuse from their female partners, they are less likely to be physically injured, frightened or upset by the experience and less likely to be subjected to a repeat pattern of abuse (Mirrlees-Black 1998). Domestic violence may also be perpetrated by another adult with whom there is a close relationship, for example a brother, son, carer or extended family member. Abuse does also take place in same sex relationships, an area that is only recently beginning to be addressed in service provision and where lesbians and gay men can find their traumatic experiences exacerbated by stereotyping, misunderstanding and homophobia. In terms of the local picture in Coventry, in the year 2000 approximately 95 per cent of incidents reported to the police were perpetrated by men against women and the strategic response in the city reflects this priority.

Domestic violence is a complex issue. It is bound up with society's norms and values, myths and stereotypes, gender roles and relationships. It is linked to identity and autonomy in intimate relationships and the misuse of power and control. The behaviour that constitutes domestic violence is wide ranging. It can include physical assault, sexual abuse, rape, threats and intimidation, humiliation, withholding money, denying physical freedom or medical care, and belittling. In the most extreme forms it leads to homicide (Domestic Violence Data Source 1999). For thousands of women the violence is frequent, repeated and life-threatening. Indeed a key issue for professionals is that domestic violence usually escalates over time and that the risks increase at the point of separation (Home Office 2000). However, the most important point in understanding domestic violence is, as Hester *et al.* (1998) noted, to listen to the accounts of survivors, as only from these can we really begin to understand how domestic violence feels, what it involves and what the implications are.

Domestic violence: the links with other forms of abuse

The links between domestic violence and child abuse are well documented and children living with domestic violence have been found to be at risk of psychological and physical harm (Hester *et al.* 1998; Mullender 1996; Hendessi 1997). In Coventry in 2001 the police recorded 5,500 incidents of domestic violence with over 2,000 children recorded as present at the time the violence took place (Coventry Domestic Violence Partnership 2001). In 2000 Coventry Area Child Protection Committee found that domestic violence had been a feature in 35 per cent of families at a child protection conference in an eighteen-month period. National research has suggested that up to two thirds of children on a child protection register live with domestic violence (Moxon 1999). We also know that recorded incidents are likely to be the tip of the iceberg as many incidents go unreported, unrecorded and are not prosecuted (British Medical Association 1998).

There is also a link between domestic violence and pregnancy, with studies finding that violence begins or escalates during pregnancy (Bewley and Gibbs 2002). Indeed there is evidence that around 30 per cent of domestic violence starts during or just after pregnancy (Lewis 2002). The Confidential Enquiry into Maternal Deaths first raised the impact of domestic violence on pregnant women in its 1994–6 report. This later became the subject of a specific chapter in the report covering 1997–9 when eight deaths were attributed directly to domestic violence (Lewis 2002). The effects of domestic violence during pregnancy have been found to include miscarriage, stillbirth, low birth weight or premature labour, as well as depression, alcohol or drug misuse and suicide (Berenson *et al.* 1994 and Lewis 2001, both cited in Bewley and Gibbs 2002). It could be argued that health care workers are in a unique position to identify and respond to domestic violence. For example, midwives and health visitors usually visit women in their homes a number of times, and have opportunities to build a rapport while assessing their client's health and well-being, as well as being well placed to assess relationship dynamics. Women who experience domestic violence may pay several visits to a General Practitioner, perhaps presenting with depression or repeated injuries. In addition, Accident and Emergency staff come into contact with women in crisis when they have been seriously injured by abuse.

Although there is still a good deal of misunderstanding, reticence, embarrassment or disbelief about domestic violence, there has also been considerable progress in providing the evidence that underpins the case for a better response. This has resulted in the Department of Health, Royal College of Obstetricians and Gynaecologists, Royal College of Midwives, the British Medical Association and other professional bodies issuing guidance and training materials on domestic violence. However, there is still a long way to go before this is matched by consistent responses on the ground; national guidance is important but it has to lead to *local* policies, procedures and most importantly *training* for staff, in order to be truly effective.

In many ways the reluctance of public bodies to consider domestic violence as core business echoes the difficulties faced in the last 20 years in forcing the issue of child abuse out into the open. Families are expected to be places of safety, love and respect and yet in some families trust is betrayed by the closest family members. Generally in society there is a belief that what takes place at home is a family matter, and that it is private business and not for public concern. The challenge for services dealing with the reality of abuse in all its forms is to challenge assumptions about the boundaries of acceptable behaviour and protect adults and children where home is no longer a place of safety.

In Coventry the domestic violence services available in the voluntary sector include a specialist refuge for Asian women and a support service for African-Caribbean women. The Asian women's project developed out of a grassroots response to violence against women and responds to a high number of incidents of abuse by other family members, as well as forced marriage and abduction of young women. These issues present a challenge to statutory and voluntary sector services, which have not yet fully grasped the complex cultural contexts of domestic violence. There has been a great deal of research about domestic violence but most studies have focused on white heterosexual relationships (Hester *et al.* 1998) and most services have developed from this perspective. Women with disabilities may also face additional obstacles in getting the help and support they need, especially if the violence is from their carer. Reporting and escaping violence is difficult enough but many services are simply not sensitive to the needs of individual women. Inadequate interpretation and translation services, poor physical access, lack of cultural understanding or fear of making things worse often compound the physical and emotional isolation women experience when seeking help. The issues faced by Black and minority ethnic women, disabled women, women with drug and alcohol dependencies, and lesbians and gay men, need to be explored by professionals if public services are to be accessible to all and not compound experiences of oppression and abuse.

In summary, there is increased understanding among people working with abuse that where one form of abuse is identified professionals should be looking for other forms; indeed it is important that people do not 'think in boxes' but understand the overlap between different forms of abuse. This is essential not just in understanding the child protection implications in families but also the connection with the abuse of vulnerable adults – an inter-relationship that began to be addressed in the Department of Health 'No Secrets' guidance on adult abuse (Department of Health 2000).

It is perhaps important to note that domestic violence also challenges professionals on a personal level, because the patterns of abuse and examples of abusive behaviour, particularly controlling, manipulative and undermining behaviour, may not be so far removed from the dynamics of the intimate relationships of some professionals. Indeed, the high level of prevalence of domestic violence in society suggests that in any sizeable staff group or organization there are likely to be both perpetrators and survivors of domestic violence. A summary of the main issues discussed above is presented in Box 8.1.

Box 8.1 Domestic violence: in summary

- Domestic violence can affect any adult in an intimate family-type relationship, although the majority of serious and repeated abuse is perpetrated by men against their female partners or ex-partners.
- Most studies suggest that one in four women will experience domestic violence at some point in their lives.
- In the UK two women every week are killed as a result of domestic violence.
- An incident of domestic violence takes place every six to twenty seconds.
- Domestic violence accounts for one quarter of all reported violent crime.
- Domestic violence often begins or escalates during or just after pregnancy.
- Risks increase at the point of separation, e.g. when the relationship breaks down.
- Individuals from minority or excluded groups and those who have additional needs can face additional barriers in getting help.
- Children who witness domestic violence are at risk of physical and psychological harm.
- There a strong correlation between domestic violence and other forms of abuse, e.g. child abuse, the abuse of vulnerable adults.

Domestic violence: the importance of partnership work

Domestic violence is a complex issue that causes complex problems in people's lives, and no single organization can respond effectively on its own. Effective partnership work is needed to share resources and information and to build the momentum to challenge the attitudes that dismiss, ignore or perpetuate violence and abuse in our society. As discussed earlier, statutory organizations have lagged behind in recognizing the social, financial and individual costs of not taking domestic violence seriously. The problem is one of responsibility: if domestic violence is not recognized as a situation in which public bodies must intervene, then the responsibility for ensuring adequate support services will continue to lie with voluntary and community groups. Yet domestic violence affects people in every aspect of their lives, it is a cross-cutting issue with significant implications for health and social care services, housing and education, voluntary and community groups, the criminal justice system and the business world. The risk with domestic violence, like all cross-cutting issues, is that it is everybody's business and nobody's responsibility.

Concern about lack of funding for refuge and other support services is no longer voiced by the voluntary sector and women's groups alone. Professionals in statutory organizations, who rely on these essential services, are also concerned about the short-fall. As domestic violence is pushed up the agenda, and public awareness raised, more people come forward for help. Similarly, once professionals are sensitive to the possibility of domestic violence, they begin to look beyond their client's presenting issues to the possibility of domestic violence as an underlying factor. This, in turn, leads to an increase in referrals to refuges and domestic violence projects. One of the dilemmas in domestic violence work is that when awareness is raised, and people feel safe enough to come forward, professionals need to be able to respond with confidence. It is important to be able to provide up-to-date information about local support services, know where to get advice from other professionals, and most importantly to give a supportive, believing response. Being part of a domestic violence forum can help organizations to do this by sharing information about services, providing access to training, establishing referral mechanisms between agencies and sharing expertise, for example, by assisting with the development of domestic violence policies and procedures.

There are currently over 200 domestic violence fora in the UK (Hague 2000), many established by the police in response to guidance from the Home Office or under the 1998 Crime and Disorder Act. The only national study of inter-agency responses to domestic violence was carried out in 1996 (Hague *et al.* 1996). The researchers found considerable variation in multi-agency fora with no easily distinguishable model or approach. They concluded that multi-agency fora offered considerable opportunities for effective co-ordination but there was a danger that they could be used as a smokescreen for inactivity or as a 'talking shop' with little actual change in practical responses.

Partnership: the Coventry response

Coventry Domestic Violence Partnership was established in the 1980s as a focus group to advise planners and commissioners in health and social care about service gaps and priorities. The impetus for the Coventry Partnership came from the voluntary sector in collaboration with the police and 'safer cities' community safety workers. Since then it has developed into a strong and dynamic multi-agency partnership with a wide remit across the spectrum of public and community services. At the time of this research, it was a closed group consisting of representatives from statutory and voluntary organizations whose core business partly or wholly involved domestic violence. This included the police, probation, magistrates, Crown Prosecution Service, social services, Primary Care Trust, education, Area Child Protection Committee, refuges and other voluntary organizations such as Victim Support and Relate. The partnership had a statutory sector chairperson with the vice chair role shared between the managers of Coventry's three specialist domestic violence services, all of which were provided by the voluntary sector. This balance of power between the voluntary and statutory sectors was perceived to have been one of the reasons for the partnership's success. While the statutory organizations, such as police, probation and social services, were powerful in structural terms, the voluntary sector women's organizations represented the voices of survivors of domestic violence and ensured the partnership remained focused on work that made a real difference to their lives. In terms of accountability, the partnership was accountable to its membership and reported to the local Crime and Disorder Partnership.

An increasingly common role in partnership work is that of a co-ordinator. Research has found that this is an important factor in successful partnership, requiring the skills to operate across service boundaries, build bridges between different interest groups, broker difference and build consensus (Webb 1991). The role of a Domestic Violence Co-ordinator is to 'oil the wheels' of partnership: facilitating communication; building bridges; networking; keeping a strategic overview; being a catalyst for action. Importantly, in Coventry this post was supported by excellent administrative staff who helped with organization and communication – vital tasks in keeping 20 organizations on board in the partnership, as well as engaging wider stakeholders in the city.

One of most effective mechanisms for partnership development in Coventry involved improvements to structure and processes within the partnership. Some of these were implemented as a result of research asking members to reflect on their experiences of the partnership and their organization's role within it. Partnership meetings moved from a time frame of monthly to quarterly meetings and were supplemented by task groups meeting more regularly. Each task group was charged with implementing part of the annual work programme drawn from priorities identified in the city's Multi-agency Strategy on Domestic Violence. Task groups were chaired by different members of the partnership according to expertise (e.g. Health, Children, Perpetrators, Diversity) and additional members were co-opted from a wide network of organizations. One of the conditions for membership of the partnership was that each member was expected to be active in at least one task group. This helped to ensure the partnership did not become a talking shop or allow organizations to 'tick the box' on domestic violence by sending a representative without a real commitment to improving services. Another significant factor was the introduction of a mentoring system, through which new members were assigned a 'buddy' to brief them about the work, explain the context of current initiatives and support them in working out how best to take forward the agenda in their own organization.

The partnership was organized in a way intended to build ownership and commitment among the representatives and their organizations. It was a closed group to avoid the difficulties of attendance changing from one meeting to the next, and numbers were restricted to around 20 members to ensure everyone had an opportunity to contribute. Organizations who had less of a key role in domestic violence work and who expressed a desire to join were encouraged to become members of task groups, and to take part in the 'City Forum on Domestic Violence' – an annual conference for anyone with an interest in the issues in the city. The process of developing a multi-agency strategy on domestic violence was also an inclusive one with organizations consulted on strategic priorities and encouraged to develop their own practical action plans. Monitoring and evaluation mechanisms were put in place to celebrate the achievements of member organizations and to hold them to account, for example, through the production of an annual report on progress in implementing the multi-agency strategy.

One of the key roles for the partnership was building momentum among communities, professionals, the media and civic leaders to create a city where violence, whatever its form, would not be tolerated. The Coventry experience showed that to get domestic violence on people's agendas it was important to do two things: to give a voice to the experiences of survivors in order for people to understand the very personal impact of abuse, and to make the social and economic case for putting a stop to the continued escalation of violence in all its forms, from school bullying to rape and sexual abuse. The partnership had a clear communications strategy and held regular seminars and conferences, published information on the Internet and worked closely with the media.

Partnership: the Coventry priorities

Detailed priorities are set out in Coventry's Multi-agency Strategy on Domestic Violence for the four key service areas of:

1. Emergency and support
2. Children
3. Prevention
4. Justice

In addition to these, the key priorities for the partnership as a whole are set out in Box 8.2.

The partnership gained a regional and national profile for its work, with recognition by the Home Office for its model of partnership (Home Office 2000). Group members regularly provided support and consultancy for new and emerging partnerships. They succeeded in getting domestic violence accepted as a political priority in the city, including the establishment by elected members of a City Council Advisory Panel on Domestic Violence. In 2002 the Lord Mayor chose the Domestic Violence Partnership children's projects as the beneficiaries of the Lord Mayor's Appeal. The high level of support among civic leaders and decision makers in the city

---

Box 8.2 Key priorities

- Secure *political* commitment from civic leaders, chief officers and senior managers in key organizations e.g. health, social care, probation services, etc.
- Secure *strategic* commitment by ensuring that domestic violence is addressed in relevant strategies and plans.
- Raise awareness among staff in statutory, voluntary and private sector organizations.
- Improve co-ordination between services.
- Improve the quality of existing services and responses.
- Identify unmet need and develop new services and responses.
- Share good practice.
- Raise awareness with the public.

---

led to additional resources for direct services and enabled the partnership to negotiate change in the statutory partner organizations. It has also ensured that when new strategic initiatives came on board, domestic violence was recognized and addressed, for example, through the Children's Fund or Neighbourhood Renewal.

The partnership led on a number of key policy and practice developments, underpinned by research. Being able to make the case for service development based on local research and data was one of the most significant factors in getting the large statutory organizations, such as health and social services, on board and begin to mainstream domestic violence into their work. The 'Voices of Children' research (Hendessi 1997) carried out in the early years of the partnership led to a whole range of initiatives aimed at supporting children living with domestic violence, including funding for children's workers in refuges, a new school-based children's counselling service and a much greater understanding about the close correlation between domestic violence and child abuse. This, in turn, led to the development of inter-agency guidance on domestic violence by the Area Child Protection Committee, which challenged the old notions in social work of 'problem families' and the value-laden judgement of women's 'failure to protect' their children. Instead the emphasis was on prevention, intervening earlier to protect women and their children, and taking steps to hold perpetrators accountable for their actions.

Members of the partnership also worked with individual organizations to develop policies and practice guidance on domestic violence, a very important step in translating research and national policy into local good practice. These included guidance for the local authority, police, Area Child Protection Committee, supported housing organizations and the primary care trust. The process of developing guidance in partnership rather than in isolation was also significant. It provided the opportunity for a group of workers from different agencies to come together, explore the dilemmas and difficulties for a particular organization, build on existing good practice, and develop a policy that would not only work in that organizational context but which would be co-ordinated across the agencies. The members of the partnership found that this brought benefits in other areas of work, for example, in dealing more generally with policing or homelessness issues, and that the relationships forged by working together around domestic violence helped establish more effective co-ordination across the board.

The development of an active partnership with the University of Warwick enabled practitioners to benefit from the knowledge and expertise of leading academics in the domestic violence field in the School of Health and Social Studies, and for members of the faculty to benefit from close contact with projects on the ground. The University of Warwick and the Coventry Domestic Violence Partnership worked on a number of projects together including: a) the 'Research into Practice' initiative developing knowledge in Health and Social Services, and focusing on mental health and domestic violence; b) a Home Office funded research project into work with non-convicted perpetrators of abuse; and c) local research into child protection and domestic violence.

The 'Research into Practice' collaboration helped pull together the research evidence on the links between domestic violence and mental health difficulties, and then ran a series of workshops for health and social care professionals to disseminate this knowledge and identify appropriate responses. A similar project was undertaken by the Coventry Domestic Violence Partnership with the Coventry Lesbian and Gay Policing Forum (established to assist the police in combating hate crime). This led to a regional seminar on the impact and implications of domestic violence for lesbian, gay, bisexual and transgender men and women, and the opportunity to disseminate information on this little known area of abuse.

The Coventry Domestic Violence Partnership has also been involved in initiating a regional network of domestic violence fora working alongside colleagues in the West Midlands. This led to the recruitment of a regional Domestic Violence strategy post, hosted by the NHS Executive, and the emerging development of e-networks for professionals in the domestic violence field to communicate, share good practice and develop regional responses to domestic violence.

Partnership: productivity or procrastination?

Partnership is very much in the spirit of the time, with new initiatives springing up throughout public services. Eradicating bureaucratic and outdated professional boundaries and establishing 'seamless' services is a clear ambition of the government's modernization agenda. In recent years, Crime and Disorder Partnerships, Drug Action Teams and Health Partnership Boards have all been established to improve service co-ordination and provide a more effective response across organizations. However, the fundamental point that government guidance and local strategies often gloss over is that partnership work is difficult. There are differences in organizational culture, terminology, practice, operational priorities and training, to say nothing of the lack of co-terminous service boundaries, for example, between health services and the police. Each partner regards the other with a degree of professional scepticism and sometimes with downright distrust. Different interests, priorities and practices in multi-agency groups make collaborative working difficult. It has been argued that trust between organizations can only be developed if based on an appreciation of divergent interests and views (Webb 1991). Practical experience suggests that providing opportunities to explore different ideological perspectives is as important as establishing common ground. Researchers have noted that one way to overcome mistrust is to take small steps early on rather than immediately set ambitious partnership goals (Webb 1991). This certainly reflects current thinking in regeneration and neighbourhood renewal where 'early wins' have been found to be very important in new and distrusting partnerships, for example, by running community clean-up campaigns, or replacing run-down play equipment in neighbourhood parks. The sense of achievement gained by working together to achieve small goals can provide the momentum for tackling more difficult, longer-term problems.

Difficulties also arise in partnerships because of the multiple organizational structures that group members come from and the fact that each representative has a different reporting arrangement and a different level of decision-making power within their own organization (Iles and Auluck 1990). Unless decision-making and reporting-back processes are clearly established, partnerships can be frustrated by their members' lack of authority, and their inability to make the decisions and agreements necessary to move the work forward.

In terms of the Coventry Domestic Violence Partnership, recognizing partnership dynamics in organizations' vested interests, conflicting priorities, different professional practices and competition over scarce resources has been important. The partnership has found that, for partnerships to work effectively, it is important to establish certain agreements (see Box 8.3).

Box 8.3 Making partnership work

The Domestic Violence Partnership has found that the following factors help to ensure productive partnership:

- Establishing shared values
- Setting common goals
- Finding champions
- Clarity of structure
- Clarity in roles and responsibilities
- Agreed work programme carried out through task groups
- Focusing on the needs of women and children

Individual members of the partnership have also identified factors to help them participate more effectively in a multi-agency context. These include the need for management commitment in their own agencies, clarity of mechanisms for communication and decision taking in their own agencies, establishment of personal and organizational goals, and opportunities to profile the work of their own agencies.

Partnership work: the future

Although there has been considerable progress in responding to domestic violence in a joined-up way, there is no room for complacency. In 2002 the Coventry Domestic Violence Partnership received funding for a training project and initiated a programme of joint training across organizations, an essential step in giving front-line staff the tools and confidence to be able to respond to domestic violence sensitively and appropriately. Another key challenge ahead is the need for more robust data to enable agencies to measure the true extent of domestic violence and to design services accordingly. This is linked to establishing systems to share information between organizations and the development of joint protocols to improve responses to individual service users. Most importantly, there are examples in the UK of joint service delivery on domestic violence, including multidisciplinary teams with co-located staff and joint budgets. Co-located staff can help break down barriers between organizations but most importantly well trained, well informed staff, who understand their roles and that of other agencies who work together to find the best solutions possible, are essential in providing an effective response to domestic violence. Finally, investigations following the death of a woman as a result of domestic violence can provide a clear indication of what is needed to change professional practice, but to date these have not been implemented in any sytematic way. However, the new Domestic Violence Bill proposes that 'homicide reviews' become a statutory requirement in the same way as 'Section 8' inquiries are carried out when a child dies. The Coventry experience has highlighted many practices that could be described as 'good practice', which are identified in the box below.

Good practice checklist

- Take on board messages from government guidance, e.g. Department of Health, Home Office
- Develop good practice guidelines
- Establish links with the local domestic violence forum
- Discuss issues about domestic violence with colleagues
- Organize training
- Consider routine questioning
- Display information about domestic violence support services
- Keep careful records
- Listen and respect service users

Conclusion

Domestic violence is set in a cultural context that has traditionally condoned, ignored or diminished the seriousness of violence and abuse perpetrated in intimate relationships. Until recently, women have typically been expected to keep quiet about their experiences of abuse, been blamed for provoking violence or conversely criticized for 'putting up' with violence. There is no doubt that considerable progress has been made in raising the profile of domestic violence and its impact on individuals, families and communities. It is safe to say that the days when brutal and systematic abuse were dismissed as 'just a domestic' by the police and other public bodies are finally over. However, there is a long way to go before women and children get the support and help they need from the organizations who should be responsible for providing it.

Domestic violence is a complex issue and no single organization has overall responsibility for providing the services that protect and support those affected. Therefore, effective partnership work is essential. As this chapter has demonstrated, a multi-agency partnership can draw on the strengths and resources of different agencies, work together to raise public awareness, challenge the attitudes that perpetuate violence and abuse, and ensure effective services are in place to deal with domestic violence. The challenge ahead is to create a society where violence of any sort is no longer the everyday life experience of many thousands of women and children. Until that situation changes, it is imperative that the services work together to protect and support women and children, and to bring perpetrators to justice.

Questions for further discussion

1. According to the evidence, which groups in society are most vulnerable to domestic violence?
2. What aspects of the Coventry experience of partnership could you apply to your organization?
3. How successful is your organization in achieving the items listed in the 'good practice' checklist?

References

Bewley, C. and Gibbs, A. (2002) Fact or fallacy? Domestic violence in pregnancy: An overview. *MIDIRS Midwifery Digest*, September 12(2).

Blyth, L. (2002) Partnership work on domestic violence: Possibilities and practicalities. *MIDIRS Midwifery Digest*, September 12(2).

British Medical Association (1998) *Domestic Violence: A Health Care Issue?* British Medical Association, London.

Coventry Domestic Violence Focus Group (2000) *Coventry's Multi-Agency Strategy on Domestic Violence 2000–03*. Coventry Domestic Violence Focus Group, Coventry.

Coventry Domestic Violence Partnership (2001) *Developing Work with Non-convicted Perpetrators of Domestic Violence*. Unpublished Briefing Paper. Coventry Domestic Violence Partnership, Coventry.

Department of Health (2000) *Domestic Violence: A Resource Manual for Health Care Professionals*. Department of Health, London.

Department of Health (2000) *No Secrets: Guidance on Developing and Implementing Multi-agency Policies and Procedures to Protect Vulnerable Adults from Abuse*. Department of Health, London.

Domestic Violence Data Source (1999) *Key Facts and Figures*. www.domesticviolencedata.org.

Frost, P.J., Moore, L.F., Louis, M.R., Lundberg, C.C. and Martin, J. (eds) (1991) *Reframing Organizational Culture*. Sage, Newbury.

Hague, G. (2000) *Reducing Domestic Violence :What Works – Multi-agency Fora*. Home Office, London.

Hague, G., Malos, E. and Dear, W. (1996) *Multi-agency Work and Domestic Violence: A National Study of Inter-agency Initiatives*. The Policy Press, Bristol.

Hague, G. and Malos, E. (1998) *Domestic Violence: Action for Change* (2nd edition). New Harion Press, Cheltenham.

Harwin, N., Hague, G. and Malos, E. (eds) (1999) *The Multi-Agency Approach to Domestic Violence: New Opportunities, Old Challenges?* Whiting and Birch Ltd, London.

Hendessi, M. (1997) *Voices of Children Witnessing Domestic Violence: A Form of Child Abuse.* Domestic Violence Focus Group, Coventry.

Hester, M., Pearson, C. and Harwin, N. (1998) *Making an Impact: Children and Domestic Violence.* Barnardos, NSPCC and University of Bristol.

Home Office (2000) *Domestic Violence: Revised Circular to the Police.* HOC 19/2000. Home Office, London.

Home Office (2000) *Multi-agency Guidance for Addressing Domestic Violence.* Home Office, London.

Home Office (2000) *Reducing Domestic Violence: What Works?* Home Office, London.

Iles, P. and Auluck, R. (1990) Team building, inter-agency team development and social work practice. *British Journal of Social Work*, 29.

Lewis, G. (2002) Domestic violence: Lessons from the 1997–99 Confidential Enquiry into Maternal Deaths. *MIDIRS Midwifery Digest*, September 12(2).

Mirrlees-Black, C. (1998) *Domestic Violence: Findings from a New British Crime Survey Self-Completion Questionnaire.* Home Office Research Study 192. Home Office, London.

Mullender, A. (1996) *Rethinking Domestic Violence: the Social Work and Probation Response.* Routledge, London.

Moxon, D. (1999) *Criminal Justice Conference: Violence Against Women.* Conference Transcript www.homeoffice.gov.uk/domesticviolence.

Stanko, E. (2000) *The Day to Count.* www.domesticviolencedata.org.

Stokes, J. (1994) Problems in multidisciplinary teams: The unconscious at work. *Journal of Social Work Practice*, 8(2).

United Kingdom Parliament (2003) Domestic Violence, Crime and Victims Bill. www.publications.parliament.uk/pa/ld200304/ldbills/006/2004006.htm.

Webb, A. (1991) Co-ordination: A problem in public sector management. *Policy and Politics*, 19(4).

Women's Unit (1999) *Tackling Violence Against Women.* Cabinet Office, London.

Women's Aid Federation of England (2000) *Directory of Multi-Agency Fora 2000.* www.womensaid.org.uk.

Women's Aid Federation of England (2004) *About Women's Aid.* www.womensaid.org.uk.

9

Working together with people who are homeless

Ruth Wyner

This chapter will explore:

- The nature and extent of homelessness.
- The needs of homeless people.
- The benefits and barriers of working together in partnership.
- Good policy and practice.

Introduction

There were 380,000 single homeless people (i.e. not families) in Great Britain in 2003, according to Crisis, a national charity for the homeless. This figure includes those living in hostels, bed and breakfast, squats, on friends' floors and in over-crowded accommodation (Crisis 2003). What it does not include is the 201,060 homeless households that approached local authorities in England in 2002/3. Local authorities have a duty to help homeless households in 'priority need' if they include children, pregnant women and single people deemed to be vulnerable, because of age or mental or physical disability, for example. Of those approaching local authorities in 2002/3, 130,000 were found to be in 'priority need' and unintentionally homeless and, therefore, entitled to re-housing. The rest were entitled to 'housing advice and assistance' only (Diaz 2003).

This chapter will focus on the single homeless, a particularly diverse and often very difficult population to work with. At one extreme there are people with few issues other than that of housing need. These are in the minority. At the other extreme there are people with a range of multiple and complex needs, such as severe mental health and substance misuse problems. This latter group tend to have chaotic lifestyles and suffer from an array of enduring difficulties. They may often be reluctant to engage with agencies offering help, wary of formal professional settings and many find it difficult to keep appointments. As a group they can appear forbidding and antagon-istic towards those trying to help them. They are a visible face of homelessness, often looking unkempt and out of control, even though they, again, represent a minority of the total homeless population. Beneath the surface they are, of course, people like the rest of us, but homeless people have, through the years, suffered from an inordinate amount of prejudice. Perhaps they remind us of our own vulnerabilities, or of the compromises we all make to accommodate the needs of society. By the very nature of their situation, homeless people tend to be dislocated and out of touch with main-stream services. Drug and alcohol problems, which give rise to much of the social denigration, can be either a cause or a consequence of homelessness, and often mask serious underlying psychological and emotional difficulties. Drug dependence, in particular, takes people into the realms of criminality, making treatment even more difficult to provide.

With such a diverse range of needs, effective partnerships and good liaison between agencies are essential if people who are homeless are going to be able to access the help they need. That is why health and social services need to consider targeted services in order to be effective with this hard-to-reach client group.

A brief recent history

The nature of single homelessness has changed considerably over the past few dec-ades. In the 1970s a number of charities set up basic night shelters for 'gentlemen of the road' alongside the largely despised government 'spikes', which can best be described as short-term 'doss houses'. The main presenting problems among this group of homeless people were alcoholism and 'eccentric behaviour'. Alienation rather than lack of accommodation seemed to be at the roots of their problems. Social relationships were few – often non-existent. As Erikson (1982) and Rutter (1971) show, young people who are under-socialized are insecure in adulthood, cannot man-age social relationships or responsibilities and avoid commitments like marriage and regular employment. Merton (1968) described homeless people as 'retreatists', in terms of being '*in* the society but not *of* it'.

Typical of these night shelters was one set up in Norwich in 1971 by St Martin's Housing Trust. The shelter was situated in a small redundant church and it offered mattresses on the floor, one cold tap and one lavatory initially for fifteen people. Such was the need that up to forty people sometimes shared these meagre facilities. In 1976 the shelter moved to a larger church which, this time, offered three toilets, one shower and a proper kitchen.

Ten years later, the shelter was still there. Chris Roberts, then director of St Martin's, described the situation thus (1986): '(The night shelter) looks like what it is: a church crammed full of beds. Eight people have to sleep on bunk beds in an area no more that 13 ft by 10 ft. This is about 12 square metres. Registered hostels have to have 10 square metres per person. Forty residents, many of them disturbed, are living in what must be some of the worst overcrowding in existence in the country.'

Many of the residents at St Martin's were no doubt 'disturbed'. By the mid-1980s, the nature of homelessness had changed dramatically. From my own experi-ence of night shelter work, one aspect of the change in the homeless population in the 1980s, that of an increase in the incidence of mental illness, appeared to be due to the large-scale closure of the old Victorian mental hospitals and the advent of

Community Care (an excellent policy provided it was properly resourced). At the outset, only a limited numbers of bed spaces were made available to cope with the influx of needy people into the community. The provision of the necessary support was variable; often little was in place. Significant numbers of people drifted away from inadequate arrangements that had been made for them and ended up sleeping rough on the streets, or in night shelters that were ill-equipped to cope with their needs. Getting these clients back into an already overloaded mental health system proved enormously difficult because services were under-resourced and often struggling. The voluntary sector sometimes had to perform minor miracles to meet the needs it was facing. For instance, surveys at St Martin's Norwich Night Shelter in the mid-1980s showed that three-quarters of their clientele had been treated previously by NHS psychiatric services. Staff described the place as 'like a psychiatric ward without the hospital around it'.

A later and more rigorous study by Pleace and Quilgars (1996), conducted when services for homeless people had been improved compared with the 1980s, as had the provision of Community Care, showed that 30–50 per cent of single homeless people had mental health problems and this included 12–26 per cent who had schizophrenia or other similarly serious mental illnesses. This figure did not generally include people with personality disorders as this condition, unless severe, was not well recognized and tended to be seen as untreatable by hospital psychiatrists at the time.

Homelessness is inevitably affected by changes in the economy as well as changes in social policy. The late 1970s saw a significant rise in unemployment, particularly among the unskilled workforce. As Crane (1999, p.68) states: 'During this period, unemployment increased in Great Britain, particularly within the manufacturing and construction industries, and the demand for unskilled manual workers fell sharply.' Alongside this, changes in the benefits led to a demise of the 'grotty bedsit', which had previously been a lifesaver for many people on minimal incomes. There was increasing regulation of the private housing sector, which cost landlords money, and over time it became harder for them to get the rental income they wanted from unemployed people who claimed housing benefit to pay for their rent, or from people on low wages. Many landlords went upmarket or just sold up. Council house tenants became eligible to buy their own homes and housing investment by local authorities virtually ceased. As a result, the private and public rental sectors diminished alarmingly. Homelessness increased, particularly among the unskilled and unqualified young who found it difficult to secure employment.

During the period of growth in the homeless sector in the late 1980s and early 1990s, many charities set up partnerships with housing associations and constructed new hostels which were more suited to the new profile of homelessness, rather than the old ad hoc night shelters. The hostels offered much better accommodation, usually in single rooms, and the better environment in itself did much to improve people's chances for resettlement into mainstream housing. More targeted services were developed along with move-on housing, in either shared supported housing or individual flats, for those who could take it on. This was a vital component in terms of getting people out of institutional living and into their own accommodation. It was also essential to prevent hostels and shelters clogging up so that beds were continually available. But such was the overwhelming level of need that night shelters continued to operate in order to give people a roof over their heads. Some shelters opened seasonally, during the coldest months when homeless people were most at risk, or over the Christmas period when homelessness has a particular emotional impact. Partnerships with health, social services and local housing authorities were key to adequate provision but practitioners, managers and politicians were frequently over-whelmed and unable to provide for unexpectedly high numbers of homeless people. Rough sleeping was a particular 'irritant' in London, where large numbers of dislocated people gathered. There were more young homeless people than ever. MPs and cabinet ministers complained about the 'inconvenience' it caused. While some were able to empathize with the plight of so many homeless people, one MP famously recounted the inconvenience of having to step over them on his way to the opera.

In 1990, in response to this growing need, the government set up the Rough Sleepers' Initiative (RSI) to provide funding for approved projects. It operated solely in London until 1997, when it took on six areas outside the capital, extending yet further to other towns and cities in the years following. Redesignated the Rough Sleepers' Unit (RSU) in 1999, it was given a focus on developing a more integrated approach to tackling rough sleeping, and aimed to reduce the total numbers of those sleeping rough by two-thirds by 2002. An important component of the RSU's work was to insist that local authorities produced a strategy on rough sleeping for their area, which encouraged improved joint working between agencies.

In 2002 the RSU controversially declared it had achieved its target: 'The target on reducing the number of people sleeping rough by two thirds has been maintained. As of June, local authority statistics show that 596 people are sleeping rough on any one night. This represents a reduction of 68 per cent since 1998.' (Homelessness Directorate 2002). There was, however, a chorus of workers claiming the figures had been manipulated through a variety of dubious methods. While street counts were going on, a Contact and Assessment (CAT) worker (doing street outreach) wrote anonymously to the *Big Issue* magazine:

> People are often not included in the government's rough-sleeping figures and the public are being gravely misled as to the seriousness of the problem . . . The Rough Sleepers' Unit is conducting a cosmetic clean-up campaign while people are in danger of dying on the streets.
>
> (*Big Issue* 2000: 44)

Thirty-five of London's 50 or 60 CAT workers were reported to have got together that winter to complain, through the Transport and General Workers Union, about the RSU's 'willingness to manipulate statistics for political ends' and accusing the RSU of demonstrating 'an authoritarian nature' (*Property People* 2000:1).

At the end of the 1990s, as well as improving and streamlining services, the government caused considerable controversy by attacking activities that they thought supported homelessness: the provision of short-term shelters, soup runs and people giving money to beggars. Homeless people did indeed become less obvious in the new millennium than they had been at the end of the old one, and more likely than before to be subject to controlling forces as well as caring ones. The government continued to drive towards making individuals responsible for their behaviour. By 2003 those considered to be behaving badly in the streets, through persistent begging, for example, or drunkenness, were now at risk of incurring one of the government's new Anti-Social Behaviour Orders (ASBOs) which, for the non-co-operative, held the possibility of imprisonment. Even so, it was obvious from continuing street counts that there were still significant numbers of homeless people sleeping rough, though in fewer numbers than five or ten years before. National homelessness charities such as Crisis and Shelter complained that definitions of homelessness must go beyond rough sleeping and must also include those in temporary, inadequate or over-crowded accommodation.

The RSU was incorporated into the new Homelessness Directorate, which was set up as part of the office of the Deputy Prime Minister. It has a continuing remit to develop a more strategic approach to homelessness generally (not just rough sleeping), to test new and innovative approaches, to encourage best practice, and help fund local initiatives working to that effect.

Analysis of the homeless population

A clear profile of the homeless population is hard to assess overall; by definition it is a fluid and transient group with a multiplicity of service needs. Overstretched voluntary agencies working in the sector often struggle to manage their services with limited resources. Some keep good data but all too often record keeping is poor and is rarely standardized, so that pooling of information is difficult, if not impossible.

Institutional living, such as being in care, in the armed forces, in hospital or in prison, does make some people vulnerable to homelessness. As Bahr and Caplow (1974, p. 74) write: 'Prolonged associations with total institutions or other environments, that provide the necessities of life with a minimum of individual initiative, may incapacitate inmates for life in more demanding contexts. They may establish patterns of behaviour incompatible with the outside.'

There are dangers for people who do not fit in. Maureen Crane spells it out:

Disaffiliation and alienation remain features of contemporary homelessness . . . (and) alienation can be seen as self-perpetuating, as a result of both the deviant behaviours of homeless people and their stigmatization and rejection by conventional society. As homeless people become entrenched in homelessness and their behaviours deviate further, they become increasingly isolated from families and social groups. They have no rights to accommodation, few social roles, are unproductive, powerless, yet visible members of society. These factors are likely to intensify alienation.

(Crane 1999: 17)

Push factors associated with homelessness are substance abuse, relationship breakdown, mental health problems, unemployment, being forced to leave home, release from prison, leaving care or the armed forces, and suffering violence, bereavement or sexual abuse (Lemos and Goodby 1999). For instance, a third of people leaving prison are homeless on release (Social Exclusion Unit 2002).

A study of the profiles of single homeless people in London was carried out in

2000 by three main agencies in London: St Mungo's, and Thames Reach Bondway housing association. They used data from outreach workers who had had contact with 4,465 people recorded as sleeping rough from April 1999 to March 2000, and from a one-night survey held on 16 August 2000, of all residents in the capital's direct-access and first-stage hostels, a total of 3,295 people in 67 hostels. Information was also taken about 1,187 attendees at 23 day centres on 11 July 2000, and about 2,300 clients who had been resettled by 64 organizations between April 1999 and March 2000. Throughout the study men heavily outnumbered women, mostly by about 4 to 1, apart from young teenagers surveyed where the women outnumbered the men. The results clearly showed that mental health and substance abuse problems were prevalent among single homeless people of all ages and in all settings. Understandably, they were most pronounced among people sleeping rough: 67 per cent of the men and 71 per cent of the women were reported to have at least one of these problems (Crane and Warnes 2001).

As was expected, alcohol was shown to be a more common problem among middle-aged and older homeless men, while illegal drug use predominated among men and women aged under 40. Among even younger rough sleepers, those aged under 25, 57 per cent of the women and 46 per cent of the men were reported to have drug problems. There was a marked increase with age in the prevalence of mental health problems among homeless women: two-thirds of women aged 50 years and over in hostels and on the streets were reported to be mentally ill. It should be noted that this study was looking at diagnosed mental illnesses that did not include incidence of depression and anxiety, which were prevalent among this client group.

In 2002 Homeless Link, a membership organization for some 700 homelessness agencies throughout the UK, conducted an independent survey looking at homeless people with multiple needs: that is, people who had two or more defined problems, such as substance abuse and a mental health problem. The results showed that almost half (47.8 per cent) of the total had multiple needs, and among rough sleepers the figure was over 50 per cent. Although there was no historical data with which to compare, the results confirmed the feeling of professionals of a high and growing proportion of homeless people with multiple needs. There was no significant difference for male or female service users. Since these surveys there has been further government attention on reducing the number of people sleeping rough. Concern remains that those left on the streets are the most vulnerable: people with the most entrenched and difficult problems (Homeless Link 2002).

While it is argued (Parker et al. 1998) that by the end of the 1990s recreational drug taking had became a normalized experience for many young people, amongst single homeless people drug dependence had become a huge problem. By the end of the 1990s Release, a UK national drugs and legal charity, estimated that between 76 per cent and 89 per cent of single people who were homeless or vulnerably housed used drugs (Flemen 1999). A survey conducted at that time stated that the projects contacted estimated that between 50 per cent and 90 per cent of their clientele used heroin, crack cocaine or amphetamines (Lemos and Goodby 1999).

According to anecdotal evidence from a frontline worker at a hostel run by English Churches Housing Group accommodating rough sleepers in a provincial city in 2003, one-third of residents had serious problems with drugs, another third had mental health problems and the final third had both. Alcohol was a problem for about 50 per cent of the residents and was on the increase, mainly due to people tackling their drug problems with some success but then reverting to heavy drinking. It was acknowledged by staff that their residents were in general self-medicating in order to cope with emotional distress, trauma and mental health problems.

Partners in homelessness: the benefits and the barriers

The voluntary and not-for-profit sectors tend to play a large role in working on the front line with homeless people and in project development. For instance, charities that were set up to provide a soup run or a basic night shelter often developed their services to better meet the local need and sometimes linked with housing associations in order to access capital funding for hostels and shared housing. There is, however, a long history of antagonism between the voluntary homelessness sectors and statutory services. Social service staff are frequently perceived by the voluntary sector as being aloof, unapproachable and not fulfilling their statutory responsibilities. They, in turn, complain that voluntary sector staff do not understand the limits of those responsibilities and fail to appreciate what they can take on within the parameters of their departments and their scarce resources. There has been, traditionally, a similar polarization between the health service and voluntary agencies. At the root of these difficulties is the way voluntary sector organizations, which are most usually charities, have been set up to provide for all-comers; that is, to offer help to homeless people who come to them without any formal assessment. This is contrary to practice in the statutory sectors where gate-keeping is the norm. But, inevitably, that gate-keeping left many homeless people out in the cold. A shift has been required from both sectors.

Many of the homelessness charities became overwhelmed by the difficulties caused by the advent of community care in the 1980s and the higher numbers of people with mental health problems, sometimes extremely serious, being discharged into the community often with inadequate support or preparation. It became common for voluntary agencies to accommodate people with mental health problems (including psychotic illnesses) with few resources to meet the needs. Many of these clients had real difficulties in even accessing a GP, let alone getting help from psychiatric services.

In recent years significant steps have been taken around the country to provide a more accessible and effective service for homeless people. For example, dedicated GP practices for the homeless have been set up as well as regular surgeries in hostels and day centres for general health or for specific problems like drug abuse. This gave clients living in temporary hostels, or in their own accommodation, a better chance of avoiding a relapse into chaotic street or night shelter living. But difficulties still remained. In the Crane and Warnes' survey (2001) the majority of the homelessness staff involved expressed concern about delays in accessing:

- specialist mental health and substance misuse treatment services;
- input from social services and community care assessments;
- suitable move-on accommodation with support.

They complained of inadequate provision for homeless people with mental health and substance misuse problems, or a history of violence, and believed that there should be more opportunities for hostel residents to develop daily living skills and to be resettled.

In the Crane and Warnes' survey staff demonstrated a widespread awareness of the intractable problems of those with dual and multiple diagnoses but the public discourse devoted little attention to the issues. Apart from references to people with drug problems, it hardly mentioned the high prevalence of alcohol problems and mental illness among homeless people, and of the entrenched difficulties and inadequate responses to these problems.

Case study – Hamden

This section explores some of the issues and tensions involved in delivering partner-ship approaches to homeless people using a case study. The inquiry was based upon interviews with health, social care and voluntary agencies operating in a UK town that will remain anonymous – we shall call it Hamden. The area had a relatively high homeless population for its size, due largely to the shortages of housing in the city and the fact that homeless people have historically gravitated there. Hamden also had high levels of employment and some homeless people came hoping that there would be some employment opportunities for them. With the severe pressures on housing, many ended up sleeping on the streets and, typically, a significant proportion of the homeless population of Hamden had additional mental health and/or drug problems. There were several key agencies concerned with homelessness in Hamden:

- Hamden City Council
- Hamden Housing Association
- Hamden night shelter
- Street outreach and mental health teams
- Community Psychiatric Nurse (hostels)
- A dedicated GP homeless service
- Drug and alcohol service

I interviewed a range of staff working in Hamden, in homelessness and health, and will give an impression of their experiences of partnership working. I also con-tacted social services, as some people were under the impression that two social workers were allocated to work specifically with homeless people, though nobody knew who they were. The social workers I spoke to (one of whom had been with the department for many years) said that this was not the case: there were no social workers assigned to work with the homeless specifically because: 'Homelessness is not a category we have a statutory responsibility for,' I was told:

'There is no social services homelessness team. If someone has a housing problem, then it goes to housing. If it's disability, it goes there. As far as I'm aware, the voluntary sector deals with homelessness as a group.'

In effect, social services had delegated the social care of people who were homeless to the voluntary sector and had formalized this arrangement by providing grant funding to some of the agencies involved: in particular, the night shelter, but also to a small hostel working with young people.

The dedicated GP for the homeless said that there used to be a named social worker for working with the homeless but now they dealt with issues on an ad hoc basis. 'The strategic input isn't there,' she said, 'and they're not really there as a presence either. If you have a concern you go to the duty social worker. It doesn't work very well. If I make a referral I make sure I follow up with a letter and keep a copy. I've learned through experience that anything can happen.' The belief that Social Services only provide a peripheral commitment to the needs of homeless people was graphically described by a manager of the voluntary Housing Association which runs the town's homelessness hostels:

'Social Services: who are they? They only figure in the most extreme cases, and only if health are screaming alongside us. Then we might, just might, get a social worker in. But frankly, we don't see them. Though we did get one assessment, for an alcoholic who was assessed as needing long-term care. It took us about six months and it'll probably take at least as long as that to find him a place in a care home. Meantime, we have to cope, though we're not a care home ourselves and have no funding for care staff.'

In common with other cities in the UK with large homeless populations, health was much more in evidence than social services. But tensions still existed. At times the statutory sector can appear to have a superior and patronizing attitude towards voluntary staff. In mid-1980s when I was working shifts at a night shelter, I remember one morning taking a resident to the local hospital's Accident and Emergency Department. When booking him in, the receptionist asked me who I was. I gave her my name. 'What's your relationship to the patient?' she demanded. I told her I was Deputy Director of the organization that ran the shelter. 'Oh, you people do give yourselves fancy titles,' she responded. I hardly imagine that a health or social worker would have met with such a response. While I have no doubt that some of the prejudice surrounding homelessness fell on the workers as well as the clientele, who were indeed often uncooperative and frustratingly difficult to treat owing to their multifarious difficulties, there is no excuse for such an attitude. Things have moved on considerably since then but some of the old stigmas and cultures remain. A voluntary sector worker described the GP in Hamden with a specific remit for working with the homeless as: caring but patronizing. One task was to identify where that feeling of being patronized came from.

A voluntary sector manager was told by an NHS commissioner that they could not call their Substance Misuse Worker that because it implied they were trained and could prescribe. 'But a substance abuse worker is what this person is,' said the manager. 'Just because they aren't health trained doesn't mean they're not professional. In the voluntary sector we just know they're going to say we're not professional and that we'll get kicked about a bit. So you have to get into the long grass and creep up on them. We are as professional as they are in our respective fields. What do they know about hostel management, for instance? We do try to make them listen. It can be hard.'

A member of the street outreach team who held a professional qualification recognized by the NHS said that the two years he had spent working in the voluntary sector had been the most stressful two years of his life. 'There is a wall of exclusion for agencies such as mine,' he said. 'If I want a response from another agency often I have to make friends with an individual in there to get a response. I find that offensive.' He felt his lack of power acutely. 'I do think I should have more power, if I've spent 90 hours with a client and I've seen them at their best and their worst. A half-hour psychiatric assessment is seen as the be-all-and-end-all. If we're going to have real partnership, there needs to be acceptance of what the others bring in, a real power balance. But the GPs and the psychiatrist rule the roost.' He complained about being excluded from a meeting about his client because it was a 'clinical' meeting: 'It's as if they own the meeting, but in fact it's the client who owns it, and he wanted me to be there. I don't get access to files, even if the client has requested it in writing. I think I get excluded because I challenge.'

However, staff from all agencies I contacted said that good partnership working was what they wanted and that things were improving. One said it was, in theory, a fantastic idea and others talked about looking at holistic solutions for individuals and providing a co-ordinated package for people which, though complex, was the ideal everyone was working towards.

'Prior to Rough Sleepers' Unit money becoming available, many voluntary sector organizations didn't deserve an equal voice because they weren't operating in a very professional way,' said a housing association manager. 'The move from housing benefits to the Supporting People regime has changed things because now you have to clearly show what work you're doing for your clients to get the higher payments. You have service level agreements and quality control. It's forced all social landlords to be professional and it imposes partnership working. There was lack of rigour before.'

Changes in the health service meant that they too had to take account of the wider picture. A new initiative from the NHS imposes a model of care on drug and alcohol services: that they must involve other organizations, such as voluntary sector agencies and housing, in their client work. There was no new money for it but if services did not comply they stood to lose funding. Even so, one worker in housing said:

'The medical service is still a fortress. Making what I see as helpful suggestions are perceived as an attack. I suggested they had a service level agreement with us and they became very defensive about that. Professionalism is just knowledge and experience. We've all got that potentially. A doctor can make a pig's ear of information just like anyone can. The assumption is that a professional's opinion means more.' But he added: 'Their edifices are breaking up because they can't do it alone. We need each other. People are learning about the parameters of each other's services and the blame culture is starting to go away.'

The health workers were certainly aware of these frustrations. The GP pointed out that homeless people were very good at arousing anxiety and could be extremely manipulative.

'With professional training you sit back and look at things in a step-wise way, and you have to be prepared to say, sometimes, that there isn't anything you can do at this particular point in time. You have to leave it and see what happens. Often there's no solution, and admitting someone to hospital can be counterproductive, though for an agency it can provide a solution for them as it gets the person off their hands. This is where the conflict can arise and then, if the patient gets involved, they think you're discriminating against them.'

A CPN working with the homeless in hostels agreed that the health service was often expected to have a magic wand type of solution to people's problems. 'Perceptions of being patronizing are to do with people's expectations about what can be done,' she said. 'If these aren't met it leads to frustration, for me as well. Knowing people want me to deliver something I can't is difficult. People become despondent but I'm bound by my rules and regulations.' She accepted that a crucially important part of her role was education, advice and support, helping staff to understand what could and what could not be done. The CPN did not, in her own mind, dismiss her colleagues in the voluntary sector.

'Residential work is the hardest thing anyone can do. It takes a special skill to manage such hard work: the slow, grinding rehabilitative work when many of the clients are so entrenched. They see these problems day in and day out. I go away and see it only on occasion. A difficulty is that voluntary sector staff often don't understand the cross-over between behaviour and illness,' the CPN explained. 'People's behaviour is sometimes seen as madness when it isn't. This can be hard to understand, even when the client is seen to be able to control the behaviour so that, for instance, they don't get arrested on the street. Frequently the behaviour is to get attention, time, or to make people frightened of you – a power thing. Then the project becomes the victim.'

The housing association manager had her own developing views on behaviour, telling me:

'We are actually shaping behaviour, doing CBT [Cognitive Behavioural Therapy] really. It's not being done by therapists but by people with a whip in their hands: if our residents want to stay they have to conform to an extent. For some people that's excellent but for others, with huge problems, it's not right, it's not enough. Even if snippets of what's happened to some of my residents had happened to friends of mine, they'd be in therapy for years.'

All the agencies accepted that drug dependency complicated matters and made it hard to assess a person's mental state; to decide what was due to the substance abuse or to what extent drugs were taken to cope with underlying mental health difficulties. 'You see people on the street in their twenties and thirties and they're quite resilient at that age,' said the CPN. 'In ten year's time it's different: the effect on their health will be apparent. It's a social issue: people who can't stop, or won't stop, or even why stop?' A hostel worker felt that more effort could be made to engage with dual diagnosis homeless people.

'A lot of the entrenched street homeless are polydrug users: they'll have crack as a treat when they get their dole money, then heroin, methadone, alcohol. They're using so much you can't tell if they have a mental health problem but health won't section them, even on a short section, to allow for an assessment. They're just not interested, and they haven't got the beds anyway.'

Most agencies agreed that there was a problem with the lack of a dedicated long-term facility for the homeless in Hamden. The main drive was to resettle homeless people but for some with high levels of need that just wasn't possible, especially the long-term drinkers, because there was nowhere for them to go. It took considerable time to get social services involved and arranging the funding was said to be enormously difficult. Even then, existing care homes were extremely reluctant to take such people on. If the local hostels were housing someone, it could let social services off the hook. As one voluntary sector worker said:

'There still seems to be a moral issue for medical people about self-harm and addictions. And then the criminal justice sector is working in another direction entirely. About half the people on the streets have refused all options. They don't want night shelter, hostel beds or keyworking. Eventually these people will end up in prison. It's about social control. It always has been to an extent but now it's more apparent.'

Everyone I spoke to accepted that the way to develop better partnership working was to meet with colleagues from different agencies and to discuss issues together. As a result, Hamden had been running a weekly agency meeting for some time. This was an information-sharing forum with an objective of improving liaison between organizations so that they could each offer an informed and unencumbered response to the clients, where overlaps were less likely to happen and staff did not work at cross purposes. There was particular concern to minimize the potential for homeless people to split and manipulate agencies, particularly for those whose lives were desperate and chaotic and who had borderline or other personality disorders, which was not uncommon. The GP explained:

'My boundaries have to be firm in order to manage what is largely a chaotic client group. I'm also concerned to avoid clients playing organizations off against each other. So at the agency meeting we spend a lot of time checking people's stories. For instance, a patient may come to me with a horrendous story about the drug and alcohol service treating them badly and ignoring their needs. You can get a completely different picture from the drug and alcohol workers themselves. If you took what the patient said on face value, you could be undoing a lot of good work, which of course is anyway for the benefit of the patient.'

The agency meeting was attended by a psychiatrist who worked one day a week with the homeless, and by the GP and her practice nurse, the CPN, and representatives from the night shelter, the hostels, the outreach service, the drug and alcohol service and the local psychiatric hospital's discharge planning team. It was a model of good practice but some staff were critical: 'There's no accountability. Verbal information is passed on but not recorded properly and the professionals can display very judgemental attitudes sometimes. I left because it was more like a gossip forum than a professional meeting. And also because they objected to me taking my own notes.' The CPN suggested that it was not possible to work effectively in this field without breaking confidentiality.

'It has to be handled very carefully. We don't have the client's permission to share information but it is done in order to help them. The more information you have the more effective you can be. The important thing is not to share that knowledge with the client. Unfortunately, staff in some organizations have taken on battles that aren't there. We all want to be advocates for the client but there are boundary issues and some workers just want to rescue, which can be dangerous.'

Even so, a voluntary sector agency pulled out because they were disturbed by the failure to maintain what they saw as good practice in confidentiality. They, and others, set up another weekly meeting specifically for referrers to housing for the homeless and the housing providers themselves. Before discussing cases, they all signed up to an information-sharing agreement and ensured the clients had signed a confidentiality waver before their cases were discussed. Health also had their own meeting, on mental health, which involved the GP, the CPN, the psychiatrist and the voluntary sector mental health team. The GP pointed out:

'Face-to-face communication is undoubtedly best: you can have a to-and-fro conversation which helps to elucidate problems. But the more you do this, the less is recorded which means there is less accountability. A balance is needed. Obviously, you don't agree with everything other services do but you weigh it up and may decide to go out a little on your own. Often, it's best to compromise a bit to preserve the relationship. Anyway, in the end, there isn't always an absolute right and wrong.'

One health worker summed up the situation thus:

'With this particular client group you have to offer them a service in a manner they'll accept. You have to be flexible, and you have to be thick-skinned. Your support is your colleagues from both the statutory and the voluntary sectors. It helps you to cope with the pressure. Sometimes you need other people to reassure you that you're doing the right thing for someone, or that nothing more can be done for a person if that's the case, however much you might want to help them.'

Conclusion

Each member of staff that I spoke to from 'Hamden' recognized the importance of partnership and wanted it to work for them and for the clientele. The main themes that emerged were the need for staff in the different agencies to understand each other's roles and to respect colleagues' professionalism, and the frustrations they felt with each other's limitations.

When looking at possible frameworks to use when developing partnerships in social care, Simon Northmore (2001) suggests a threefold focus: communication, training and assessment. Communication in the homelessness sector is essential, but it is not easy. Homeless people are often in touch with a number of agencies due to the multiplicity of their needs. Co-ordination and communication is crucial to ensure that work is not duplicated and that people do not work at cross purposes. Regular multi-agency meetings, such as Hamden's Agency Meeting, are important in this respect. The meetings need to be set up on a basis that all can accept. If people agree, procedures can be written down and reviewed at regular intervals. Decisions made outside the meetings, as will inevitably happen, should be brought back into them through proper reporting. There can be difficulties if one agency dominates the proceedings or if key organizations opt out. These difficulties need to be addressed by the whole group and, sometimes, compromise solutions have to be reached.

Effective communication also involves establishing good relations with individuals in the different agencies. Staff may well do all they can to work to set criteria, but the fact is that, in the real world, it is easier to negotiate with a person if some basic trust and understanding has already been built up through previous contact: attendance at meetings, perhaps, or at assessments or training sessions.

Joint training is an excellent way to develop understanding of each other's services, and the roles and restrictions that different agencies are bound by. Staff can develop common knowledge of legislation and requirements and what it means for different organizations. Work exchanges between agencies can also be arranged, so that workers learn first-hand about the way other services operate.

With regard to assessment, it is essential to bring in everyone involved with an individual and to include non-medical and voluntary sector workers as well as those from the statutory sector. That step alone could make an enormous difference to ongoing perceptions in the voluntary sector of being denigrated by statutory sector staff. Proper assessments are instrumental in ensuring a containing and well-boundaried holistic package for some of the complex cases in the homelessness field.

Homeless people tend to be a low priority for statutory services. The multi-layered and polymorphous problems they present with make it difficult to identify which service would be most appropriate for individuals to be referred to if they suffer, for instance, from a combination of poly-drug and alcohol abuse, mental health problems and physical illnesses, as is often the case, on top of their need for accommodation. Add to this a chaotic lifestyle, which makes it hard for people to even keep appointments, and the chances of success seem slim. Agencies sometimes fear opening a Pandora's Box should they take on the homeless population in addition to their normal workload. With the pressures of limited resources there is often, understandably, a strong defence against working with them. Good liaison between agencies can help to counter that defence.

The homeless tend to be seen as outsiders by society and anyway often place themselves in that role, acting out their disaffection. The social exclusion of homeless people all too often feeds these existing feelings of alienation, feelings that frequently have a genesis in early attachment problems, traumas and deprivations. Thus initial difficulty in engaging can, once overcome, turn around to become an over-attachment to a particular worker or a constant demand to meet their multifarious needs. Individual members of staff cannot manage this single-handedly.

Homeless agencies themselves can, through association, be placed in the outsider position by mainstream organizations, often as a result of anxieties about the client group or in response to the fears of the community as a whole. To counter this, agencies should support rather than belittle, and everyone in the sector needs to be clear about the responsibilities and boundaries of their work. Strategies need to be drawn up collaboratively, involving housing, social and health care, and the police and the probation service as well as the voluntary sector.

In cities where there is a concentration of homeless people, specific services need to be instituted. GP surgeries that work solely with the homeless have a significant impact, especially when they have mental health and substance abuse workers attached, or coming in for dedicated sessions. Agency staff can go out to meet the client in their own settings, such as hostels, night shelters and day centres, either informally or to run organized surgeries on those projects. Street outreach work is an essential component in areas where people are sleeping rough. Good liaison is crucial and the three areas mentioned above, of communication, training and assessment, should be thought through. Some areas set up umbrella bodies to offer training in homelessness issues, give advice and further good liaison and networking. The statutory sector needs to involve itself in such worthwhile bodies and help to fund them.

In smaller towns and rural areas, where there are fewer homeless people, there needs to be a similar approach whereby staff go out to meet homeless people and attempt to engage them in their own environments. It may not be possible to set up designated services, due to unpredictable local need, but it can be helpful to designate named individuals within each agency who have specific responsibility for the homeless. Small hostels and shelters that meet local needs and have designated routes out into move-on accommodation should be encouraged, supported, properly resourced and linked in with statutory agencies.

This may go some of the way towards meeting the concerns in 'Hamden'. It may, if properly resourced, also meet the needs identified in the Crane and Warnes' survey (2001), that is: for targeted input from specialist mental health and substance abuse services, the involvement of social service and community care assessments and the provision of supported move-on accommodation.

Homelessness is a problem that is unlikely to disappear from our society. There will always be people who don't quite fit the community they find themselves in, who become displaced through circumstance, and who at certain points in their lives suffer crises and traumas, often repeatedly. Like all of us, they are entitled to receive services appropriate to their situation, condition and need.

Questions for further discussion

1. What are likely to have been the main causes of homelessness in single people?
2. In this chapter, examples are given of negative attitudes towards voluntary workers, on the part of statutory workers. Do you have any examples of this from your own practice?
3. What lessons can we learn about collaboration between statutory and voluntary services from the examples in this chapter?

References

Bahr, H. and Caplow, T. (1974) *Old Men Drunk and Sober*. New York University Press, New York.

Big Issue (2000) issue no. 416, December.

Crane, M. (1999) *Understanding Older Homeless People*. Open University Press, Buckingham.

Crane, M. and Warnes, A. (2001) *Single Homeless People in London*, SISA.

Crisis (2003) *How Many, How Much*. Crisis, London.

Diaz, R. (2003) *Housing and homelessness in England, the facts*. Shelter factsheet.

Erikson, E. (1982) *The Life Cycle Completed, A Review*. W. W. Norton, New York.

Flemen, K. (1999) *Room for Drugs – Drug Use on Premises*. Release, London.

Homelessness Directorate (2002) *Homelessness Statistics June 2002, Policy Briefing 1*. the Office of the Deputy Prime Minister, London.

Homeless Link (2002) *Supporting People with Multiple Needs*. Homeless Link.

Lemos, G. and Goodby, G. (1999) *A Future Foretold – New Approaches to Meeting the Long-term Needs of Single Homeless People*. Crisis, London.

Merton, R. (1968) *Social Theory and Social Structure*. (3rd edn) Free Press, Glencoe, IL.

Northmore, S. (2001) in S. Balloch and M. Taylor (eds) *Partnership Working* The Policy Press, Bristol.

Parker, H., Aldridge, J. and Measham, F. (1998) *Illegal Leisure: The Normalisation of Adolescent Drug Use*. Routledge, London.

Pleace, N. and Quilgars, D. (1996) *Health and Homelessness in London: A Review*. King's Fund, London.

Property People (2000) issue no. 268, December.

Roberts, C. J. R. (1984) The New Jerusalem, *Nighlight, The Night Shelter Magazine*. St Martin's Housing Trust, Norwich.

Rutter, M. (1971) Parent-child separation: psychological effects on the children, *Journal of Child Psychology and Psychiatry*, 12.

Social Exclusion Unit (2002) *Reducing Re-offending by Ex-prisoners*, Social Exclusion Unit.

10

Partnership approaches to working with people with HIV

Ruth Wilson

This chapter will:

- Present an overview of how and why multidisciplinary and multi-agency working are essential in caring for people with the Human Immunodeficiency Virus (HIV).
- Explore the specific issues that confront staff in this rapidly changing and developing area.

Introduction

There are currently 49,500 people living with HIV in the UK and numbers continue to rise with new diagnoses increasing by 20 per cent between 2002 and 2003 (Health Protection Agency 2004). Each year since 1999, the number of new HIV diagnoses in heterosexuals has exceeded the number of new diagnoses of homosexual/bisexual men, with a threefold increase from 1996 to 2002 of infections that were heterosexually acquired – now accounting for 57 per cent of the total number. Three-quarters of the total of heterosexually acquired infections were probably acquired in Africa and two-thirds were in women. However, the number of infections acquired as a result of sex between men also continues to rise steadily, with 1,671 diagnoses in 2002. Further, more up-to-date reports have been subject to delays (Health Protection Agency 2003).

For many people living with HIV, treatment with Highly Active Antiretroviral Therapy (HAART) has led to dramatic health improvements. HIV, a disease once considered uniformly fatal, has become a chronic illness (Carpenter *et al.* 1997; Brashers *et al.* 1999). The combined use of Viral Load and CD_4 monitoring and HAART have revolutionized HIV treatment, with consequent declines in morbidity and mortality (Gazzard 1996; Carpenter *et al.* 1997). People who were once given limited life expectancy are returning to work and leading full lives once again. The treatment consists of combinations of antiretroviral drugs that require strict adherence in order to suppress viral replication and prevent resistance developing (Chesney *et al.*

1999; Carr and Cooper 2000; Paterson *et al.* 2000). For some people HAART has given them a renewed life and a future, for others, drug resistance, side effects and treatment failures have brought increased difficulties. Recovery remains fragile, the future uncertain and the psychological ramifications unclear (Rabkin and Ferrando 1997; Sowell *et al.* 1998; Anderson and Weatherburn 1998; Brashers *et al.* 1999).

The multidisciplinary team model of HIV care has evolved out of necessity due to the social impact of the disease, clinical needs and diverse characteristics of people with HIV (Pinching 1998; Sherer *et al.* 2002). The recommended standards for NHS HIV services set out by MedFASH (2002) clearly state that services should be person-centred, developed in partnership, equitable, integrated and outcome orientated, and stress the importance of drawing on the knowledge and skills of health and social care professionals across a multidisciplinary HIV health care team, including primary, social and specialist services. However, as Molyneux (2001) points out, there are challenges when working together in teams – disagreement, confusion, lack of cohesion, professional jealousy and poor communication. Inter-professional teams work well when there is good communication; respect for other professions; committed, professional staff; and when the opportunity is available to develop creative working methods from within the team. This relies on the professional maturity of members within the team. Staff who are sufficiently confident in their own role and professional identity are able to share ideas and expertise within the team and work effectively together in a user-focused way, allowing flexible boundaries to develop within the team. It is difficult to form collaborative ties when one is unsure of one's professional identity (Dombeck 1997), whereas an egalitarian working style allows trust and confidence to develop.

Working in a multidisciplinary way with people with HIV therefore presents a number of challenges for professionals as indicated in Box 10.1.

Box 10.1 Challenges facing professionals working with people with HIV

- The challenge for the multidisciplinary team of caring for people with HIV across the boundaries of primary, secondary and tertiary care.
- The challenge of conception, pregnancy and childbirth faced by the multidisciplinary team.
- The challenge of treatment with Highly Active Antiretroviral Therapy (HAART).
- The challenge of adherence to HAART.
- The challenge of developing and maintaining partnerships between organizations involved in the monitoring, care and treatment of people with HIV.

This chapter will address each of the above challenges in turn.

The challenge of caring for people with HIV across the boundaries of primary, secondary and tertiary care

HIV is the only chronic and potentially fatal condition for which a patient is able to attend a hospital clinic directly, bypassing the GP. This may mean that the useful information the GP has about the home situation and other social and psychological issues is unavailable. Community nurse specialists/liaison nurses have the unique opportunity to cross the boundaries of primary and secondary care and into the patient's home. Gay men and drug users often have poor links with primary care services due to stigma and attitudes towards their lifestyle, as well as being a highly mobile population. Fears about medical reports for life insurances and mortgages may cause some patients to decline shared care. This means that issues of confidentiality need to be discussed and resolved within the primary care multidisciplinary team to create a 'safe' environment for the patient.

The multidisciplinary team may include the following members (depending on individual circumstances) when working with people with HIV:

- Community/liaison nurses
- General Practitioners
- Health advisors
- Dietitians
- Occupational therapists
- Physiotherapists
- Clinical psychologists
- Mental health nurses
- Psychosexual counsellors
- Social workers
- Chaplains
- Consultant physicians
- Sexual health clinic nurses
- Health visitors
- Midwives
- Pharmacists
- Welfare rights advisors
- Complementary therapists
- Voluntary organizations
- Housing departments

The role that each member or organization plays when working with people with HIV is discussed within this chapter.

Education, training and support from the HIV specialist services will enable skill sharing and staff with any uncertainty should feel at ease in asking for help from specialists. Moreover, according to Theobald (2002), patients respect this and feel more confident if it is done. In fact, although GPs may have few contacts with HIV-positive people, well-managed shared care with good communication can reduce hospital outpatient visits and the length of any inpatient stays (Theobald

2002). If primary care staff have had little or no involvement prior to the terminal stages of the illness, there is little opportunity for any relationships to develop, which creates difficulties for both staff and patients. Community nurses may be involved in the administration and supervision of medication, care of dressings and medium- and long-term intravenous access sites, parenteral feeding and personal care, when necessary.

As well as their involvement in primary care, the team is also involved at the hospital outpatient clinic during routine visits and with any inpatient admission. In addition, each team member possesses valuable information regarding dimensions of HIV care that are necessary in planning, implementing and evaluating a patient's individualized care. Health advisors, for example, provide advice on safer sex and sexual health screening, as well as dealing with the sensitive issue of contact tracing. Health care professionals also help patients come to terms with their diagnosis and reveal it appropriately to others, in particular sexual partners they may put at risk. Trust is ultimately more powerful than any coercion and is essential in helping people work through the shame, guilt and fear associated with HIV infection and in dealing with any rejection and broken relationships that may result from disclosure. However, establishing trust may be difficult due to suspicion and fear, particularly with patients from different ethnic backgrounds.

Dietitians have an important role in assessing the patient's nutritional status and ensuring they have an adequate, nutritious and culturally appropriate diet. Dietitians regularly monitor weight, size and shape, using the Body Mass Index to give an accurate guide to any significant wasting. If nutritional support is needed they will advise on dietary supplements, appetite stimulants, anti-emetics and anti-diarrhoeals, as well as discussing food safety with patients who are susceptible to food poisoning because their immune system is compromised (i.e. if CD_4 is below 200). This would include advice on the safe purchase and storage of perishable foods, hand washing and kitchen hygiene generally, ensuring all fish, meat, poultry and eggs are thoroughly cooked and tap water is boiled for one minute before drinking or using to wash salads and so on, and to avoid water-borne infections such as cryptosporidiosis. Dietitians also advise on dietary requirements of HAART and give advice on metabolic abnormalities that may occur as side effects (Morlese 2002). Any facial lipoatrophy and lipodystrophy (body fat redistribution) detected may require changes to treatment and referral for specialist treatment. Discussion with the wider multidisciplinary team may highlight financial difficulties which impact on the individual's ability to buy appropriate food, which can be addressed in the short term by applications to local and national HIV charities and by referral to welfare rights organizations such as the Citizens' Advice Bureau and also to social services, the Benefits Agency or asylum services, if appropriate. Local churches and other faith groups may also offer financial and practical assistance. For very sick and weak patients the dietitian may advise artificial feeding through an appropriate route. This could be via a nasogastric tube that goes through the nose and directly into the stomach, or a tube through the abdominal wall into the stomach (a gastrostomy) or other part of the gut. Patients whose gut is not functioning properly may be given total food replacement through a central venous catheter. This may be very traumatic for the patient and the involvement of a psychologist or counsellor may be required in accepting this treatment.

Another important member of the multidisciplinary team is the occupational therapist, who will assess whether adaptations are necessary to the home and procure equipment (such as bath rails, level access showers, etc.) to facilitate activities of daily living. Any mobility difficulties will also be assessed by a physiotherapist. Such difficulties might result from side effects of medication, such as peripheral neuropathy, or following a period of artificial ventilation and immobilization, enabling the person to develop strength and confidence in their own ability again. Physical and psychological causes of loss of libido and erectile dysfunction also need to be investigated and treated. These may be side effects of medication or result from the psychological impact of HIV. The person may fear transmitting the virus and, therefore, a clinical psychologist or sexual health counsellor would help them to explore and resolve these issues. The clinical psychologist can also offer psychological assessment of HIV-related brain impairment and assessment of safety issues in HIV dementia and confusional states. Recognizing the spiritual dimension to every person is essential but particularly for people who have been given a potentially life-threatening diagnosis. Involving the appropriate chaplain in the ongoing care of patients is, therefore, important.

Social services staff will also be involved in planning the discharge of patients from the inpatient setting. They will ensure appropriate home care services are in place and assess access requirements to accommodation, as well as the needs of any children in the family. Social worker involvement varies between centres, with some having a dedicated specialist social work team and others using generic social workers for the hospital or community. Encouraging patients to allow a referral to generic social services remains a challenge for health care staff due to patients' fears regarding confidentiality and where and how information about them may be stored. In cases where a *specialist* social worker attends the multidisciplinary team meetings within the health care setting, patients normally see them as part of the team and needs can be identified and met appropriately.

Confidentiality may present particular problems for the multidisciplinary team when dealing with a gay man whose family have little or no knowledge of his lifestyle, living arrangements or his HIV diagnosis. For the inpatient this may be a particular problem regarding next of kin. In these circumstances a living will may be a useful tool in defining a person's wishes about who is consulted with regard to their care. If the man decides to disclose to his family, having appropriate people within the multidisciplinary team, such as a psychologist or a specialist mental health worker, who are able to talk to them sensitively, listen to their fears and anxieties and answer their questions is essential.

The nursing care of someone with HIV is no different to the care of any other person with a chronic illness with periods of acute exacerbation. The differences arise because of the external factors such as stigma, fear and contagion, and attitudes towards sexual orientation associated with HIV. All nurses have the appropriate skills to care for the person with HIV. The HIV specialist staff need to support generic staff, enhancing their knowledge and skills rather than deskilling them. The wider multidisciplinary team can have an important role in addressing the fears and concerns above and to enable assessment of how HIV is affecting the whole person. It is important to see the patient in relation to their illness, not as a person with an illness.

Palliative care

Death is part of life and the process of dying is living the end of life. People need acceptance, love, the ability to give love, refuge or sanctuary, safety, comfort and belonging. The multidisciplinary team needs to facilitate this process for the person who is dying with HIV/AIDS. There may be particular difficulties for the person rejected by their family because of HIV or those living alone in a foreign country, separated from friends and family and unable or unwilling to disclose their condition to them. The person will need support from different members of the multidisciplinary team, such as the psychologist or counsellor as well as the nursing team, as they attempt to come to terms with dying. There may also be cultural aspects of death and dying that need to be identified and accommodated. It is important for the staff team to have adequate facilities to debrief, such as regular clinical supervision, when working with people who are dying. Multidisciplinary meetings, with input from a clinical psychologist, counsellor or mental health nurse, can help facilitate discussion of feelings aroused by patient deaths or if there is a conflict between medical opinion and the patient's wishes, either in person or through a living will (also known as an advance directive). A living will that is completed when the person is competent, outlining their wishes for treatment and care if they become incompetent to make that decision, should be adhered to (Department of Health 2001a).

The challenge of conception, pregnancy and childbirth faced by the multidisciplinary team

In the case of a couple where one partner is HIV positive and the other is HIV negative, consideration should be given to the options to prevent transmission of the virus when they are trying to conceive. The HIV-positive woman who has a negative partner can inseminate herself using sperm from her partner thus avoiding unprotected sexual contact. For the HIV-positive man with a negative partner there is the option of sperm washing and insemination at specialist centres. These challenges indicate how HIV intrudes into the intimate life of patients, making something that is usually private and special into something that has to be discussed openly.

In 1999 the government introduced targets to increase the uptake of antenatal testing for HIV to 90 per cent of all pregnant mothers by the end of 2002 and to reduce mother-to-baby transmission of HIV by 80 per cent. Accurate figures are not yet available due to reporting delays, but it is currently estimated that HIV detection rates in 2002 were as follows:

London	75 per cent
England and Wales	85 per cent
Scotland	73 per cent

This increase in detection has reduced the number of children infected vertically in London from 19 per cent in 1997 to 8 per cent in 2002, and from 22 per cent to 6 per cent in the rest of the United Kingdom (Health Protection Agency 2003). In order to facilitate antenatal testing, midwives have been trained in pre- and post-test counselling. Mothers who are found to be HIV positive are offered interventions that can reduce transmission of the virus to between 1 and 2 per cent of babies. Guidelines giving up-to-date information on interventions to reduce the risk of mother-to-child transmission of the virus have been drawn up using best evidence (and expert opinion where limited evidence exists) by a multidisciplinary group of clinicians and lay workers active in the management of pregnant women infected with HIV. These include taking antiretroviral therapy, either AZT monotherapy or combination therapy in the latter weeks of pregnancy (dependant on Viral Load and CD_4 results); intravenous AZT during delivery by elective bloodless caesarean section; AZT syrup for the baby for the first six weeks of life and not breastfeeding (Lyall *et al.* 2001). It is extremely traumatic for the woman diagnosed as HIV positive in pregnancy. She not only has to deal with her own diagnosis and its implications for herself and her partner, but also decisions regarding treatment and delivery of her child. Liaison with obstetricians and paediatricians is essential with regard to antenatal care, delivery and postnatal care of mother and baby. Community midwives and health visitors have an important role in supporting mothers not to breastfeed, which may be extremely difficult for some mothers to contemplate or explain, particularly if their family is unaware of their diagnosis or if there is a strong cultural expectation to breastfeed.

Children who are found to be HIV positive are referred to tertiary centres often some distance from the District General Hospital. For this partnership to be successful it is vital that clear, effective lines of communication are established between the different centres in order to provide efficient and safe management of patients and accurate dissemination of information regarding treatments. The tertiary centre can share its knowledge and expertise while local workers can identify the appropriate local services (White 2001). Any referral for shared care highlights concerns about confidentiality and disclosure for the family. The family's confidence needs to be gained by health care staff so they are open to referral to appropriate services and can gain benefit from shared care. The family affected by HIV may have experienced previous losses to HIV and more than one family member may be infected. Parents of a child with HIV have to cope with their guilt at transmitting HIV to their child and face the difficult decision of what, when and how to tell their child about their condition. They will therefore require skilled workers to explore the options open to them and their implications. HIV is a complex burden for a young person who is developing his or her own sexual identity to carry and requires sensitive handling by parents and specialist staff.

The challenge of treatment with Highly Active Antiretroviral Therapy (HAART)

The introduction of HAART has led to longer life expectancy and dramatic reduction in death rates for people with HIV. However, uncertainty remains about the long-term effectiveness of treatment and patients' ability to continue treatment and tolerate side effects (Sowell *et al.* 1998; Brashers *et al.* 1999; Bogart *et al.* 2000; Rabkin *et al.* 2000). No studies have been followed long enough to determine what the eventual improvement in prognosis will be, although death rates remain low nine years after the introduction of antiretrovirals used in combination therapy (Gazzard 2002). Given current knowledge, people will have to stay on antiretrovirals for the remainder of their lives, which is very difficult to do (Bertholen *et al.* 1999). Concomitant infection with hepatitis or tuberculosis may mean additional treatment, with great potential for drug interactions (Pratt 2003) requiring input from other specialists. Excellent communication between services is, therefore, essential in monitoring treatment effectiveness and adherence.

The change of HIV from a fatal illness to a chronic disease as a result of HAART demands dramatic psychological changes for individuals as they face the challenge of restructuring an unexpected future (Sowell *et al.* 1998; Brashers *et al.* 1999; Klyma *et al.* 2001). People who had been contemplating their own death may now be facing returning to work, rebuilding relationships and having to redefine their identity (Kalichman and Ramachandran 1999). Unexpected revival also has financial implications. People who were aware of their limited life expectancy and had relied on state benefits, cashed in their insurance policies and lived what they believed was the last part of their life to the full. They are now facing giving up the security of these entitlements and returning to work, despite having limited evidence of the long-term effects of these medications (Rabkin and Ferrando 1997). This uncertainty, the magnitude and duration of improvement, the burden of an unremitting and onerous drug regime, anxiety about lapses in adherence and also the complex issues that an unanticipated future brings means the psychological burden of the illness remains (Anderson and Weatherburn 1998; Sowell *et al.* 1998; Trainor and Ezer 2000; Rabkin *et al.* 2000). A second life brings with it complex issues that seem largely irrelevant when there seems to be little time left and people are faced with balancing the idea of life being worth living now and in the future against sinking into a narrowing existence due to the limitations HAART and its side effects may put on their life.

Prior to HAART, Kaposi's Sarcoma, which causes purplish-black lesions on the skin, mucous membrane or internal organs, was for many a visible sign of HIV disease. This has largely disappeared due to the restoration of people's immune systems. However, as the length of time people have been taking HAART increases, the emergence of longer-term side effects of treatment, such as lipodystrophy, are causing similar problems for patients (Collins *et al.* 2000; Martinez *et al.* 2001). Lipodystrophy is a visible marker of HIV disease creating a similar look in many people to that of the HIV wasting, particularly in the face, common prior to treatment with HAART. It can also lead to the development of a hump on the back of the neck, as well as increased chest and trunk fat with shrinkage of the buttocks, arms and legs. This easily identifies a person taking antiretrovirals to many of their peers and can have a negative effect on individuals' psychological and social lives, which can also impact their quality of life causing low self-esteem, isolation, depression and narrowing of the patients' social world (Collins *et al.* 2000; Power *et al.* 2003).

Peripheral neuropathy is another disabling side effect of some HIV medication. It is important that the patient is aware of this and monitors for its development alongside the physician and specialist nurse so that a change in treatment can be instigated if necessary. Some patients may require the involvement of a neurologist, pharmacist and physiotherapist in its management and treatment.

People with HIV are seen regularly for follow-up, usually at three-monthly intervals when the Viral Load, CD_4 count and other routine tests are measured. For those on treatment there is the constant fear of treatment failure, raised lipids and abnormal liver function tests. Attendance at the outpatient clinic is a reminder of HIV and the ongoing need for monitoring of the disease process. The response to treatment failure is influenced by the patients' treatment history. A person who has had a number of regime changes as a result of failure becomes psychologically prepared (Kalichman and Ramachandran 1999), but they may need help to grieve, mourning the loss of hope and expressing anger, guilt and resentment.

The challenge of adherence to HAART

Since the advent of HAART we have seen dramatic improvements in CD_4 counts, Viral Loads and mortality among HIV-positive people, but these benefits are contingent on patients' adherence to treatment. Adherence in chronic diseases ranges from 15 to 93 per cent with average estimates of around 50 per cent (Meichenbaum and Turk 1987; Singh *et al.* 1996; Dunbar-Jacob *et al.* 2000). Regimes of antiretrovirals are relatively inflexible and the need to maintain adequate levels of drug in the bloodstream means that patients must achieve near perfect adherence in order to give themselves the best possible chance of sustained viral suppression (Carr and Cooper 2000; Chesney 2000; Paterson *et al.* 2000). If adequate adherence is not maintained, the patient is likely to develop resistance to some or all classes of antiretrovirals and not only face treatment failure but also may transmit resistant virus to any people he or she subsequently infects. As Rabkin and Chesney (1999) state, adherence is, therefore, not only a personal but also a public health issue. Combination therapy for HIV illness is perhaps the most rigorous, demanding and unforgiving of any oral outpatient treatment ever introduced, and may be prescribed for some patient without any current symptoms (Rabkin and Chesney 1999). To be effective HAART has to maintain the balance between quality of life and quantity of life. People need to be able to live their life on therapy and live well.

Barriers to adherence

The literature indicates that adherence to treatment is difficult in the following circumstances:

- if the regime is complex;
- if there are side effects;
- if the demand is long-term;
- if the regime interferes with daily living routines;
- where support and communications are non-optimum.

HAART fulfils all these criteria (Sherr 2000). Adhering to medication is more difficult when the illness is chronic and the treatments are largely prophylactic (Loveday 2003). Patients who have never been ill as a result of HIV, but started treatment as a result of their CD_4 and Viral Load test results reaching the treatment range (BHIVA 2003) may not realize the significance of adherence to their treatment, or have the same commitment as someone who has been very ill as a result of HIV. It is difficult to gain a sense of the seriousness of their illness with only blood test results and the doctor's advice to rely on and when viral resistance seems unreal. Those who have 'returned from the dead' as a result of HAART are more focused on their treatment. There is a need for excellent patient education and follow-up to facilitate the best adherence possible and to ensure patients are aware of the virological consequences of poor adherence (Anderson and Weatherburn 1998 and 1999).

Patients with little or no social support are more likely to have difficulties with adherence (Anderson and Weatherburn 1999) and, therefore, may rely heavily on the team caring for them. For many, professionals involved in their care are the only people aware of their diagnosis and the burden of secrecy they are carrying. There are also many barriers to adherence evident within the literature, as indicated in Box 10.2.

Box 10.2 Potential barriers to adherence to HAART

- Depression
- Current drug use
- Homelessness
- Alcohol use
- Concerns about confidentiality at home or work
- The constant reminder of HIV
- Dietary restrictions
- The nature and severity of side effects
- Medication being too large to carry conveniently
- Inconvenient dosing schedules
- Difficulty remembering
- Ethno-cultural factors such as a differing world view or lack of understanding of cultural influences
- Lack of knowledge or understanding about treatments
- Immigration difficulties
- Irregular working patterns
- Time and family pressures
- Financial insecurity
- Scepticism

(Chesney et al. 1995; Singh et al. 1996; Crespo-Fierro 1997; Rabkin and Chesney 1999; Catz et al. 2000; Mellins et al. 2003)

Multidisciplinary teamwork can, however, improve adherence, and research has shown that patients who received help from social services, transportation, mental health and chemical dependency were more likely to remain in contact with the HIV services (Sherer et al. 2002). Many African people receive an AIDS diagnosis alongside their HIV diagnosis as they often present late for testing (Del Amo 1996) and need to start treatment quickly. They, therefore, have little time to build trusting relationships with health care staff. They may perceive their illness from a religious or spiritual standpoint in which it is a manifestation of evil or a sign from God (King 1999). They might, therefore, reject any HIV care, believing that God will cure them through prayer. Plans to encourage and enhance adherence must incorporate person-specific variables and be tailored to individualized needs (Crespo-Fierro 1997) – the multidisciplinary team is well placed to do this.

Promoting adherence

The best combination for every patient is the combination they are willing and able to take (Catz *et al.* 2000), and efforts to maximize adherence must be started before the prescription is dispensed (Daar *et al.* 2003). Patients need to be *ready* to start treatment (Enriquez *et al.* 2004) and will be more likely to adhere if they have a clear understanding about HIV disease (Rabkin and Chesney 1999; Weiss *et al.* 2003). Reducing the pill burden increases the level of adherence (Altice and Friedland 1998; Anderson and Weatherburn 1999; Chesney 2000), and doctors will aim for the fewest tablets at the fewest dosing times. However, research has shown that it is the ease with which the regime is accommodated into the patient's daily routine that is crucial (Singh *et al.* 1996; Stone *et al.* 2001).

Multidisciplinary discussion prior to treatment commencing enables potential barriers to adherence to be identified and appropriate referrals and action to be taken. An example of this in practice is shown in the case study in Box 10.3.

Box 10.3 Case study of adherence to treatment

Alice lives alone and none of her family, friends or colleagues is aware of her HIV diagnosis. She works two nights a week in a nursing home and also for a care agency on four or five other days each week but doesn't have a regular shift pattern.

Due to her declining test results the medical consultant planned to start Alice on HAART, however, following discussion in the multidisciplinary team meeting it became clear from other team members, combined with knowledge of Alice's work pattern and the potential side effects of Efavirenz, that the regime initially considered would be very difficult for Alice to adhere to.

An alternative regime was suggested taking into consideration Alice's blood test results and social requirements and the specialist nurse worked with Alice to identify the times she could take it 12 hours apart and on an empty stomach as the regime required. Incorporating her work, eating and sleeping pattern and the need to take her medication in secret, Alice decided to take it at 6 a.m. and 6 p.m.

Despite having to set her alarm to wake her at 6 a.m. when she is not working a night shift, Alice continues to adhere well to her regime, having been part of the decision-making process and committing herself to taking her medication at these times.

N.B. Names have been changed to protect patient confidentiality.

The Department of Health has identified the need for patients to become 'experts' about their own health. Doctors, nurses and other health professionals who undertake long-term follow-up and care of people with chronic diseases have recognized for many years that their patients understand their disease better than they do, and this knowledge and experience has been an untapped resource. Today's patients with chronic diseases need not be mere recipients of care – they can become key decision makers in the treatment process. By ensuring that knowledge of their condition is developed to a point where they are empowered to take some responsibility for its management and work in partnership with their health and social care providers, patients can be given greater control over their lives (Department of Health 2001b).

Multidisciplinary working encourages collaborative treatment decision making and physician–patient partnerships lead to greater satisfaction and higher adherence for patients (Anderson and Zimmerman 1993; Chesney *et al.* 1999; Paterson 2001). Through talking with the patient about what they understand about HIV, its spread and treatment, multidisciplinary team members can begin to understand and work with the patient to build on this knowledge, thus enhancing the patient's autonomy. Mutual respect and trust develops between the team and the patient, encouraging people to participate as equal partners in decisions about the health care they receive (Opie 1998). The goal of treatment plans is not to hand over the decision making to the patient, but rather to promote non-judgemental dialogue and negotiation between patients and the team (Lerner *et al.* 1998).

Time spent with the doctor is usually limited and patients are often daunted, feeling more able to talk and confide in a nurse or social worker that they may meet for longer and perhaps in their own home. The nurse–patient relationship is a powerful tool that greatly affects adherence. In most settings it is the nurse who provides patient education surrounding treatment regimes and who is often privy to patients' reported challenges associated with adherence (Crespo-Fierro 1997; Halkitis and Kirton 1999). The community nurse specialist also has insight into the real home situation and can evaluate how this will impact on adherence. A genuine collaboration between patients and their health care providers regarding preferences and available options is essential. Identifying potential side effects of medication enables discussion with the individual about what they are prepared to tolerate. For example, one antiretroviral – Efavirenz (Sustiva ©) – can cause vivid dreams and nightmares. For some people this is not a problem, others are unable to tolerate them. It is essential for the multidisciplinary team to address the behavioural aspects of HIV therapies, taking account of optimal meal schedules, dietary considerations and dosing schedules, particularly with regard to holidays and travel (Kalichman and Ramachandran 1999) and to identify the difficulties patients face in their lives and to try to resolve them. This may involve referring them to a drug treatment programme, nutritionist, psychiatrist, pharmacist, case manager, welfare rights adviser, immigration solicitor or housing department (Gerbert *et al.* 2000). Partnership with HIV support centres is important as they can provide valuable information, advice, peer support, counselling and often therapies such as reflexology and aromatherapy massage that are important in enabling patients to maintain adherence to medication.

There are many ways in which adherence can be enhanced, as indicated in Box 10.4, adapted from Rabkin are Chesney 1999 and Loveday 2003.

In addition to the techniques in Box 10.4, referral to a psychologist for relaxation and guided imagery training and cognitive restructuring to focus on positive aspects

---

Box 10.4 Techniques to improve adherence

- Use of weekly or daily pill boxes
- Printed medication charts
- Alarms on watches or key fobs
- Identification of lifestyle triggers and cues
- Designing a draft plan that integrates pill doses to established daily activities (e.g. keeping pills by the kettle or at the bedside)
- Using dummy pills or jelly sweets for trial runs
- Identification and resolution of dysfunctional attitudes

---

of treatment is also useful. Culturally appropriate leaflets and information using CD-ROMs and videos about how pills are to be taken and possible side effects are useful tools provided by various HIV charities and information services and regular feedback of CD_4 and Viral Load test results by medical staff encourages continued adherence.

Confidentiality can be breached inadvertently, particularly when people live in close-knit communities (Gorna 1994), which leads to reluctance to fill in prescriptions in their home neighbourhood and hiding or relabelling medications to maintain secrecy within the home (Working Group on Antiretroviral Therapy and Medical Management of Infants, Children and Adolescents with HIV Infection 1998). Lack of disclosure of HIV creates specific problems, for example, having to store drugs in a refrigerator that may be available to others, or in a situation where a wider or extended family are living together. Finding appropriate, secret storage for medicines and disposal of packaging, continually hiding the process of taking medication at specific times and making plans and excuses for having medication are ongoing difficulties facing people on treatment for HIV and has the potential to interfere with adherence to treatment. An example of how staff can help patients to deal with this is shown in Box 10.5 opposite.

The challenge of developing and maintaining partnerships between organizations

Treatment for HIV is commenced when a person's blood test results and clinical picture reach limits set out in the BHIVA guidelines (BHIVA 2003). The British HIV Association is a 600-member association with a commitment to provide excellence in the care of HIV-infected individuals. Their aims are the relief of sickness, and protection and preservation of health through the development and promotion of good practice in the treatment of HIV and HIV-related illnesses, and to advance public education in the subjects of HIV and the symptoms, causes, treatment and prevention of HIV-related illnesses through the promotion of research and the dissemination of the useful results of such research (www.bhiva.org.uk 2004). Members are drawn from all disciplines and have also formed the Children's HIV Association of UK and Ireland (CHIVA), the Dietitians HIV Association (DHIVA), the National HIV Nurses Association (NHIVNA) and the HIV Pharmacists' Association (HIVPA),

---

Box 10.5 Case study of adherence to treatment

Grace is a 23-year-old Zimbabwean who came to England to study two years ago. She lives in a shared house with her two sisters and others from her home town. She shares a room with her older sister. Her parents and wider family remain in Zimbabwe.

Grace was diagnosed HIV positive as part of a routine sexual health screen. She was very shocked at her diagnosis and has decided not to tell anyone outside the clinic about her diagnosis, stating that her sisters would not be able to cope if she told them and they would in turn disclose to her family back in Zimbabwe.

Unfortunately Grace's results showed she needed to start on medication fairly soon after diagnosis. Because of the difficulties in maintaining confidentiality at home, she initially declined medication saying she was unable to hide anything from her sisters as they shared many possessions and had little or no privacy. She also often had to lie in order to attend the outpatient clinic. She began to develop symptoms of depression.

The consultant discussed this within the multidisciplinary team meeting and referral was made to the specialist community mental health nurse and they arranged to meet.

Grace was started on an antidepressant and seen regularly for counselling and monitoring of her mood. She expressed great fear of disclosure but also recognized her need to start medication. Through discussing her fears and developing trust in the specialist nurse, she was able to identify a way she could use a dermatological problem as a reason to explain her need for medication to her sisters.

Grace is now established on her antiretroviral therapy, her confidentiality remains intact and her mental health has improved.

N.B. Names have been changed to protect patient confidentiality.

---

thus providing a breadth of experience and knowledge. Through critical examination of the research and through personal experience, the organization produces clear guidelines that are regularly updated and easily accessible on the internet for the treatment and care of people with HIV. This is essential in disseminating knowledge and sharing best practice to clinical staff, particularly those working outside large treatment centres, ensuring best possible treatment for patients. Due to the rapid changes and developments in treatments and care in HIV this partnership between clinicians and these associations is essential.

Stigma associated with HIV continues and fears, misconceptions and negative attitudes to people with HIV remain prevalent (Alonzo and Reynolds 1995; Anderson and Weatherburn 1998; Katz 1996; Bunting 1996; Brashers *et al.* 1999; Barroso and Powell-Cope 2000; Taylor 2001). Fear of the disintegration of family relationships inhibits patients disclosing their status, even when it is necessary to access services (Anderson *et al.* 2000). HIV disease does not occur in a social vacuum, people who develop HIV infection often belong to a group that has experienced previous social rejection such as gay men, intravenous drug users and people from other ethnic groups (Catalan *et al.* 1995). Many are multiply disadvantaged, particularly those who are migrants to the UK having witnessed or experienced rape, torture or other severe trauma in their home country and have come as refugees with an uncertain future. As a result many are living in poor housing and become isolated due to cultural and language differences and fears about confidentiality. Refugees may take little interest in their health when their prime concern is for their relatives left behind or how they are going to negotiate the asylum system or pay their bills. Mental health problems are common (Himid *et al.* 1998). Counselling and support needs to be made available to help people to deal with the ongoing stigma of HIV and the effects of HAART, as well as managing uncertainty and living with a chronic illness. Many have seen friends and family members with HIV dying and fear the same for themselves, reflecting the situation for many gay men who have seen many of their friends, living and dying with HIV, struggling with adherence to their medication, side effects and drug resistance. These multiple bereavements have a profound effect on the individual who then discovers they are HIV positive themselves. Fear of breach of confidentiality is the most common reason for Africans not accessing HIV services due to the continuing high level of stigmatization of HIV in African communities (McMunn *et al.* 1997). If their diagnosis is discovered, they fear abandonment by their family and social exclusion from previous sources of support such as friends, social networks and cultural groups. Many people do not disclose their diagnosis to anyone outside the health care provider setting and may become isolated as a result.

People with HIV draw their support from a variety of sources, both formal and informal, depending to a large extent on whom they trust, who is around and who makes a difference (Anderson *et al.* 2000). National support agencies such as Terence Higgins Trust, Positively Women, Body and Soul and others offer support groups, information and advice to HIV-positive people. These partners in supporting and caring for the individual with HIV can offer support and provide services in ways that health care professionals are unable to. One important area is in peer support and self-help groups where patients can share personal stories and experiences and learn from each other. For many people, finding a safe place where they can be open about their diagnosis and discuss their fears, hopes, dreams and expectations with others who are facing the same situation is a lifeline. HIV support centres also fulfil an invaluable role in bringing together families affected by HIV to share experiences. Body and Soul, in particular, runs a youth club for teenagers with HIV, enabling them to relate to young people of their own age in a safe environment. There are also many local support centres and networks for people to access – ensuring that patients receive contact details and information about groups is important in maintaining this partnership. Self-referral to the group avoids any conflict over disclosure of confidential information, although an introduction to staff, volunteers or members of the group/centre can facilitate easier integration. The health care team will provide a letter confirming an HIV-positive diagnosis, if required, and may discuss patients' needs with staff with the patient's permission.

For those who have experienced revival as a result of HAART, a crucial decision is whether to give up disability benefits, which, although limited, are secure and predictable, and return to work. Although feeling physically well enough to work, fear of employers' attitudes and trying to explain gaps in their CV due to periods of illness may make them reluctant to apply for jobs and training opportunities, again highlighting the impact of continuing stigma surrounding HIV. However, uncertainty about the durability of treatment response means people are attempting to reconcile the hope of regaining normal relationships, returning to work and having a future with the fear that their improved health may prove only transitory (Brashers *et al.* 1999). Advocacy programmes, advice on state benefits and 'back-to-work' and career counselling, are important facilities provided by many HIV support centres to help people cope with this uncertainty and take control of their life again.

Terence Higgins Trust, Avert and the National AIDS Manual provide excellent written information, covering a wide range of relevant topics, many of which are free to the HIV-positive person. These include a series written for gay men, young people and African men and women, recognizing that different groups require information written in culturally sensitive or age appropriate language. These organizations also provide excellent internet web sites that give accurate information on medical, treatment, and social and welfare issues, enabling people to access information in the privacy of their own home or through one of the local support groups. Magazines such as 'Positive Nation' and '+ve' provide excellent information and social contact details for patients. These are available at most treatment centres and HIV support centres and are free by post to individual patients.

Conclusion

HIV remains a complex and stigmatized disease that challenges professionals to work together to provide holistic, individualized care for patients. Significant advances in treatment mean that HIV, once considered uniformly fatal, is now regarded as a chronic disease. However, treatments are complex and require almost perfect adherence to achieve viral suppression. The rapid developments in treatment and psychosocial knowledge about HIV mean that health care staff need to constantly keep themselves updated in order to incorporate the latest evidence in their work. Being able to call on the knowledge and expertise of specialists and the guidelines produced through BHIVA, CHIVA, DHIVA and NHIVNA is essential in keeping on track with the latest developments. The role of the multidisciplinary team in being able to assess and treat each person as a whole person and from different perspectives has been highlighted, as has the importance of developing a partnership with the patient to enhance adherence to treatment. The need for multi-agency working to enable people to cope with the psychosocial impact of HIV and of treatment with HAART has been discussed and the valuable role support groups and information organizations play in the care of people with HIV has been identified. Many organizations have ceased during recent years due to withdrawal of funding. It is essential that those that remain continue to fulfil this function because of the stigma, prejudice and discrimination related to HIV.

Questions for further discussion

1. The treatment of HIV with HAART has led to increasing complexities of medical treatment. How can members of the multidisciplinary team ensure that they do not lose sight of the patient in the midst of the rapid developments?

2. HIV remains a stigmatized and largely secret disease and further changes of funding away from support and information agencies and towards treatment will leave people even more isolated and vulnerable. How can the multidisciplinary team respond to this challenge?

3. HIV care has largely led the way on holistic, patient-centred care. How are other areas of medicine and social care responding to the challenge?

References

Alonzo, A.A., and Reynolds, N.R. (1995) Stigma, HIV and AIDS: An exploration and elaboration of a stigma trajectory, *Social Science and Medicine*. 41(3): 303–15.

Altice, F.L. and Friedland, G.H. (1998) (Editorial) The era of adherence to HIV therapy, *Annals of Internal Medicine*, 129(6): 503–5.

Anderson, L.A. and Zimmerman, M.A. (1993) Patient and physician perceptions of their relationship and patient satisfaction: a study of chronic disease management, *Patient Education and Counselling*, 20(1): 27–36.

Anderson, W. and Weatherburn, P. (1998) *The Impact of Combination Therapy on the Lives of People with HIV*. Sigma Research, London.

Anderson, W. and Weatherburn, P. (1999) *Taking HAART?: The Impact of Combination Therapy on the Lives of People with HIV*. Sigma Research, London.

Anderson, W., Weatherburn, P., Keogh, P. and Henderson, L. (2000) *Proceeding with Care: Phase 3 of an Ongoing Study of the Impact of Combination Therapies on the Needs of People with HIV*. Sigma Research, London.

Barroso, J. and Powell-Cope, G.M. (2000) Metasynthesis of qualitative research on living with HIV infection, *Qualitative Health Research*, 10(3): 340–53.

Bertholon, D.R., Rossert, H. and Korsia, S. (1999) The patient's perspective on life with antiretroviral treatment: Results of an 887-person survey, *The AIDS Reader*, October, pp. 462–9.

BHIVA Writing committee on behalf of the BHIVA Executive Committee (2003) British HIV Association (BHIVA) guidelines for the treatment of HIV-infected adults with antiretrovirals, *HIV Medicine*, 4(1): 1–41.

Bogart, L.M., Catz, S.L., Kelly, J.A., Gray-Bernhardt, M.L., Hartmann, B.R., Otto-Salaj, L.L., Hackl, K.L. and Bloom, F.R. (2000) Psychosocial issues in the era of new AIDS treatments from the perspective of persons living with HIV, *Journal of Health Psychology*, 5(4): 500–16.

Brashers, D.E., Neidig, J.L., Cardillo, L.K., Russell, J.A. and Haas, S.M. (1999) 'In an important way, I did die': Uncertainty and revival in persons living with HIV or AIDS, *AIDS CARE*, 11(2): 201–19.

Bunting, S.M. (1996) Sources of stigma associated with women with HIV, *Advances in Nursing Science*, 19(2): 64–73.

Carpenter, C.C., Fischl, M.A., Hammer, S.M., Hirsch, M.S., Jacobsen, D.M., Katzenstein, D., Montaner, J.S., Richman, D.D., Saag, M.S., Schooley, R.T., Thompson, M.A., Veella, S., Yeni, P.G. and Volberding, P.A. (1997) Antiretroviral therapy for HIV infection in 1997: Updated Recommendations of the International AIDS Society, *Journal of the American Medical Association*, 277(24): 1962–9.

Carr. A. and Cooper, D.A. (2000) Adverse effects of antiretroviral therapy, *Lancet*, 356(9239): 1423–30.

Catalan, J., Burgess, A. and Klimes, I. (1995) *Psychological Medicine of HIV Infection*. Oxford University Press, Oxford.

Catz, S.L., Kelly, J.A., Bogart, L.M., Benotsch, E.G. and McAuliffe, T.L. (2000) Patterns, correlates and barriers to medication adherence among persons prescribed new treatments for HIV disease, *Health Psychology*, 19(2): 124–33.

Chesney, M., Wall, T., Sorensen, J.L., Batki, S.L., Delucci, K.L. and London, J.A. (1995) Adherence to zidovudine (AZT) among HIV infected methadone patients: A pilot study of supervised therapy and dispensing compared to usual care, *Drug and Alcohol Dependence*, 37: 261–9.

Chesney, M.A., Ickovics, J., Hecht, F.M., Sikipa, G. and Rabkin, J. (1999) Adherence: a necessity for successful HIV Combination Therapy, *AIDS 13* Supplement A S271–8.

Chesney, M.A. (2000) Factors affecting adherence to antiretroviral therapy, *Clinical Infectious Diseases*, 30(2): S171–6.

Collins, E., Wagner, C. and Walmsley, S. (2000) Psychosocial impact of the lipodystrophy syndrome in HIV infection, *The AIDS Reader*, 10(9): 546–51.

Crespo-Fierro, M. (1997) Compliance/adherence and care management in HIV disease, *Journal of the Association of Nurses in AIDS Care*, 8(4): 43–54.

Daar, E.S., Cohen, C., Remien, R., Sherer, R. and Smith, K. (2003) Improving adherence to antiretroviral therapy, *AIDS Reader*, 13(2): 81–90.

Del Amo, J., Goh, B.T. and Forster, G.E. (1996) AIDS defining conditions in Africans resident in the United Kingdom, *International Journal of STDs and AIDS*, 7: 44–7.

Department of Health (2001a) *Reference Guide to Consent for Examination or Treatment*. Department of Health (Crown Copyright), London.

Department of Health (2001b) *The Expert Patient: A New Approach to Chronic Disease Management for the 21st Century*. Department of Health (Crown Copyright), London.

Dombeck, M. (1997) Professional personhood: training, territoriality and tolerance, *Journal of Interprofessional Care*, 11: 9–21.

Dunbar-Jacob, J., Erlen, J.A., Schlenk, E.A., Ryan, C.M., Sereika, S.M. and Doswell, W.M. (2000) Adherence in chronic disease, *Annual Review of Nursing Research*, 18: 48–90.

Enriquez, J., Lackey, N.R., O'Connor, M. and McKinsey, D. (2004) Successful adherence after multiple HIV treatment failures, *Journal of Advanced Nursing*, 45(4): 438–46.

Gazzard, B. (1996) What we know so far, *AIDS*, 10 (Supplement): S3–S7.

Gazzard, B.G. (2002) Natural History of HIV infection, in B.G. Gazzard (ed.) *AIDS Care Handbook*. Mediscript, London.

Gerbert, B., Bronstone, A., Clanon, K., Abercrombie, P. and Bangsberg, D. (2000) Combination antiretroviral therapy: health care providers confront emerging dilemmas, *AIDS Care*, 12(4): 409–21.

Gorna, R. (1994) *Positive Practice* (1st edn). Health Visitor's Association, London.

Halkitis, P.N. and Kirton, C. (1999) Self-strategies as a means of enhancing adherence to HIV antiretroviral therapies: a Rogerian approach, *Journal of the New York State Nurses Association*, 30(2): 22–7.

Health Protection Agency (2003) *Renewing the Focus: HIV and other Sexually Transmitted Infections in the United Kingdom in 2002*. Health Protection Agency, London.

Health Protection Agency (2004) Health Protection Agency warns of impending HIV crisis (Press statement) Health Protection Agency, London.

Himid, K.A., Zwi, K., Welch, J.M. and Ball, C.S. (1998) The development of a community based family HIV service, *AIDS Care*, 10(2): 231–7.

Kalichman, S.K. and Ramachandran, B. (1999) Mental Health Implication of New HIV Treatments, in D.G. Ostrow and S.C. Kalichman (eds) *Psychosocial and Public Health Impacts of new HIV Therapies*. Kluwer Academic/Plenum Publishers, New York.

Katz, A. (1996) Gaining a new perspective on life as a consequence of uncertainty in HIV infection, *Journal of the Association of Nurses in AIDS care*, 7(4): 51–60.

King, B. (1999) Caring for African clients with HIV, *Nursing Management (London)*, 6(6): 14–17.

Kylma, J., Vehvilainen-Jlkunen, K. and Lahdevirta, J. (2001) Hope, despair and hopelessness in living with HIV/AIDS: A grounded theory study, *Journal of Advanced Nursing*, 33(6): 764–75.

Lerner, B., Gulick, R.M. and Dubler, N.N. (1998) Rethinking nonadherence: Historical perspectives on triple-drug therapy for HIV disease, *Annals of Internal Medicine*, 129(7): 573–8.

Loveday, H. (2003) Adherence to antiretroviral therapy in R. Pratt, *HIV & AIDS. A Foundation for Nursing and Health Care Practice*, Arnold, London.

Lyall, E.G.H., Blott, M., de Ruiter, A., Hawkins, D., Mercy, D., Mitchla, Z., Newell, M-L., O'Shea, S., Smith, J.R., Sunderland, J., Webb, R. and Taylor, G.P. (2001) Guidelines for the management of HIV infection in pregnant women and the prevention of mother-to-child transmission: British HIV Association, *HIV Medicine*, 2(4): 314–34.

Martinez, E., Garcia-Viejo, M.A., Blanch, L. and Gatell, J.M. (2001) Lipodystrophy syndrome in patients with HIV infection: Quality of life issues, *Drug Safety*, 24(3): 157–66.

McMunn, A.M., Mwanje, R. and Pozniak, L. (1997) Issues facing Africans in London with HIV infection, *Genitourinary Medicine*, 73(3): 157–8.

Medical Foundation for AIDS and Sexual Health. (2002) *Recommended Standards for NHS HIV Services*. MedFASH, London.

Meichenbaum, D. and Turk, D.C. (1987) Treatment and adherence: terminology, incidence and conceptualisation, *Facilitating Treatment Adherence*. Plenum Press, New York.

Mellins, C.A., Kang, E., Leu, C.S., Havens, J.F. and Chesney, M.A. (2003) Longitudinal study of mental health and psychosocial predictors of medical treatment adherence in mothers living with HIV disease, *AIDS Patient Care and STDs*, 17(8): 407–16.

Molyneux, J. (2001) Interprofessional teamworking: What makes teams work well? *Journal of Interprofessional Care*, 15(1): 29–35.

Morlese, J. (2002) Abnormalities of lipid metabolism and body fat distribution in B.G. Gazzard, (ed.) *AIDS Care Handbook*. Mediscript, London.

Opie, A. (1998) 'Nobody asked me for my view': Users' empowerment by multidisciplinary health teams, *Qualitative Health Research*, 18: 188–206.

Paterson, B. (2001) Myth of empowerment in chronic illness, *Journal of Advanced Nursing*, 34(5): 574–81.

Paterson, D.L., Swindells, S., Mohr, J., Brester, M., Vergis, E.N., Squier, C., Wagener, M.M. and Singh, N. (2000) Adherence to protease inhibitor therapy and outcomes in patients with HIV infection, *Annals of Internal Medicine*, 133: 21–30.

Pinching, A. (1998) In it together, *Nursing Standard*, 12(47): 18.

Power, R., Tate, H.L., McGill, S.M. and Taylor, C. (2003) A qualitative study of the psychosocial implications of Lipodystrophy Syndrome on HIV positive individuals, *Sexually Transmitted Infections*, 79(2): 137.

Pratt, R. (2003) *HIV & AIDS. A Foundation for Nursing and Health Care Practice*. Arnold, London.

Rabkin, J.G., Ferrando, S.J., Lin, S., Sewell, M. and McElhiney M. (2000) Psychological effects of HAART: A 2-year study, *Psychosomatic Medicine*, 62(3): 413–22.

Rabkin, J.G. and Chesney, M. (1999) Treatment adherence to new HIV therapies, the Achilles heel of the new therapeutics, in D.G. Ostrow and S.C. Kalichman (eds) *Psychosocial and Public Health Impacts of new HIV Therapies*. Kluwer Academic/Plenum Publishers, New York.

Rabkin, J.G. and Ferrando, S. (1997) A second life agenda. Psychiatric research issues raised by protease inhibitor treatments for people with the Human Immunodeficiency Virus or the Acquired Immunodeficiency Syndrome, *Archives of General Psychiatry*, 54 November, pp. 1049–53.

Sherer, R., Stieglitz, K., Narra, J., Green, L., Moore, B., Shott, S. and Cohen, M. (2002) HIV multidisciplinary teams work: Support services improve access to and retention in HIV primary care, *AIDS Care*, 14 (1): S31–44.

Sherr, L. (2000) Adherence – sticking to the evidence, *AIDS Care*, 12(4): 373–6.

Singh, N., Squier, C., Sivek, C., Wagener, M., Hong Nguyen, M. and Yu, V. (1996) Determinants of compliance with antiretroviral therapy in patients with HIV: Prospective assessment with implications or enhancing compliance, *AIDS Care*, 8: 261–9.

Sowell, R.L., Phillips, K.D. and Grier, J. (1998) Restructuring life to face the future: the perspective of men after a positive response to protease inhibitor therapy, *AIDS Patient Care and STDs* 12(1): 33–42.

Stone, V.E., Hogan, J.W., Shuman, P., Rompal, A.M., Howard, A.A., Korkontzelou, C. and Smith, D.K. (2001) Antiretroviral regimen complexity, self-reported adherence and HIV patient's understanding of their regimens: survey of women in HER study, *Journal of Acquired Immune Deficiency Syndromes*, 28: 124–31.

Taylor, B. (2001) HIV, stigma and health: integration of theoretical concepts and the lived experience of individuals, *Journal of Advanced Nursing*, 35(5): 792–8.

Theobald, N. (2002) Caring in the community, in B.G. Gazzard (ed.) *AIDS Care Handbook*. Mediscript, London.

Trainor, A. and Ezer, H. (2000) Rebuilding life: The experience of living with AIDS after facing imminent death, *Qualitative Health Research*, 10(5): 646–60.

Weiss, L., French, T., Finkelstein, R., Mukherjee, R. and Agins, B. (2003) HIV-related knowledge and Adherence to HAART, *AIDS Care*, 15(5): 673–9.

White J. (2001) Sharing the care of children with HIV infection, *Nursing Standard*, 15(20): 42–6.

Working Group on Antiretroviral Therapy and Medical Management of Infants, Children and Adolescents with HIV infection (1998) Antiretroviral therapy and medical management of pediatric HIV infection (report), *Pediatrics*, 102(4 Supplement to Pediatrics, Part 2 of 2): 1005–62.

Resources and information

Avert
(AIDS Education and Research Trust)
4 Brighton Road
Horsham
RH13 5BA
Tel: 01403 210202
www.avert.org

Body and Soul
9 Tavistock Place
London
WC1H 9SN
Tel: 020 7383 7678
www.bodyandsoul.demon.co.uk

BHIVA
Tel: 020 8446 9194
www.bhiva.org

i-Base
3rd Floor
Thrale House
44–46 Southwark Street
Bankside
London
SE1 1UN
Tel: 0808 800 6013

National AIDS Helpline
1st floor
8 Matthew Street
Liverpool
L2 6RE
Tel: 0800 567123

National AIDS Manual Publications
16a Clapham Common Southside
London
SW4 7AB
Tel: 0207 627 3200
www.aidsmap.com

National AIDS Trust
New City Cloister
196 Old Street
London
EC1V 9FR
Tel: 020 7814 6767
www.nat.org.uk

+ve Magazine
Eton House
156 High Street
Ruislip
Middlesex
HA4 8IJ
Tel: 01895 637878
www.howsthat.co.uk

Positive Nation Magazine
250 Kennington Lane
London
SE11 5RD
Tel: 020 7564 2121
www.positivenation.co.uk

Positively Women
347–349 City Road
London
EC1V 1LR
Tel: 020 7713 0444

The Terrence Higgins Trust
52–54 Grays Inn Road
London
WC1X 8JU
Tel: 020 7831 0330
www.tht.org.uk

11

Drug misuse and safeguarding children: a multi-agency approach

Julian Buchanan and Brian Corby

This chapter will:

- Explore the social context in which 'problem drug users' and 'inadequate parents' are constructed.
- Outline key issues and difficulties involved in working with problem drug users whose children are considered to be at risk of abuse or neglect.
- Draw on research carried out with social workers, health visitors, drugs clinic workers and parents to examine the barriers of working together to assess children's needs where parents misuse drugs.
- Explore blockages and strategies for better partnership approaches.

The problem of 'drug misuse'

A major difficulty for professionals working with drug misusing parents is that the combination of problem drug use and child neglect heightens fear for the worker and brings considerable stigma to the client. Illicit drug users (as opposed to legal drug users) who develop drug problems have become a pariah group and are seen as a disgrace to their family and community. This is somewhat contradictory given the serious criminal, social and medical problems arising from the use of legal substances such as alcohol and tobacco. A legal drug user who develops a problem is unlikely to face the hostility or exclusion that will confront an illegal drug user in the same circumstances.

Alcohol and tobacco are embedded within everyday life in Western society, and are responsible for serious psychological and physiological damage to individuals, their families and the wider community. In the UK 120,000 people are killed every year as a result of tobacco use, and the health-related problems it causes costs the NHS up to £1.7 billion every year (HMSO 1998). The social and health costs from alcohol in the UK amounts to a staggering £3.3 billion a year (Alcohol Concern 2000). The US Institute of Medicine (1998) asserts that alcohol causes more damage to the developing foetus than any other substance (including marijuana, heroin and cocaine) and the irreversible effects of Foetal Alcohol Syndrome now affects one baby in every 500 born in the UK (FAS 2004). Excessive alcohol and tobacco use are seen as extensions of, or even part of normal behaviour (particularly alcohol). Indeed, in Western culture drinking alcohol (often to excess), is seen as a fitting way to celebrate a special occasion. However, imagine the reaction to a person celebrating a successful driving test by becoming intoxicated with an illicit drug – this would be seen as dangerous, deviant and highly irresponsible. It is important that professionals who are responding to drug-misusing parents understand this contradictory and confusing division between legal and illegal drugs. Otherwise, there is a risk that professionals will be assessing behaviour and parental capability through the 'tinted lenses' of prejudice, ignorance and fear.

Successive British Crime Surveys (BCS) indicate that over the past thirty years there has been a significant growth in the percentage of the population using illicit drugs. In the 1998 BCS, 49 per cent of 16–29-year-olds indicated they had taken a prohibited drug at some time in their life (Ramsey *et al.* 1999). There are now large numbers of illegal drug users (many of whom will be parents of young children) who use a range of drugs on a recreational basis and seem neither to develop problems nor come to the attention of the statutory or voluntary agencies. Indeed, it has been estimated (Edmunds *et al.* 1998) that only 3 per cent of illegal drug users could be categorized as problem drug users. It has been argued (Parker *et al.* 1998) that for most young people, illicit use of drugs has become a normalized risk-taking activity that is part of everyday life.

Those that become long-term problem drug users tend to have a history of multiple disadvantages before they developed a drug problem, with a high number having been 'looked after' as children, with poor educational experiences and patterns of chronic unemployment (Buchanan and Young 2000; SEU 2002). For many of these 'problem' drug users, drug taking is partly a symptom of an underlying problem often caused by difficult personal, social and/or economic circumstances. Already marginalized, the development of a drug problem only further exacerbates their plight and with the UK's punitive approach to drugs and crime, many end up in prison – hence the ever increasing UK prison population. There is a rapidly growing female prison population, many of whom would be sole carers for their children. At Scotland's only all-female prison, 94 per cent of the women on admission tested positive for illicit drugs (HMIPS 2001). The Social Exclusion Unit research into the social circumstances of prisoners in England and Wales provides further evidence of the link between multiple disadvantage, problem drug use and crime. It found that:

> Many prisoners have experienced a lifetime of social exclusion. Compared with the general population, prisoners are thirteen times as likely to have been in care as a child, thirteen times as likely to be unemployed, ten times as likely to have been a regular truant, two and a half times as likely to have had a family member convicted of a criminal offence, six times as likely to have been a young father, and fifteen times as likely to be HIV positive. Many prisoners' basic skills are very poor. 80 per cent have the writing skills, 65 per cent the numeracy skills and 50 per cent the reading skills at or below the level of an 11-year-old child. **60 to**

70 per cent of prisoners were using drugs before imprisonment. Over 70 per cent suffer from at least two mental disorders. And 20 per cent of male and 37 per cent of female sentenced prisoners have attempted suicide in the past.

(SEU 2002: 6, *emphasis added*)

Government policies that 'declare war on drugs' (Buchanan and Young 2000a) have further served to isolate and exclude this group, portraying them as an 'enemy within', blaming them for the problems within their community, resulting in added stigma and hostility from individuals, communities and agencies. This 'otherness' ascribed to problem drug users has reinforced their 'apparent' difference and often led to their isolation from families, the community and wider society. This isolation makes problem drug users more vulnerable to relapse and makes rehabilitation and reintegration extremely difficult. Given this approach to problem drug users, it is easy to understand how the emphasis of the statutory agencies may shift away from rehabilitation, care or social inclusion, and instead focus upon the assessment of risk, monitoring and protection of others. Where children are involved, the fear and need to protect is multiplied and it may be assumed wrongly that any parent who uses illegal drugs places their children at risk.

The climate surrounding illicit drug misuse is likely to have a negative impact on professionals. It may lead to doubts about the value and validity of rehabilitative work being done with problem drug users, or the setting of unrealistic expectation for change. It is likely to lead to mistrust between professionals and parents. Those working with drug users need to make sense of the complicated and sometimes contradictory messages about the effects, risks and dangers of illegal drugs, in order to engage with drug users in a properly informed manner. This problem of misinformation inevitably affects the relationships between different agencies working with illegal drug users, and alienates the client. It is possible for a problem drug user to be exposed to numerous agencies each having a different attitude and understanding of the risk posed by their illicit drug taking. A pregnant drug-using parent could be discussing her drug habit with her GP, midwife, social worker, community psychiatric nurse (from the local Drug Dependency Clinic), health visitor, probation officer, drug counsellor (from the voluntary organization) and housing support workers, and each one could be giving different messages about how best to tackle drugs and what the risks are to the baby. Getting these professionals to work collaboratively in partnership to provide the most effective service is not easy.

Child protection

Social attitudes have also had a major influence on work done with children and families where there are concerns about abuse and/or neglect, though in a somewhat different way to that in the drugs field. While it is clear that society has little sympathy for adults who ill-treat their children, perhaps even greater criticism has been levelled at professionals who have 'failed' to ensure their protection. This has been a consistent issue from the time of the Maria Colwell inquiry (DHSS 1974) right up to the present day. Social workers have borne the brunt of this criticism, but it should be noted that other professional workers have also been included. What has particularly exercised many public inquiries into child deaths by abuse has been the failure of all the professions and agencies with responsibilities in the child protection field to collaborate and communicate effectively. Although formal systems have been set up to improve this aspect of child protection work, nevertheless the findings of inquiries and serious case reviews have consistently pointed to poor information sharing and role confusion as key factors in events leading up to the child deaths they have been looking into (Corby *et al.* 1998). Most recently, in the Victoria Climbie inquiry (Laming 2003), there has been extensive criticism of those responsible for managing child protection agencies for failing to ensure that front-line workers are properly overseen and supervised in their activities.

A key consequence of this critical atmosphere has been to promote among child protection professionals a defensive mentality about their work, resulting in greater emphasis being placed on procedures and processes. Research conducted in the 1990s concluded that child care workers were over-focused on child protection issues and that child protection agencies were targeting all their resources on cases where risks of child abuse were deemed to exist (Dartington Social Research Unit 1995). As a consequence, the much larger number of families where children were in need received less attention and services than they warranted. This analysis led to a policy shift placing greater emphasis on the need to support families with a view to preventing abuse. There is still much ambivalence about how to get the balance right between working to support families while at the same time remaining vigilant to the possibilities of abuse (Corby 2003). Another key factor emerging from the Dartington research was the fact that many parents saw child protection workers as officious and unhelpful in the way in which they dealt with them. To date there seems to have been little change in perception on the part of parents as to the roles and purposes of social work intervention – they are still seen by many as people with authority to protect children by removing them from parents and placing them in care.

Drugs misuse and child protection

The link between drug misuse and children protection remains a contested one (as will be seen from our empirical study). Until relatively recently, there has been little written on this subject, and knowledge in this area has been described as 'woefully inadequate' (McKeganey *et al.* 2002: 244). While social workers are dealing with many more drug-using parents than before, there has been little serious estimation of overall numbers. This has led to a request by the Advisory Council on the Misuse of Drugs for agencies to ensure that details are recorded of all children of dependent drug users (ACMD 2003: 70). They estimate that between 250,000 and 350,000 children have at least one parent with a serious drug problem (ibid p. 30) and, on average, parental problem substance use was identified as a feature in 24 per cent of cases of children on the child protection register (ibid p. 54).

Despite this prevalence, there is limited specific guidance about what weight to place on drug misuse as a child protection risk issue. Although the ACMD report offers a useful examination of the nature and extent of the problem (ACMD 2003), much has been left to the judgement of practitioners in terms of risk assessment and how best to proceed. A Department of Health publication (Cleaver *et al.* 1999) has highlighted research findings about the links between child neglect, drug and alcohol misuse and mental illness, emphasizing the risks to children. Jo Tunnard (2002) has provided an informative overview to distil the key messages from a wide range of research in the drugs and child protection field. There are also some recent social work texts on the subject (Harbin and Murphy 2000; Kroll and Taylor 2003), which while trying to achieve as balanced a view as possible, have tended to see parental drug misuse as providing an ongoing risk to children's development.

There are now a few detailed research accounts of the way in which child protection work with drug-using parents is carried out in England (see Forrester 2000; and Klee *et al.* 1998, 2001). However, the amount of researched information about inter-professional issues, while extensive in the child protection field generally (see Birchall and Hallett 1995; Corby 2001), is limited in relation to the combined issues of drug misuse and child protection.

A perennial dilemma is how to support the parent and the child at the same time when it seems that the parent is not motivated or able to give up drugs and may be continuing with patterns of behaviour that make the child more vulnerable. Marina Barnard's research study highlights the difficulties this places upon carers and relatives, with many in her study expressing concern that supporting the parents may inadvertently be facilitating their ongoing drug use (Barnard 2003: 296). Kroll suggests a shift of focus towards the child is needed, in order to develop a better understanding of the impact of parental drug misuse. She advocates the importance of interviewing the children of drug-using parents: 'Communication between professionals needs to be made open and the child's perspective needs to be brought more firmly into the entire assessment process so that workers can gain a sense of what children's lives are really like' (Kroll 2004:138).

This challenge illustrates the complexity of engaging with the combined and interrelated issues of drugs and child protection, and the difficulty in juggling with the distinctively different needs of the parent to that of the child.

Interprofessional issues

In England, Wales and Scotland, Drug Action Teams (DATs) or similar bodies have been established at local authority or health authority level with the explicit purpose of enabling services to work together. However, when combined with child care there are a wide range of different agencies involved in providing services. These include:

- The Probation Service, who supervise offenders on court orders and can make proposals in Pre-sentence Reports for a range of sentencing options including Drug Treatment and Testing Orders, and Abstinence Orders.

- Social Services Departments who, with their statutory responsibility to protect children from abuse and neglect, employ social workers, family support workers and family centre workers.

- The Health Service, which has a significant responsibility to oversee all substitute prescribing services and provide health promotional advice and treatment.

Within the NHS there is a range of health professions who will come into contact with drug-using parents – GPs, DDU Clinic staff, Drug Action Team workers, midwives, health visitors, community psychiatric nurses and nursing staff involved in inpatient detoxification facilities.

- Education and Careers Departments, which include school teachers, learning mentors, Connexions advisers and youth and community workers.

- A variety of other agencies including the police, Crown Prosecution Service (CPS), courts, Sure Start, voluntary agencies and private bodies.

While attempts have been made to draw these agencies together through DATs and Area Child Protection Committees (ACPCs), policy and practices between the different agencies in respect of problem drug use and child protection too often remain parochial and unco-ordinated.

Professionals from different agencies are not immune from prevailing prejudicial societal values, but in this difficult field of work they need to be careful not to embrace such prejudices: 'practitioners and policy makers need to be vigilant about the biases they bring to their work' (Tunnard 2002: 43). As already noted, problem drug users experience stigma and isolation from the legal drug using population. This is intensified in the case of drug-using parents and even more so for drug-using mothers, who are seen to be failing their maternal responsibilities ascribed by gender stereotypes. This unfair and inappropriate response should not be perpetuated by agencies, despite their need to be vigilant about the possibilities of child neglect: 'Many drug misusing parents are already consumed with guilt about the effect their drug use may be having on their child, and it is important to maintain a non-judgmental approach while being firm and precise about the limits of adequate child care' (Keen and Alison 2001: 299).

Stereotypical views are likely to become tempered by ongoing contact with drug-using parents – indeed professionals whose key role is to work with the parents in these situations will not be able to do their job effectively without getting alongside them and developing a degree of empathy, this may not always be easy for professionals whose primary role is to protect and care for the child. As we have seen, child protection social workers have experienced considerable criticism for not being sufficiently authoritative and proactive in intervening in risk situations. It would be surprising if they did not, therefore, think and act defensively in the case of children whose parents are misusing drugs. On the other hand, they are also social workers and, as such, have a professional commitment to respect each human being regardless of their behaviour, and to be non-judgemental in their approach. Hence, there are a range of complex and at times contradictory values and attitudes that professionals must bring to their work with drug-using parents, but also to the inter-professional system.

Lessons from research – attitudes

In our qualitative study (Bates *et al.* 1999), we asked professionals from three different agencies involved in working with drug-using parents in Liverpool about their value positions in relation to drug misuse and child protection issues. We interviewed 11 specialist drug workers from an inner-city-based Drug Dependency Unit, 15 child protection social workers based in three different field teams and one based at a maternity hospital, and 15 community-based health visitors. We also interviewed ten known drug-using parents, to ascertain their perceptions of how professionals viewed and responded to them. The DDU workers were the most experienced of the professional groups we interviewed in relation to working in the drugs field. Their main commitment was to working with the drugs users themselves in a positive and rehabilitative way, to reduce the harm arising from illicit drug dependence. Most of the drug workers seemed to have sympathy for the parents they worked with and a strong awareness of the stigma attached to drug using and being a parent:

'Drug using parents have to live with stigma. Society considers them very low down the ladder. A lot of work needs to be done to help them get their confidence back. Drug users are made to feel they are bad parents from the outset.'

Many of the drug workers felt that other professionals tended to be more judgemental than they were. In particular, they felt that social services department workers' narrow concerns with child protection could, at times, result in stereotyping of drug-using parents:

'(they) should be looking at the specific issue of concern rather than the fact that someone uses drugs.'

Several of the Drugs Dependency workers commented that parents who used drugs could also be responsible parents:

'if drug use is managed properly, i.e. taking place privately and the after effects don't interfere with child care, then the parents can't be considered a poor role model.'

Most social workers were convinced that parental drug misuse was bound to impact negatively on children, largely because of the lifestyle and poverty that dependence on an illicit drug created. Some, however, held views similar to the DDU workers:

'I do not like making a judgement on families just because they use drugs. Every family is different. The risk is not necessarily greater.'

Nine of the fifteen health visitors felt that drug-using parents were poor role models for their children. One health visitor was clearly appalled by her experiences and felt particularly strongly about the issue:

'I would strongly agree that they are poor role models. It is the psychology of evil – the violence the children have to witness – the comings and goings that goes on.'

There were some clear differences between the three agencies in relation to values and attitudes, reflecting to some degree their different roles in dealing with drug misuse and child protection. DDU workers were overall more positive about the potential of drug-using parents to care reasonably for their children, reflecting the fact that they work mainly with and on behalf of parents. Social workers, on the other hand, were more circumspect, probably because of their focus on the needs of the child. Health visitors were overall least positive about drug-using parents, possibly reflecting their focus on the child, being referrers on behalf of at risk children, and their lack of sustained contact with drug-using parents. While these attitudinal differences between professions have significant implications for partnership work, it should be noted that there was encouragingly a good deal of common ground.

Lessons from research – knowledge

Not surprisingly the DDU workers in our study had the most detailed and informed knowledge about the impact of drugs and this was recognized among other the agencies:

'people from the DDU are well informed, well organized and usually very good to talk to when working with drug using families.'

This level of competence in respect of drugs led DDU workers to be more considered and less likely to panic about situations where children were involved. From their point of view, other professions tended to overreact as a result of their lack of knowledge:

'Some midwives told parents that methadone leads to deformed babies, or your baby will withdraw, or if it sneezes five times, we will need to take it to hospital.'

On the other hand, the drug workers had limited knowledge of child protection matters. As one worker put it:

'Some drug agencies can be quite blasé. If we are not careful, we can become over-confident about drug users' capability of parenting.'

The situation was almost reversed for social workers, who had considerable knowledge about child protection. While several social workers had received some training about drug misuse, most felt that it was inadequate given the extent of drug taking amongst their client group:

'I don't think the department supports us enough in training. Most of my experience comes from working with families where drug use is involved.'

Social workers, however, felt that lack of knowledge of child care and child protection issues was a weakness for some drugs dependency workers:

'Drugs agencies tend to put their clients' interests first before that of the clients' children, which is fair enough to a certain extent unless those children are at risk. I feel that they need more knowledge as to what degree of neglect is acceptable.'

Only two of the fifteen health visitors in this study had received drugs-specific training, although most had received some child protection training. As a whole, health visitors felt they had less expert knowledge than professional workers from the other two agencies, in that they were neither drugs nor child protection specialists. In some ways, they saw their generalist approach as being more balanced than that of the other two agencies:

'(DDU workers) are still not keyed up to looking at issues of child care. They are looking at issues of drugs and not at the wider family.'

Social workers were seen by health visitors to have too high a threshold of concern about child protection and, therefore, did not respond sufficiently to what health visitors considered to be 'worrying' cases. It seems that the knowledge differences, combined with the different roles and focus, created differences in perception between the three professional groups about what is acceptable and unacceptable behaviour from drug-misusing parents.

Lessons from research – roles

As can be seen from the two preceding sections, the roles and responsibilities of the different agencies seem to play an important part in the values, attitudes and views of their workers. In this section, the roles of the three sets of agency workers interviewed in our study are considered in more detail. DDU workers who were concerned more directly with the needs of the adults using drugs estimated that less than a quarter of their work involved parents with families. Their attention focused on helping chaotic drug users, to encourage them to stabilize their habit with substitute drugs (reduction or maintenance), reduce health and social harms, and support them once they had become stable. In this respect, parental care of children was not their main priority and they felt that drug misuse did not necessarily put children at risk:

'The only problem with drug users is what they have to do to get drugs. Most are decent families just like any other person.'

DDU workers did recognize the need to protect children and some were critical of workers from other agencies (those more involved with drug counselling and support) for not being sufficiently aware of the need to protect children.

'Some voluntary agencies [don't take child protection seriously] . . . seem to think "confidentiality" is paramount.'

The commitment to respect confidentiality of information between the worker and client cannot be allowed to become paramount in all circumstances. The complex task of engaging with social problems requires the worker to understand when other values, such as the rights of a child, or the rights of others, override a commitment to maintain confidentiality with the client. Several of the social workers interviewed had a fair amount of experience of working with drug-using parents and, despite their primary child protection concern, saw that their allegiances were to the whole family not just the child. Health visitors saw their allegiances as being most closely with the children, more so than did the social workers. They were more likely for instance, to be critical of drugs workers for failing to take into account the needs of children in the families with which they were working:

'Drugs workers . . . [they] do not see risk as they tend to look at their client and not the child.'

Lessons from research – interprofessional collaboration and training

Given the clear differences between the agencies, we were interested to explore what each of the professional groups felt about working in partnership. All felt that inter-agency collaboration and training was important for different reasons. DDU workers felt that health workers (including health visitors) were ill-informed and ill-trained in relation to illegal drug use. They felt that many in these professions, and some social workers, were not sufficiently discerning in the way in which they worked with drug-using parents. They welcomed more informal methods of collaboration with other professionals as a means to improve this situation, and core group meetings for the key professionals responsible for ongoing work with families were seen as more effective than child protection conferences. The need for all agencies to operate along shared, agreed guidelines was stated as important by the DDU workers. In particular, the emphasis given to confidentiality was seen as a thorny issue, which needed greater clarification and consistency in application.

Social workers shared many of these views. They too felt that health workers needed to be better informed and realistic in their attitudes to drug-using parents. Many commented on the lack of good communication between all agencies. In particular, they were critical in this respect of drugs workers, GPs, health visitors, school teachers and the police. The impression gained was that communication and collaboration was a lottery given the vast range of views, knowledge and anxiety that existed over the issue of parental drug misuse and child protection. Another concern raised was the fact that in the absence of clear policy practice guidelines, individual views about illicit drug taking could have considerable negative influence on the way in which families were assessed and treated:

'Sometimes you are working with drug users and you come across a health visitor or a doctor who really does have a problem with drugs. This is also the case with some social workers. You can't work together when some people have their own personal agendas.'

Many of the social workers felt that specialized drug training was essential to improving the situation and that this should be carried out jointly on an interpro-fessional basis with all the key agencies together. This level of exchange may also address the need to improve knowledge among the professions of each other's roles, priorities and responsibilities. Training concerning child protection may also benefit from being interprofessional, as most of the health visitors had concerns about the lack of attention to child protection by DDU workers:

'Drug agencies are adult-centred and keying their service to the needs of the individual who is an older person and not necessarily looking at issues around whether they are or are not involved with families. I think that in Liverpool it has become enlightened that they should seek information but they are still not keyed up at looking at issues of child care. They are looking at issues of drugs and not at the wider family.'

Several of the health visitors considered that they were not properly informed of what was happening in cases where there were concerns about drug misuse and child care. They considered that some drugs agencies' focus on confidentiality provided a barrier to good communication. They felt marginalized by the other professionals, particularly GPs, who, in their view, were not sufficiently aware of the potential risks to children that drugs present. They considered that social workers were too crisis-oriented and failed to give serious attention to their referrals, which were often centred on emerging need requiring preventive action. Most of the health visitors felt dissatisfied with the quality of interprofessional work:

'No one seems to understand each other's professional role. There is a long way to go. When I was first health visiting we used to make social contact with all the social workers, so you used to know who they were and they used to know who you were. You could pick up a telephone and it was much easier to make a referral. Now that we are coming out of clinics and we are all separate, I think it is a negative move – you don't know each other.'

Health visitors, like social workers, felt that matters could only be improved by a much greater emphasis on joint training.

The following case study illustrates the potential issues that can arise and how they could be resolved by greater inter-agency partnership practice.

Case study

The probation service, social services, the education authority and the health service each had specialist workers with a remit to specialize in substance misuse. However, each had different perspectives, different philosophies and language to understand and describe the drug problem; 'addicts', 'users', patients, clients, service users. Some agencies saw methadone as a dangerous drug only to be prescribed as a last resort on a four-week reducing programme; others believed methadone maintenance should be freely available. Some felt that 'addicts should be left to hit rock bottom' before any help should be given. It became apparent that clients were seen by a number of agencies with limited co-ordination or exchange of information, and were being given conflicting advice and information. The agencies got together, and after almost 18 months of careful planning and preparation exploring different philosophies, policies and practices and understanding and appreciating the different roles and focus, they united together by locating their staff into a single centrally-located building to form a specialist drugs team for the borough.

When Michelle, who was six months pregnant and dependent upon street heroin, came to the newly-created team for help she was extremely anxious and fearful of losing her child. However, the partnership approach meant that with Michelle's permission, the CPN was able to ring her GP, explain the situation and immediately arrange a methadone maintenance prescription. The social services drug counsellor was able to speak to the social worker at the local hospital to explore the likely outcome and the need for hospital support, and the probation officer was able to clarify the situation with their colleague, who was supervising Michelle on a twelve-month Community Rehabilitation Order following an offence of theft from a local shop.

Throughout the pregnancy Michelle was taking 30 mls of methadone linctus daily and not using any street drugs. Just after the birth of the baby a case conference was held. The mood of the conference was that Michelle should immediately be placed on a four-week methadone reduction programme to become drug free, the baby placed on the at risk register and arrangements made to systematically monitor her child care capabilities – despite the fact that she already had a happy and well adjusted four-year-old son. However, specialist members of the drugs team representing two different agencies were able to argue against this pressurizing strategy, which they believed was in danger of asking too much of Michelle and 'setting her up to fail'. After some debate the decision was eventually made to keep the baby in hospital for an extra three days to monitor possible withdrawal symptoms, not to make any demands to reduce Michelle's current levels of substitute prescribing, and to allow informal support from the drugs team to continue. There was not felt to be sufficient concern to warrant placing her child on the at risk register. Had it not been for the authority and consistent expert knowledge and guidance from the recently established specialist multi-agency drug team who spoke at the conference, the outcome of the case and the ultimate future care of the baby may have been very different.

Feedback from drug-using parents

Understandably, engaging with professionals who have a concern for the needs of the child raises real anxiety for many drug-using parents and some difficult encounters:

'I lied to social services and told them that I didn't know nothing about it, because the vibes I was getting from the situation was that H. could be whisked away into care.'

'I said you're not getting your hands on this one . . . what I don't agree with is that the baby's not even born yet and as soon as it's born, even if it's born in the night, these have got to phone child protection to let them know I've had the baby so that it can go on the at risk register straight from birth. Now I don't think that's right. I think you should be given a chance like, a couple of months, six weeks' trial, to see whether the baby does need to go on the at risk register or whatever. Know what I mean?'

Clearly, health and social care workers have to be prepared for this type of resistance. Parents who are subject to child protection investigations are sometimes antagonistic and resentful, particularly drug-using parents who consider the interventions to be based too often on judgemental attitudes about the way they live rather than on the way they care for their children. The parents who had attended child protection conferences felt intimidated and threatened by the process:

'I didn't like it . . . it was scary. It was very intimidating. I was sitting there and everybody was looking at me as if I couldn't look after my own children . . . and I felt so annoyed.'

'Worse than a court . . . you haven't got a jury. It was scary.'

'It was awful . . . it was awful . . . we just ended up screaming at them, giving them all loads of abuse, verbal abuse, and walking out. I was in tears . . . it was awful.'

However, drug-using parents were not generally dismissive of agency staff. They were critical of those who they believed were patronizing and excluded them from an open dialogue, whereas many parents spoke highly of those staff that dealt with the process of monitoring and social control in a manner that was open and honest, yet retained respect and dignity for the parent as well as the child.

'Some are better than others. That last one I had – Derek – he was brilliant. He always used to tell us up front. The last time everything was done behind your back.'

A key message here is that it is not so much what is done but how it is done that matters. This is further supported by a research study that centred exclusively on the views of drug-using clients about agencies: 'judgemental attitudes are also criticised by service users and it is clear that the type of service and the way people are treated is more important than the model of treatment' (Jones *et al.* 2004: 36).

Conclusion

It is important to reiterate that working in the field of drug misuse and child protection is not an easy task. The context within which the work is done, as has been noted, is exceptionally difficult. Most people in society distance themselves from drug misusers and parents who ill-treat or neglect their children. Policies and practices for dealing with service users reflect and augment this stigmatization. In the field of drugs, apart from the reclassification of cannabis, there seems to have been little shift in thinking over the past two decades. All illegal drug misuse is seen as dangerous, and there is limited tolerance towards, or help for, users who do not commit themselves to working towards abstinence. In the child protection field there have been some shifts in approaches. Since the mid-1990s, there has been greater emphasis placed on responding more supportively to families where children are seen to be in need or at risk of neglect or ill-treatment with a view to prevention. However, social workers and other child protection professionals are only adapting slowly to these changes (see Corby 2003), while at the same time facing constant reminders of the dangers of not responding sufficiently actively to risk situations (see Laming 2003). Indeed, greater emphasis has been placed on drug and alcohol misuse as a threat to children's welfare in recent government publications (Cleaver *et al.* 1999). In a climate such as this not only are professionals put on the defensive but so are the local community, family and service users. It is hardly surprising then, that drug-using parents tend to avoid contact and open dialogue with child protection professionals. They might be willing to work more cooperatively with professionals if low threshold intervention was offered in a sympathetic, helpful and supportive manner. If honest and realistic dialogue is to be achieved, it does not just depend on the client – it also depends upon the attitudes, values and responses of professional workers.

The importance of achieving a positive interprofessional collaboration in this field to deliver high quality, shared care to all drug users is widely recognized (Keen and Alison 2001) though it is not as straightforward as it seems. Child protection work generally has been dogged by this problem – as has already been noted, the recommendations of public inquiries into child abuse have consistently pointed to the need to improve communications between professionals (Corby *et al.* 1998). With the added ingredient of drug misuse and the interprofessional issues associated with this field of activity, improving collaboration where drugs and child abuse are interlocking issues is that much more problematic. However, McKeganey argues strongly for partnership work in this area, suggesting there is a need for: 'radical developments in the provision of services to drug-using parents and their children. We need much closer links between children's services and adult drug services, we need much greater flow of information between services' (McKeganey *et al.* 2002: 244).

The situation is not helped by the fact that there are no satisfactory agreed guidelines for this area of work. The safeguarding children guidelines (SCODA 1999) are too broad and lack specificity, while the useful insights offered by the ACMD (2003) and Tunnard (2002) have not been widely implemented. The main issues arising from our research to be addressed in respect of policy and practice are:

1. The wide variations in knowledge between professions and, in some cases, within professions about drug misuse and its impact on families;
2. The lack of shared values and attitudes about drug misuse between and within professions;
3. The different roles played by different professions, with some having more allegiance to and responsibility for adults and some for children;
4. The lack of shared training and opportunity for developing interprofessional understanding;
5. The lack of guidance and shared understanding regarding acceptable and unacceptable risk behaviour.

There was sufficient evidence in our study to show that most drugs workers and social workers occupied enough shared ground to fuel optimism about the potential for developing better partnerships. While some health visitors we interviewed seemed to be more anxious about working with drug-using parents, several of them held values and attitudes similar to the other two groups of professionals. A key issue of difference between the professionals was in relation to risk assessment. While almost none of the professionals we spoke to were of the view that drug use per se placed children at risk, the variation in views was sufficiently wide to be of concern. Clearly there is much work to be done to ensure that assessments about child welfare where drugs are present are accurate, appropriate and informed.

There is also much work needed to achieve greater consistency among the different professions, and the issue of confidentiality needs to be properly aired. Establishing ongoing interprofessional training will help to address many of these issues. Another tool for achieving consistency between professions is that of second-ment across agencies. Areas of sufficient size should consider the example illustrated in the case study and the setting up of specialist interprofessional teams with remits for developing interprofessional policy/practice guidelines and working with drug misusing parents:

> Developments of this nature cannot succeed without positive liaison between different disciplines and between adult and children's services . . . There are examples of good practice along these lines developed in the UK. One offered parents misusing drugs a one-stop shop.
>
> (Tunnard 2002: 40)

This task must be given priority by Area Child Protection Committees or their successors. A significant proportion of child protection cases now involve drug mis-use, therefore, there will be a need to employ professionals who can be strong enough to provide positive help and support to both parents and children, in spite of what might at times be hostile and negative external conditions. In circumstances like this professionals need to develop mutual trust, understanding and respect for each other's roles and judgement. This can only be achieved by shared training and the development of ongoing dialogue and communication.

Our interviews with drug-using parents in this study, all of whom had had contact with drugs workers and child protection professionals, are highly instructive and, while they are by no means the sole criteria for organizing and developing policy and practice, they do, in our view, provide a rich source of understanding, which should be given particular emphasis in interprofessional training. It was notable that style and approach were seen by these parents as the key factors in their acceptance of professional intervention. Interestingly, they were not as critical of the way in which professional related to them as might have been expected, given the gravity and repercussions of the intervention upon their lives. They emphasized:

1. The importance of professional consistency.
2. The importance of open and honest communication.
3. The need for workers to be comfortable with the issue of drugs.
4. The need to be viewed realistically and not harshly or negatively.

All of these factors require professionals to work together in a collaborative way and to share their views and attitudes in order to achieve the sort of consistency that both parents want and children need in order to ensure their future health and well-being.

Questions for further discussion

1. To what extent is a parent who regularly uses illicit drugs a poor role model?
2. What drug-related behaviours would you identify in relation to child protection as posing 'low' risk and what drug-related behaviours pose a 'high' risk?
3. What practical steps can be taken to help agencies work more closely together?

References

Advisory Council on the Misuse of Drugs (ACMD) (2003) *Hidden Harm: Responding to the Needs of Problem Drug Users*. Home Office, London.

Alcohol Concern (2000) *Britain's Ruin*. Alcohol Concern, London.

Barnard, M. (2003) Between a rock and a hard place: the role of relatives in protecting children from the effects of parental drug problems, *Child and Family Social Work*, 8(4): 291–9.

Bates, T., Buchanan, J., Corby, B. and Young, L. (1999) *Drug Use, Parenting and Child Protection: Towards an Effective Inter-agency Response*. University of Central Lancashire.

Birchall, E. and Hallet, C. (1995) *Working Together in Child Protection: Report of Phase Two, a Survey of the Experience and Perceptions of Six Key Professions* (Studies in Child Protection). The Stationery Office, London.

Buchanan, J. and Young, L. (2000) Examining the relationship between material conditions, long term problematic drug use and social exclusion: A new strategy for social inclusion, in J. Bradshaw and R. Sainsbury (eds) *Experiencing Poverty*, pp. 120–43. Ashgate Press, London.

Buchanan, J. and Young, L. (2000a) The war on drugs – a war on drug users, *Drugs: Education, Prevention Policy*, 7(4): 409–22.

Buchanan, J. and Young, L. (2001) Child protection and social work views, in Klee *at al.* (eds) *Issues in Motherhood and Substance Misuse*. Routledge Press.

Cleaver, H., Unell, I. and Aldgate, J. (1999) *Children's Needs – Parenting Capacity: The Impact of Parental Mental Illness, Problem Alcohol and Drug Use and Domestic Violence on Children's Development*. The Stationery Office, London.

Corby, B. (2001) Interprofessional cooperation and inter-agency co-ordination and child protection, in K. Wilson and A. James (eds) *The Child Protection Handbook* (2nd edn) Bailliere-Tindall, London, pp. 272–87.

Corby, B. (2003) Supporting families and protecting children – assisting child care professionals in initial decision-making and review of cases, *Journal of Social Work*, 3(2): 195–210.

Corby, B., Doig, A. and Roberts, V. (1998) Inquiries into child abuse, *Journal of Social Welfare and Family Law*, 20(4): 377–96.

Dartington Social Research Unit (1995) *Child Protection: Messages from Research*. HMSO, London.

Department of Health and Social Security (1974) *Report of the Committee of Inquiry into the Care and Supervision Provided in Relation to Maria Colwell*. HMSO, London.

Department of Health (2000) *Framework for the Assessment of Children in Need and Their Families*. The Stationery Office, London.

Edmunds, M., May, T., Hearnden, I. and Hough, M. (1998) Arrest Referral: Emerging Lessons From Research, DPI Paper No. 23. Home Office DPI, London.

FAS (2004) Foetal Alcohol Syndrome Aware UK web site accessed 6th June 2004 http://www.fasaware.co.uk/pics/FASleafletA4.pdf.

Forrester, D. (2000) Parental substance misuse and child protection in a British sample: a survey of children on the Child Protection Register in an Inner London District Office, *Child Abuse Review*, 9: 235–46.

Harbin, F. and Murphy, M. (eds) (2000) *Substance Misuse and Child Care: How to Understand, Assist and Intervene when Drugs Affect Parenting*. Russell House Publishing, Lyme Regis.

Hayden, C., Jerrim, S. and Pike, S. (2002) *Parental Substance Misuse – The Impact on Child Care Social Work Caseloads*. Report No. 47, Social Services Research and Information Unit (SSRIU), University of Portsmouth.

HM Government (1998) *Tackling Drugs to build a Better Britain*.

HMIPS (HM Inspectorate of Prisons for Scotland) (2001) Report on HMP and YOI. Cornton Vale, Edinbrurgh.

HMSO (1998) *Smoking Kills: A White Paper on Tobacco*. Cm 4177, HMSO, London.

Hogan, D. and Higgins, L. (2001) *When Parents Use Drugs – Key Findings from a Study of Children in the Care of Drug-using Parents*. The Children's Research Centre, Trinity College, Dublin.

Institute of Medicine (1996) *Fetal Alcohol Syndrome Diagnosis, Epidemiology, Prevention, and Treatment*. National Academy Press, Washington, D.C.

Jones, S., Drainey, S., Walker, L. and Rooney, J. (2004) *Collecting the Evidence: Clients' Views on Drug Services*. Addaction, London.

Keen, J. and Alison, L.H. (2001) Drug misusing parents: key points for health professionals *Archives of Disease in Childhood*, 85: 296–9.

Klee, H., Jackson, M. and Lewis, S. (eds) (2001) *Drug Misuse and Motherhood*. Routledge, London.

Klee, H., Wright, S. and Rothwell, J. (1998) *Drug Using Parents and Their Children: Risk and Protective Factors*. Report to the Department of Health. Centre for Social Research on Health and Substance Use, Manchester Metropolitan University.

Kroll, B. and Taylor, A. (2003) *Parental Substance Misuse and Child Welfare*. Jessica Kingsley Publishers, London.

Kroll, B. (2004) Living with an elephant: Growing up with parental substance misuse, *Child and Family Social Work*, 9(2): 129–40.

Laming, Lord (2003) The Victoria Climbié Inquiry. Cm 5730, HMSO, London.

McKeganey, N., Barnard, M. and McIntosh, J. (2002) Paying the Price for their Parents' Drug Use: The Impact of Parental Drug Use on Children, *Drug Education, Prevention and Policy*. 3: 233–46.

Parker, H., Aldridge, J. and Measham, F. (1998) *Illegal Leisure: The Normalisation of Adolescent Drug Use*. Routledge, London.

Ramsay, M., Partridge, S. and Byron, C. (1999) Drug Misuse Declared In 1998: Key Results From the British Crime Survey Research Findings No. 93. Home Office, London.

SEU (2002) *Reducing Re-offending by Ex-prisoners*. Social Exclusion Unit, London. http://www.socialexclusionunit.gov.uk/reduce_reoff/rr_main.pdf

Standing Conference On Drug Abuse (SCODA) (1997) *Drug Using Parents: Policy Guidelines for Inter-agency Working*. Local Government Association Publications, London.

Tunnard, J. (2002) Parental Drug Misuse: a review of impact and intervention studies. Research in Practice. http://www.rip.org.uk

12

Interprofessional communication in child protection

Brian Corby

This chapter will:

- Discuss key problems associated with the safeguarding of children by various professionals.
- Exemplify professional errors in safeguarding children by drawing on the Victoria Climbie inquiry.
- Consider the key roles of the main professions involved in safeguarding children, and how good practice can be achieved.
- Review central government proposals for the development of safeguarding procedures following the Climbie inquiry and analyse how these may impact on communication between professionals working in this field in the future.

Introduction

Since the first of the modern-day inquiries into child abuse deaths, that of Maria Colwell (DHSS 1974), to the most recent, that of Victoria Climbie (Laming 2003), one of the key problems associated with safeguarding children has been seen to be inadequate communication and co-operation between the various professionals involved (see DoH 1991a; Corby *et al.* 1998, 2001). Between these two landmarks, almost all inquiries and published reviews have, with the advantage of hindsight, looked back at the situations in which child deaths have occurred and highlighted missed opportunities by social workers, NSPCC workers, police, health visitors, nurses, paediatricians, teachers, probation officers and housing officials to pass on information to each other which, if pooled together, could have heightened concern and perhaps have led to protective intervention before a child died. This was most graphically demonstrated in two Part 8 reviews carried out by the Bridge Child Care Consultancy, which were subsequently made publicly available, one into the death of a girl named Sukina in the county of Avon (The Bridge 1991), and the second into the death by neglect of a child named Paul in the London borough of Islington

(The Bridge 1995). The authors of these reports, using the material found in the case files of key involved agencies (health, social services and education), showed how the cumulative information in these documents painted a far more worrying picture than that provided by examination of one agency's files only. The inference is that, had all agencies been privy to and shared the details of each other's records, they would probably have acted sooner to safeguard the children in question.

The Victoria Climbie inquiry

The Victoria Climbie inquiry (Laming 2003) points to similar conclusions. In the short time in which Victoria was involved with health, housing and social work agencies (she died only ten months after coming to live in England), there were several occasions where the sharing of information between professionals could have led them to have been more concerned about her safety. The most glaring example of this was when she was brought to North Middlesex Hospital on 24 July 1999 with scalds to her head and face. Doctors there were told by her aunt that Victoria had scabies and that she had poured hot water over herself in order to relieve the itching. This, of course, was a highly dubious explanation, made even more suspect by the fact that there had been a five-hour delay between the time of the alleged incident and Victoria being brought into the hospital. Indeed, the doctors who examined her were rightly concerned and, in accordance with agreed procedures, the matter was communicated to the social services department in which the child was resident. As all this took place on a Saturday, it was referred on to the emergency duty social services team, who in turn passed it on to the relevant district office on the following Monday. A strategy meeting was held on the subsequent Wednesday. It was attended by a hospital social worker and police and social services personnel, and a decision was reached that there was a need for protective measures of intervention. However, the degree of concern was still not a strong one, and it was suggested in the inquiry that the hospital social worker might not have sufficiently emphasized the concerns of the hospital staff because she did not attend ward meetings and, therefore, had not had direct contact with them. One of the hospital staff who was particularly concerned was the consultant paediatrician who had examined Victoria. She was adamant at the inquiry that she had expressed her views robustly, but social services department social workers did not think this was the case. It is notable that her communications were by letter and there was no face-to-face meeting with social services department personnel. Nurses in the hospital witnessed worrying changes in Victoria's behaviour when visited by her aunt on the ward, but did not communicate their concerns sufficiently strongly to other professionals. In addition to this, no one had collected information about Victoria's previous contacts with other hospitals, social services departments and the police. The net outcome was that Victoria was returned to the care of her aunt and that she was viewed as a child in need of help and support rather than as one who was either being abused or at risk of being abused.

This particular incident highlights many of the reasons why communication in safeguarding children can go wrong, as indicated in Box 12.1.

What is evident from this box is that failure of communication between professionals was one of the main reasons why Victoria was not protected from abuse.

Box 12.1 What went wrong for Victoria Climbie?

1. There were a wide range of people from different professions involved in the case and, as is well known, the more people that are involved in a communication chain, the greater the likelihood of the original message being altered in the process.
2. There was little face-to-face contact between key professionals, with a good deal of communication depending on letters and messages being passed on by third parties, which again is likely to influence the integrity of the original message.
3. Some professionals (e.g. the nurses on the ward) did not realize the significance of their observations and, therefore, did not ensure that they were communicated.
4. There were difficulties in gathering and collating past information sufficiently quickly to influence current decision making.

Certainly had there been better communication in this case, it is likely that the pooled concerns would have aroused greater suspicion and, possibly, Victoria could have been properly safeguarded at this time. For a detailed account of these events see Chapter 10 of the Climbie inquiry (Laming 2003 paras 10.1–10.163, pp. 255–78).

Communication in context

Of course, communication is not the only issue in safeguarding children cases. There are many other factors that have a part to play in making this area of work problematic. Lack of adequate resources is a key issue. An audit of health, police and social services arrangements for safeguarding children following on from the Climbie inquiry (Commission for Health Improvement 2003) found that there was a high level of unallocated registered child protection cases in several areas. Another key factor is that the quality of staff involved in safeguarding children work, in terms of knowledge and experience, is very mixed. In particular, interprofessional training seems to have been very variable over the past decade, according to the post-Climbie audit just referred to. Also the child protection system is a complex one with a wide range of health, welfare and police personnel involved, and in some parts of the country, particularly in large urban areas like inner London, there is a bewildering overlap of occupational boundaries and the added complication of disadvantaged and transient families. Furthermore, policy developments since the mid-1990s have made the task of safeguarding children even more uncertain, in that they have required social workers to be more careful about pursuing investigations and more focused on the needs for family support (Dartington Social Research Unit 1995; Spratt 2001; Corby 2003). Bearing these contextual factors in mind, however, this chapter will single out interprofessional communication for examination.

In what follows, the key roles of the main professions involved in safeguarding children will be considered with focus on how good practice can be achieved. This will be followed by a review of central government proposals for the development of safeguarding procedures following the Climbie inquiry and an analysis of how these may impact on communication between professionals working in this field in the future.

Social services departments and child protection

There is both a duty and an expectation on the various agencies involved in safeguarding children to work together. The duty is set out in Sections 47(9)(10) and (11) of the 1989 Children Act, which stress that where a local authority is carrying out an inquiry into suspected child abuse, it is the duty of other local authorities and of the local education, housing and health authorities to assist with the inquiries if called on to do so, by providing information or advice. Subsection (10) provides the caveat that no person is obliged to offer this assistance where doing so would be unreasonable in all the circumstances of the case. In addition to the Children Act itself there is an abundance of guidelines – *Working Together to Safeguard Children* (DoH 1999), the *Framework for Assessing Children in Need* (DoH 2000) and *Safeguarding Children: What to do if you're worried a child is being abused* (DoH 2003). In theory, then, although it has not always been the case, there are now few legal barriers to the full sharing of information in safeguarding children cases. While confidentiality remains an issue for most professions, and particularly for doctors, it is now clear that safeguarding children concerns override these. However, in practice, as the Climbie case shows, there can be many barriers to good communication between professionals. How best to overcome these is a very important issue in the aftermath of this inquiry, but before looking at these developments, consideration will be given to the current situation.

The agency with primary responsibility in the field of child protection is the social services department, which has a statutory duty to safeguard children and to support families in need. It has powers to seek emergency protection of children, and holds key responsibility for setting up child protection conferences, for the registration of abused children and for carrying out need and risk assessments. It also normally provides the key worker for the continuing conduct of safeguarding cases. Finally, social services departments have duties in relation to commencing care proceedings and providing ongoing care for looked after children. It is in many ways, therefore, a hub agency in that other professionals are required in the various guidelines for practice to refer matters to it as soon as possible, so that a co-ordinated response can result.

The centrality of social work in child protection is both a strength and a weakness. On the one hand, it is important for there to be an agency with ultimate responsibility for dealing with abused and disadvantaged children, in that it can be a source of real support to others with a wider range of duties and responsibilities. On the other hand, there is a danger that other agencies may refer on too quickly and that social services departments can become a dumping ground. In that case, the expectations of those agencies might well not be met because of the inability of social services agencies to deal with the numbers involved.

Research in the early nineties showed that, in fact, social services departments operated like a large filter, sifting out the vast majority of cases referred to them and concentrating on a relatively small minority, i.e. 15 per cent (Gibbons *et al.* 1995). Buckley (2003), in a study which, though carried out in Ireland in the 1990s, still has resonance for our safeguarding children system and demonstrates how this works in practice. She shows how social workers, driven mainly by the need to make their workloads realistically manageable, are as keen to eliminate potential cases from the system, as they are to accept them. There are two likely negative consequences of this process – first, families with broader child care needs tend to be overlooked for service provision and, second, because such a large number of cases are referred, it may make it harder to pick out the more risky cases. A recent Social Services Inspectorate (2001) study estimated that about 6 per cent of worrying cases referred to social services departments are not being properly responded to.

In terms of interprofessional communication, this process is also problematic. Other agencies may refer cases to social services departments expecting action but, in fact, nothing happens and, more often than not, the reasons for this may not be communicated back. From the viewpoint of social services departments they may be sent what they consider to be a large number of inappropriate referrals with which they feel unable to deal. In this way, communications can become seriously problematic between agencies over time.

Central government has been active in recent years in ensuring that children in need (who are not at risk) are properly screened and responded to. Its rationale is that this has been a statutory requirement since the implementation of the 1989 Children Act (though a fairly neglected one) and also that meeting the needs of deprived children may well prevent deterioration resulting in abuse or neglect. As a result, since 2001 social services departments have been required to assess all referrals made to them about children in need, to check whether there are services they or other agencies could provide. It is intended that such assessments be contributed to by all agencies, but that the key responsibility should lie with social services departments. This, in turn, should improve some of the more negative communication processes referred to above. However, a major worry for social workers in social services departments is one of resources, in terms of person power, to handle the number of assessments required (see Corby *et al.* 2002). Yet a further concern is that spreading the focus across families in need as well as across safeguarding children, may mean more serious cases slipping through the child protection net. This may well have played a part in the Climbie case – for the most part she (and her family) were seen to be 'in need' rather than at risk of serious abuse.

Health professionals and child protection

Unlike teams of social workers, who focus almost exclusively on deprived families where children are either in need or at risk, health workers – such as community nurses, midwives, GPs, paediatricians, hospital nurses and doctors – have a wide range of responsibilities for meeting the health needs of children. With the possible exception of health visitors and paediatricians, most health professionals will have minimal involvement in child protection. In such circumstances, it is hard to develop expertise and knowledge of procedures and to maintain vigilance, and often heavy reliance is placed on referral to social services departments in the manner outlined earlier. One way of developing expertise among health professionals is to appoint specialists who have an educational function within their own agency and a liaison/communication function with social services departments, and this has been happening in the health service both in community settings and hospitals over the last decade.

Another way is to participate in interprofessional training. Health visitors have made considerable strides in this respect. On the other hand, GPs have tended to play a peripheral role in child protection work. They have always battled with the notion of breaking confidentiality with their adult clients/patients, despite direction from the General Medical Council of the need to do so in child protection cases. It is notable that post-Climbie, GPs will be required to follow the model being adopted in other parts of the health service; that of appointing child protection lead persons for their profession in each primary care trust.

Health visitors are also frequently concerned about breaching confidentiality in cases of child protection. This often arises from the length of time they spend building up a trusting relationship with parents – a relationship that can easily be destroyed if the health visitor is perceived by parents to be in danger of 'reporting' them to social services. Health visitors are encouraged to discuss a referral with the family so that it is agreed with all concerned. However, if the family does not wish to have social services involved and the health visitor makes a referral anyway, this can result in problems for all concerned, as indicated in Box 12.2.

Paediatricians who played a pioneering role in the development of child protection work in the 1960s and 1970s have taken quite a battering in the past decade or so.

Box 12.2 A case of protecting the client–professional relationship

The Brown family had enjoyed a good relationship with their health visitor since the birth of their twins, Jack and Sam. They were both unemployed and had struggled to make ends meet, normally running out of money before weekly benefits were due. The health visitor had noticed recently during her visit that Mr Brown was rather aggressive towards his wife and on more than one occasion Mrs Brown had bruises on her arms. Although the health visitor asked discretely how she had come by these bruises, Mrs Brown seemed reluctant to discuss them. Three months later, when the twins were ten months old, she noticed that Jack had two black eyes. When she asked his parents what had happened, they said he had fallen and banged his head on the chair arm. They reported that he had recently started to climb from a crawling position to grip the chairs to stand and often fell in the process. The health visitor felt that this would explain one black eye, but not two. She had spent months attempting to build a good relationship in what she thought might become a precarious situation and was reluctant to damage this by suggesting a referral to social services.

Key questions

1. Should the health visitor discuss referral with the family?
2. If yes, what might be the consequences of this and how should she deal with them?
3. Should the health visitor refer to social services without the family's knowledge and/or consent?
4. If yes, what might be the consequences of her actions?
5. Should the health visitor discuss the case with her manager?
6. If yes, what will be the likely outcome?
7. What lessons are there here for joint working?

The Cleveland inquiry (Butler-Sloss 1988) was a low water mark for this profession as a result of the reliance placed on the reflex anal dilatation tests. Since then there have been concerns raised about use of covert video surveillance to gain evidence of parental abuse of children in Munchausen's syndrome by proxy cases (Thomas 1996) and, most recently, the furore over the links between cot deaths and child abuse and the questioning of the advice given in criminal court cases by Sir Roy Meadow, a leading paediatrician in this field (Sweeney 2003). Another example is illustrated in the Victoria Climbie case, in which there was much concern about the diagnosis of scabies made by Dr Ruby Schwartz when Victoria was taken to the Accident and Emergency Department of Middlesex Central Hospital on 14 July 1999. Such weight is given to the judgement of senior doctors that her diagnosis led to an immediate reduction in concern about Victoria's safety and a police protection order that had been deemed to be warranted when she was admitted to hospital was left to run out without a proper follow-up ensuing. The task of paediatricians is certainly not an easy one. Often they are unable to produce the type of evidence that is sufficient to satisfy a court of risk to a child, or of the culpability of a parent. On the other hand, their judgement can be crucial in determining the course of a child protection case. Following the Climbie inquiry, there is likely to be more questioning of paediatricians' diagnoses. While it is important to ensure that there is no undue reliance on the judgement of single professionals, it will be concerning if the effect of this is to reduce the commitment of paediatricians to taking a high profile in child protection work.

In general, however, it is vital that health and social care professionals work closely together to safeguard children. Health visitors and GPs, in particular, have considerable information and expertise about babies and infants that is crucial to the assessment of children in need and at risk, and to decision making about and monitoring of ongoing cases. The key question, however, is how best to do this. The professional cultures of health workers, doctors and social workers are very different (Barr 1997), and although over time there has been more convergence in this respect and improved communication (Cooper et al. 2001), as the Climbie inquiry has shown, it is an area that needs constantly working at.

Police and child protection

Police involvement in safeguarding children has increased quite considerably since the late 1980s. In the early days of the rediscovery of child abuse, the police played a relatively minor role, only becoming involved in cases where serious abuse was taking place and there was need for a criminal charge to be brought. The Cleveland (Butler-Sloss 1988) and Orkney (Clyde, Lord 1992) cases, however, had a big impact on the role of the police, giving them much more central involvement in child sexual abuse cases and, in theory, in all cases where a criminal offence was suspected. Joint interviewing of children by police and social services department workers, where there is likelihood of a criminal hearing to follow, is now an established part of child protection procedures (Home Office/Department of Health 1992). All police forces now have Child Protection Teams with officers specializing in this area of work, and because of this they are potentially better equipped to work in co-operation with other professionals involved in the child protection field. However, there was little evidence of this happening in the Victoria Climbie case.

Although police and social work staff in Brent and Haringey were working together, the quality of co-operation was poor, certainly in Haringey, where a police report noted that social workers were 'extremely powerful within the child protection network and some social workers work hard to actually prevent police involvement' (Laming 2003, para.14.17). The inquiry was particularly critical of the fact that, despite Victoria being assessed for being a victim of child abuse, there was never any sense of the police considering that a crime might be taking place. Victoria's aunt, Mrs Kouao, was never questioned by the police – indeed the police officer involved when Victoria was diagnosed as having scabies refused to do a home visit for fear of infection. The Climbie inquiry painted a picture of poorly-resourced police child protection teams, which had low status within the wider police force, lacked proper supervision and management, and collaborated with other agencies in a superficial way only. How widespread such poor practice is remains unclear. However, a recent self-audit prompted by the government in response to the Climbie inquiry suggests that there are areas of deficiency across many police authorities. Significantly, several police forces report finding it difficult to find sufficient adequately trained officers for joint interviewing and they also report not being able to provide supervision for all cases of child abuse being dealt with by front-line officers (Commission for Health Improvement 2003).

Education and child protection

Schools play a major part in the lives of most children from the age of three or four onwards. Children of school age in Western societies probably spend more direct time with their teachers than they do with their parents (Corsaro 1997). Of course, this was not the case with Victoria Climbie who was never registered at school while she was in England, a fact that seemed to go unnoticed by all the agencies that crossed her path. Educational services have normally tended to play a very limited role in child protection work in the past, despite their centrality in children's lives. Since 1991, following the implementation of new child protection guidelines (Department of Health 1991b), all schools now have liaison teachers with a specific role for communication with social services departments about safeguarding the needs of children. Education welfare officers can act to facilitate this process. Thus, there are better procedures than before and also a greater awareness of abuse than used to be the case. Nevertheless, there are still very difficult issues for teachers in making referrals. With younger children in particular, there may be fears that parents with whom the school will in all likelihood continue to work following a referral, will become alienated. Older children who choose a teacher to divulge abuse to may feel that their confidences have been betrayed.

Individual teachers may have little ongoing contact with social workers and, therefore, be uncertain about trusting them to act appropriately. In these circumstances, it is obvious why it is of key importance to have a well-informed and trained link worker who maintains regular contact with social workers and other professionals. Good communication depends on trust and a sense of predictability about the way in which others will respond to information passed on.

Other professionals and child protection

There are, of course, many other professionals involved in safeguarding children – probation officers, housing officials, youth and community workers and social workers from a wide range of voluntary agencies and associations. A recent addition to the already wide range of professionals are Sure Start and Children's Fund project workers and Connexions personal advisors. Probation officers have a key role in respect of offenders with histories of violence and sex offences. Housing officials often hold important information passed on by other tenants. Youth workers and Connexions advisors work closely with adolescents and their advice and help is often sought as a result. Social workers in voluntary child care agencies and those working in the new Sure Start and Children's Fund agencies are in constant touch with families whose children are in need. The NSPCC retains statutory powers under the 1989 Children and Young Persons Act to issue emergency protection orders and to initiate care proceedings, but in practice now leaves these duties almost exclusively to social services department social workers. All these professional people need to have at least a working knowledge of the child protection system – the recent government publication on how cases should be referred on to key child protection personnel will no doubt help in this respect (Department of Health 2003). Some need to be more fully involved in joint training and developing closer ongoing contacts with the main agencies – certainly this is the case with regard to the relative newcomers to the scene, that is those working in Sure Start, Children's Fund and Connexions agencies.

The current situation

It is not easy to come to a clear assessment of where we are now in terms of interprofessional communication in safeguarding children. In some ways, there have been considerable improvements. For instance, the level of awareness of child abuse is much higher than it was 20 years ago. Also the systems now in place to aid professional communication are more fully developed. However, five key factors have acted as barriers to doing much better as indicated in Figure 12.1.

The five factors indicated in Figure 12.1 overlap and impact on each other. For instance, the fact that we have complex systems and large numbers of cases referred through these systems has implications for resources. Nevertheless, for the sake of clarity they will be considered separately.

Any analysis of the development of the child protection system will conclude that it has become far more complex over time. The procedures for responding to child protection cases today are labyrinthine compared with those in the 1970s. There are a whole host of guidelines, assessment frameworks and procedures across all the agencies involved. Area Child Protection Committees have taken on a wider range of responsibilities over time, including the conduct of serious case reviews in cases where children die or are seriously harmed as a result of child abuse. A major consequence of this is that at front-line worker level, the demands of the systems result in the likelihood of less face-to-face contact with service users.

The extent and range of cases coming into the child protection system has mushroomed over time. It now deals with physical abuse and neglect, emotional abuse

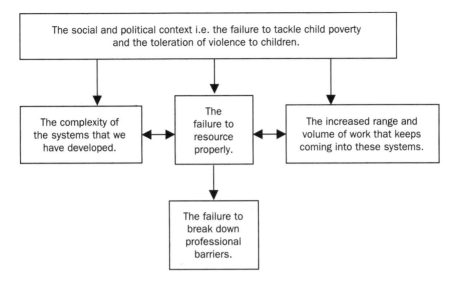

Figure 12.1 Barriers to professional communication

and neglect, organized abuse, institutional abuse, child prostitution, young sex offenders, abuse on the Internet and bullying (Department of Health 1999) – a far cry from the single focus on battered children in the 1960s (Kempe *et al.* 1962).

Resourcing this 'industry' has proved problematic. Throughout the late 1980s and 1990s there have been regular reports of unallocated cases on child protection registers, echoed, as we have seen, in the recent post-Climbie audits. Social services departments in the 1990s were criticized for allocating the bulk of their community child care resources to child protection cases and for not providing services and support for children and families in more general need of help. Training of professionals has also been variable, and, as has already been noted, has not been sufficiently interprofessional.

Breaking down the barriers between professionals has not been achieved as well as it might have been. While the failure to communicate, evidenced in the Climbie inquiry, may be a worst-case scenario, there are, as post-Climbie audits attest (Commission for Health Improvement 2003), similar situations (in terms of type) in many other parts of the country. Two remedies that might be applied are as follows. First, there is a need for more joint training, which focuses specifically on communication and barriers to it, such as stereotyping and ignorance of the roles and duties of others. Second, more consideration should be given to the notion of interprofessional teams. They seem to be working in relation to youth offenders, but have not been considered as a solution by Lord Laming (Laming 2003). In the absence of such a development, much greater attention should be given to improving the opportunities for key child protection professionals to meet face-to-face on a regular basis (not just in crises). Such contact is vital to the development of the sort of trust and understanding that is required to maintain good communication between professionals.

The issue of the political and cultural context in which child abuse and safeguarding takes place, while not directly related to day-to-day practice, is important in the long-term. The present Labour government has made a strong commitment to reducing child poverty and this commitment is reflected in its policy towards safeguarding children. However, it has been much more ambivalent in relation to the issue of parental corporal punishment, which many child protection professionals consider to be crucial to the goal of reducing the incidence of child abuse (see Freeman 1999).

Conclusion

In this concluding section, consideration will be given to the measures being introduced post-Climbie in order to improve working together between agencies in safeguarding children. Autumn 2003 has seen the publication of a range of key documents, including the Green Paper, 'Every Child Matters' (House of Commons 2003a), the Government's response to the Victoria Climbie report (House of Commons 2003b) and new guidelines about referring safeguarding children concerns (Department of Health 2003).

Many of the recommendations of these reports are at policy and systems levels, and there is a strong emphasis on the development of universal services, such as Sure Start, Children's Fund and Connexions, as a means of reducing the need for safeguarding interventions. Two measures are seen as likely to improve inter-agency co-operation at the level of policy – the bringing together under one ministerial department responsibility for children's education and social services needs (this took place in summer 2003), and the establishment of Children's Trusts at a local authority level. There is no blueprint for the latter and, at the time of writing, it is unclear exactly how this change will impact on interprofessional co-operation. Another change in the offing is the replacement of Area Child Protection Committees with Local Safeguarding Children Boards. However, again at this stage it is not clear how these will differ from their predecessors. Key agencies such as social services, the police and health authorities have been required to review all their practices and procedures for safeguarding children and to set performance standards to be reached. There are recommendations for improving communication at the front-line level. These include the development of electronic health and social care records, which will give key professionals common access to data held about children in need of safeguarding. It is also being recommended that all agencies use a unified assessment form for the evaluation of children's needs, to replace the proliferation of separate methods currently existing. Key to the usefulness of these changes is the development of the appropriate technology and the training of staff to use it.

It is clear, therefore, that the concerns raised by the Climbie inquiry are being given serious consideration by central government. The issue may well be, however, whether all these systemic and technological changes will have any significant impact on co-operation between agencies at the cutting edge. As already noted, the child protection system at present suffers from being over complex, resulting in less direct contact between service users and professionals (and between professionals). There is a danger that the changes being proposed could make matters worse. Clearly this needs to be borne in mind and guarded against.

There are several ways of developing better working together relationships at the front-line level, which are crucial to the process of safeguarding children. Most of these have been indicated already in this chapter and are as follows:

1. The need for joint training for professionals to establish a common purpose and sympathetic evaluation and understanding of each other's roles. Ideally, such training should be built into professional qualifying courses, as well as taking place during practice.
2. The need to give further consideration to the development of interprofessional, specialist child protection teams along the lines of the youth offending team arrangements.
3. The need for positive ongoing contact between professionals in the form of discussions about policy and practice at a general rather than crisis level. Meetings of this kind might be used to discuss concerns raised over the handling of cases, with a view to developing clearer practice.
4. The need for secondments between agencies to facilitate better communication and understanding of respective roles.
5. The development of respect for the roles of others and the need to check on stereotyping.

The biggest barrier to developments of this kind is that they are time-consuming and costly, and could be seen as an unaffordable luxury. However, time spent in reflection and careful discussion with others about cases is, in my view, not wasted. Returning to the Climbie inquiry, one gets a sense of decisions being made quickly, assessments being carried out on the hoof and follow-up work not being done because staff were busy moving on to the next problem at breakneck speed. There is need for more careful consideration of issues and for a more questioning, critical approach to the work of safeguarding children (see Munro 2002). To achieve these goals, in addition to time, there is also a need to retain good quality and experienced practitioners at the front line. Measures of this kind are every bit as important as the development of sophisticated tracking systems – indeed they are crucial to their effective use.

Questions for further discussion

1. What are the major challenges in recognizing that a child may be in danger of abuse?
2. Besides the issue of cost what other barriers exist to prevent joint working?
3. How can these barriers be overcome at local level?

References

Barr, O. (1997) Interdisciplinary teamwork: consideration of the challenges, *British Journal of Nursing*, 17: 1005–10.

Bridge, Child Care Consultancy Service (1991) *Sukina: An Evaluation of the Circumstances Leading to her Death*. The Bridge, London.

Bridge, Child Care Consultancy Service (1995) *Paul: Death from Neglect*. The Bridge, London.

Buckley, H. (2003) *Child Protection Work: Beyond the Rhetoric*. Jessica Kingsley, London.

Butler-Sloss, Lord Justice E. (1988) *Report of the Inquiry into Child Abuse in Cleveland 1987*. DHSS Cmnd 412 HMSO, London.

Clyde, Lord (1992) *Report of the Inquiry into the Removal of Children from Orkney in February 1991*. HoC 195. HMSO, London.

Commission for Health Improvement (2003) *The Victoria Climbie Inquiry Report: Key Findings From the Self Audits of NHS Organizations, Social Services Departments and the Police*. Commission for Health Improvement, London.

Cooper, H., Carlisle, C., Gibbs, T., and Watkins, C. (2001) Developing an evidence base for interdisciplinary learning: a systematic review, *Journal of Advanced Nursing*, 35: 228–37.

Corby, B., Doig, A. and Roberts, V. (1998) Inquiries into child abuse, *Journal of Social Welfare and Family Law*, 20: 377–96.

Corby, B., Doig, A. and Roberts, V. (2001) *Public Inquiries into Abuse of Children in Residential Care*. Jessica Kingsley, London.

Corby, B., Millar, M, and Pope, A. (2002) Assessing children in need assessments – a parents' perspective, *Practice*, 14(4): 5–16.

Corby, B. (2003) Supporting Families and Protecting Children: Assisting Child Care professionals in Initial Decision-Making and Review of Cases, *Journal of Social Work*, 3: 195–210.

Corsaro, W. (1997) *The Sociology of Childhood*. Sage, London.

Dartington Social Research Unit (1995) *Child Protection: Messages from Research*. HMSO, London.

Department of Health (1991a) *Child Abuse: A Study of Inquiry Reports 1980–1989*. HMSO, London.

Department of Health (1991b) *Working Together under the Children Act 1989: a Guide to Arrangements for Inter-agency Cooperation for the Protection of Children from Abuse*. HMSO, London.

Department of Health (1999) *Working Together to Safeguard Children: a guide to inter-agency working to safeguard and promote the welfare of children*. The Stationery Office, London.

Department of Health (2000) *Framework for the Assessment of Children in Need and their Families*. The Stationery Office, London.

Department of Health (2003) *Safeguarding Children: What to Do if You're Worried a Child is being Abused*. Department of Health, London.

Department of Health and Social Security (1974) *Report of the Committee of Inquiry into the Care and Supervision Provided in Relation to Maria Colwell*. HMSO, London.

Freeman, M. (1999) Children are Unbeatable, *Children & Society*, 13: 130–41.

Gibbons, J. Conroy, S. and Bell, C. (1995) *Operating the Child Protection System: A Study of Child Protection Practices in English Local Authorities*. HMSO, London.

Home Office/Department of Health (1992) *Memorandum of Good Practice on Video-recorded Interviews with Child Witnesses for Criminal Proceedings*. HMSO, London.

House of Commons (2003a) *Every Child Matters*. CM5860. House of Commons, London.

House of Commons (2003b) *Keeping Children Safe: The Government's Response to the Victoria Climbie Inquiry Report and Joint Chief Inspectors' Report Safeguarding Children*, CM5861. House of Commons, London.

Kempe, C., Silverman, F., Steele, B., Droegemuller, W. and Silver, H. (1962) The battered child syndrome, *Journal of the American Medical Association*, 181: 17–24.

Laming, Lord (2003) The Victoria Climbie Inquiry: Report of an Inquiry by Lord Laming. CM5730. House of Commons, London.

Munro, E. (2002) *Effective Child Protection*. Sage, London.

Social Services Inspectorate (2001) *Developing Quality to Protect Children: SS Inspections of Children's services, August 1999–July 2001* (author K. Adams). Department of Health, London.

Spratt, T. (2001) The Influence of Child Protection Orientation on Child Welfare Practice. *British Journal of Social Work*, 31: 933–54.

Sweeney, J. (2003) Meadow: the Unseen Victims, in the *Observer*, 14 December.

Thomas, T. (1996) Covert video surveillance – an assessment of the Staffordshire protocol, *Journal of Medical Ethics*, 22: 22–5.

13

Across the Great Divide: creating partnerships in education

Thoby Miller

This chapter will:

- Evaluate the educational needs of young people in its broadest sense; challenging the preoccupation with academic excellence at the expense of personal and social development, and proposing the delivery of a more holistic form of education.
- Examine the professional insularities that exist between teachers and youth workers and consider how their respective inputs into the lives of young people might be developed into a partnership.
- Discuss the human tendency to identify by difference rather than focusing on a clearer understanding of our fundamental commonalities and whether placing concepts like emotional intelligence and eco-literacy more centrally might make us all more generally aware of our mutual interdependence.

Introduction

Teachers and youth workers both spend time working with young people, engaging in various kinds of focused activity. Although there is some collaboration between the two, for many teachers and youth workers, there still exists a perceived distance in terms of practice and often a mutually critical attitude towards each other's style of engagement with young people.

The present discussion tries to look at how partnerships between teachers and youth workers might benefit young people. It considers some of the advantages that might be gained from a more integrated system of education; one in which a greater commitment to the principles of social education might enhance more formal approaches. It could be said that there exists a 'Great Divide' between formal and social education, and there is a case for increasing co-ordination both at the level of theory and practice, expanding the breadth of the education that we offer young people. It is argued here that young people may benefit from both groups being willing to cross that 'Great Divide'; though crossing the boundaries may involve an uncomfortable journey into unfamiliar surroundings. However, it could be worth it, in terms of the benefits that might accrue for young people, by way of a closer fit to their actual needs. That, after all, is the central concern of both groups. In the past, too much energy has been expended on the negative practice of identifying differences between the two professional areas; areas which have more in common than is generally accepted. Perhaps it is time for those commonalities to be recognized and developed. In the words of Michelle Erina Doyle:

> The split between formal and informal education is part of the problem. We would all do better if we concentrated on being in the same field – education – rather than trying to convince ourselves and others of our differences. Learning involves process *and* product not process *or* product.
>
> (Doyle 2001: 6)

The following discussion operates on three levels. First, it examines the relationship between teachers and youth workers and how this might be made more effective for young people. While it is not usual to discuss students/pupils as service users, it may be useful to do so in order to explore some of the ways in which the service they receive from education professionals could be improved through better co-ordination. If we are serious about promoting the rights of young people, as well as their responsibilities, we might be led to consider whether they deserve more choice in the topics covered and consultation over other issues that significantly affect their learning. To do so would require a re-examination of the service being provided and a consideration of whether professional insularities might be compromising the overall outcomes.

Second, and more generally, an examination of the relationship between teachers and youth workers suggests a need to look at the balance between formal and social education in the lives of young people, and to consider whether there is a case for a more holistic approach. We need to question the kind of preparation we are giving successive generations and whether it is appropriate to their needs, in terms of their personal and social education, as well as a preparation for future employment. The current policy initiative launched around citizenship is unlikely to succeed while it comprises just another segment of a formal curriculum; especially when it is part of an education agenda that denies students the right to express their views on key issues. Far better surely, to integrate more securely the principles of social education into formal practice, so that citizenship becomes an element within a developed focus on personal and social education, and a springboard for a subsequent pattern of lifelong learning.

Most speculatively, we will consider our innate tendency as human beings to delineate and conceptualize ourselves as separate from others, despite the overwhelming evidence of our interdependence on each other and of our being a part of the natural environment. It is a feature of modernist discourse that we more readily identify points of difference rather than points of commonality. Maybe this is the root of professional rivalries.

As modern societies steadily take on more of a multi-cultural character, we may need to be mindful of how far we continue this differential delineation. Bryan Turner argues that modern society has outlived its need for the 'thick' solidarities and hot commitments that currently generate so much nationalist fervour and ethnic hatred: '. . . modern democracy . . . presupposes large nation states, mass audiences ethnic pluralism, mass migrations and globalized systems of communication . . . (so) modern societies probably need cool cosmopolitans with ironic vocabularies' (Turner 1999: 99). So, while recognizing and valuing points of difference, we should not allow our sensibilities to overheat into a kind of insularity that it is negative and exclusive, particularly so for educators who are directly responsible for much of what is learned by subsequent generations.

At a deeper, third, level then, this present discussion is a consideration of the boundaries that divide us. Borders and boundaries are inevitably points of interface. They are as much sites of potential conflict and incursions, as they are of agreements and resolutions. These points of resolution could be developed into a productive space where new syntheses can be generated. Teachers and social educators could create such a synthesis around the concepts of sustainable development and eco-literacy. The conclusion to the discussion will suggest that the integration of such concepts into education practice would constitute a legacy that could be crucial, not only to the current generation but to many generations to come; an introduction to a pattern of lifelong learning that transcends individual lives and makes a fundamental contribution to life in the future.

Teachers and the formalization of schooling

The protagonists on this educational boundary are engaged in proposing apparent alternative visions of what young people need in the way of education. Teachers are part of a formal education system, focused primarily on a finite product. Eraut (1994) identifies five features of formal learning:

- a prescribed learning framework;
- an organized learning event or package;
- the presence of a designated teacher or trainer;
- the award of a qualification or credit;
- the external specification of outcome.

All of these are characteristics of a secondary school. We might add to the above features the concept of intentionality from the perspective of the learner. For our present purpose, this is a significant addition. Do all students in secondary school follow their studies with intentionality? This is hardly the case, considering the number of disaffected students currently being identified and 'managed' so that they do not impact on the school's position in the league tables.

Until recently, the main focus of secondary education has become the achievement of more passes, with better grades for as many students as possible. The learning process that young people go through has not been valued in the same way as the product; a pursuit of the Holy Grail of summative assessment. The difficulties those students may have overcome in order to get good grades and the informal learning that may have taken place along the way, have only been given marginal consideration.

However, recent initiatives have begun to indicate a positive change, with increasing recognition of learning achieved outside the formal curriculum. The Department for Education and Skills policy document, *Investment for Reform* (2002), outlines an intention to 'transform secondary education . . . (making) . . . a decisive break with the old comprehensive system . . . (and) . . . radically reforming working practices in schools.' This radical agenda includes a reform of teaching and learning, ensuring that the learning needs of individual students are met, as well as reforming partnerships beyond the classroom.

Working in partnership with teachers, social educators are well placed to drive forward such an initiative, collaborating on inclusive strategies. Meeting the individual needs of students could, for example, involve a re-evaluation of the importance of conversations with their students or, again, could include the development of emotional literacy. In this way, education policy might move beyond an instrumentalist concern for future employment into improving personal awareness and social skills.

The DfES Green Paper on extending opportunities and raising standards for 14 to19-year-olds provides a promising basis for subsequent partnerships:

> The best education is far more than the acquisition of knowledge, skills and qualifications. It also helps young people develop attitudes and values that provide the basis for a successful and rewarding life at home, at work and in the community. Young people in this new century should have self-confidence, the ability to be self-critical, the drive to take on new challenges and take risks and the capacity to relate to others in positive, constructive ways. Today's generation of young people need these skills.
>
> (2002: 1.20)

This statement virtually comprises a definition of the aims of social education and, as such, seems to suggest a significant shift in education policy and one that is much overdue. Over the past 20 years or more, secondary schools and the practice of teachers who work in them, have been made increasingly accountable. While this culture of accountability has achieved overall increases in the quantifiable elements of education, and in particular improved exam results for the majority of students, it has done less to reduce the sense of exclusion experienced by less able and less motivated students.

During the 1960s and 1970s, British education went through a process of liberalization, which focused increasingly on the needs of the child. Along with the introduction of comprehensive secondary education and the abolition of physical punishment came developments in both the substance and delivery of the curriculum, which made the experience of schooling more user-friendly. When Margaret Thatcher and Keith Joseph initiated a rejection of these changes in the 1970s, they presented their reforms as a more accurate way of assessing the effectiveness of current education practice. There were certainly instances of indifferent teaching and even downright incompetence and there was a case for teachers to become more accountable and to be encouraged to demonstrate good practice. However, the Thatcherite project was also driven by an innate mistrust of the power of professional bodies and the ways in which their power could be used to challenge central government.

In a climate that places such emphasis on the pursuit of excellence, it has been harder for schools to follow inclusive methods of education. Intensive support for students who are experiencing difficulties is much harder to justify in an environment focused primarily on exam success, mainly because investing extra time on a student who is only likely to achieve a moderate grade, may not register in the league table. There is little external recognition for the educational value of helping less able students to gain a bare pass, even when that achievement comprises a considerable personal journey. Perhaps this kind of success is considered too difficult to reduce to statistical analysis.

Mike Tomlinson, ex-head of Ofsted, gave an indication that things might be about to change. Following his explicit criticism of the way Ofsted inspectors under Chris Woodhead carried out their inspections, he offers a strong hint of a move away from reductionist forms of analysis:

> . . . there were cases where staff in schools were not treated . . . as professionals . . . any inspector who thinks that behaving in an off-handed, curt and rude way is doing Ofsted's business is wrong. We must make sure that we look at parts of education which are not susceptible to simplistic measurements . . . For some schools, their achievements and the pride they have in them, are very often more associated with the non-quantifiable aspects than with the quantifiable.
>
> (*Guardian*, 28 August 2001)

If Tomlinson is right, then it is additional evidence to support the idea that teachers already value the inclusive characteristics of social education and perhaps only need a shift in education policy to build on these values and the partnerships that could be developed.

The new culture of accountability, which developed during 18 years of Conservative government, brought with it a huge increase in the amount of paperwork that teachers were supposed to deal with, complicating tasks unnecessarily and generating a perception among the profession that current practice was perceived by central government to be unsatisfactory unless teachers had demonstrated otherwise. Hardly surprising then, that teachers responded by seeking early retirement in their droves and that recruitment to the profession declined to the point where schools were soon to face their worst ever shortage of teachers.

The Labour landslide of 1997 did little to improve the situation, endorsing the heavy-handed criticisms voiced by the head of Ofsted and its aggressive use of inspections. The new legislation carried on a process that went beyond an audit of education practice. It consolidated the Conservative's move towards a more centralized control of education and carried out a massive re-structuring project, policed by a system of inspection, which has questioned the integrity of teachers and demoralized the profession. It is hard then, not to see teaching as a beleaguered profession, compromised and ground down by increasing formalization, inadequately resourced and viewed by successive governments with suspicion and a lack of respect for their professional integrity.

However, developing partnerships with social educators could point the way towards a more holistic and negotiable curriculum that engages more precisely with the needs of all young people. Issues like anti-social behaviour, drug use and bullying could be dealt with as part of an active critical evaluation of education that involved students as well as teachers. If we begin to look at students more as service users, we would be more likely to accept the legitimacy of their responses to the service they are being offered. At present, their opinions are seldom sought and still less often responded to.

If such partnerships were successful in reducing the problems caused by those issues identified above and others, not only would the curriculum be enhanced to give a greater breadth of education but the delivery of formal elements would be more effective.

Youth and community work: a profession in transition?

Compared to the number of full-time teachers currently employed, the numbers of full-time youth and community workers is small, although these numbers are supplemented by a large number of part-time workers. Some youth and community practitioners feel it is important to defend the 'unique' character of their practice but this can create what could be seen as artificial divisions with others who are also involved in young people's education.

While teachers and pupils are brought together as part of the legal requirement for young people to take part in a period of compulsory education, social or informal education carried out by youth and community workers is normally based on a voluntary relationship. From the young person's point of view, this is intended to help them to develop and express themselves in a less prescribed way. However, the voluntary nature of this relationship means that social educators' access to young people is limited. Youth provision is often restricted in its ability to engage with young people. Its purpose is often misunderstood and the value of its impact undervalued by young people as well as adults. The result of this is that relatively few young people experience its benefits. It needs to extend beyond its current tendencies towards involvement with 'marginalized youth' and into mainstream society.

Over the past 20 years, there has been a trend towards emphasizing the problematic nature of young people, since funding for youth projects has been readily available to finance a range of solutions to these problems. Jeffs and Smith (1999) refer to youth workers exhibiting a 'huckster's desire for easy funding', resulting in a proliferation of activities which, in turn, can tend to characterize young people by the problems they experience. The needs of those young people who do not present the school with any particular problems can get overlooked. It is indicative of the demand for social education that when a youth worker initiates a 'drop-in' provision within a school, the take-up in terms of numbers of students is often so enthusiastic as to be almost unmanageable. As service users, these students are articulating a felt need. As educators, we have a duty to respond to it.

First though, we need to be more explicit about the terms we are using to describe this non-formal area of practice. Youth and community professionals often use the term 'informal education' to describe their style of practice. I have used the term 'social education' as a more explicit and positive term (in line with European models of social pedagogy), although I also use 'informal' to contrast more precisely with formal settings.

This model of social education is one that aims to enable individuals within communities to regain a level of control over their learning and is based on the fundamental principles of democracy, equality and dialogue. Social education practice in Scandinavia provides a useful example of this, emphasizing as it does, the importance of an equal and ongoing dialogue between students and educators, with learning seen as an active process, enabling students to gain a greater understanding of themselves and others. This process is activated by ensuring that the substantive content of learning is always seen by learners as relevant to their individual aspirations; students are encouraged to negotiate with the educator in a critical examination of suitability, both of the subject being taught and of the way in which learning is taking place.

Perhaps the most important element in this, and its sharpest point of contrast with formal education, is the active engagement of the learner in the process of learning. We might associate the absence of such an involvement on the part of the learner with a disaffected attitude towards the whole idea of education and one from which that person never recovers, negating the possibility of their establishing a pattern of lifelong learning. The open access policy that underpins the Youth and Community Education degree at NEWI encourages applications from many people whose experiences of school range from the uninspiring through to the completely intolerable. In most cases, they speak of being obliged to study subjects that seemed to have no meaning for them and being taught in ways that required their passive acceptance, whether learning was achieved or not. Together, these two factors comprise a potent means of generating disaffection with the whole idea of education.

Although the experience of formal education may not be a positive one for all school students, the mode of practice is generally understood. In contrast, fewer people understand the meaning of social education and even amongst professionals working in the field, there is considerable dispute over terminology and contexts. Colley, Hodgkinson and Malcolm (2002) have provided a comprehensive summary of the different discourses that exist in areas outside formal education and argue that the boundaries between different kinds of learning can only be understood within particular contexts. They experience difficulty with the large number of different classifications of the kinds of education practice carried on outside formal settings. This is complicated by a tendency in many texts to imply that one particular form is superior, either morally or in its effectiveness, as a means of learning. They use data from two ongoing research projects; one looking at schoolteachers' work-based learning and another examining learning cultures in further education:

This revealed that, in what would almost always be assumed to be formal educational settings (FE courses), informal learning was very important, whilst for schoolteachers' workplace learning, normally regarded as informal, some formal elements were present. In both cases, it was the *blending of formal and informal that was significant, not their separation.*

(Colley *et al.* 2002:2, emphasis added)

This supports my contention that formal and social educators need to co-ordinate their activities both within formal settings and elsewhere. If the 'blending' that Colley *et al.* refer to is a feature of the kind of learning that *actually* occurs in formal settings, there needs to be a more direct recognition of the importance of social education within that learning process.

Furthermore, such a recognition might encourage a greater public awareness of the importance of social education. David Bell, the director of Ofsted, has called for parents to prepare their children better for school. He appears to be talking about social education, a lack of which could cause the kind of anti-social behaviour that he is so concerned about. Perhaps some parents do not understand how best to manage their children. It is unlikely that they will have been helped to learn such skills when they were in school themselves. It may be that an input of good social education practice into schools would enable generations of parents to see how they could include elements of it in day-to-day interactions with their children.

In a society characterized by rapid change such an understanding becomes even more necessary. A world that Jock Young sees as defined by its uncertainty: '. . . where . . . market forces which transformed the spheres of production and consumption relentlessly challenged our notions of material certainty and uncontested values, replacing them with a world of risk and uncertainty, of individual choice and pluralism . . .' (1999: 1). If the principles of social education were integrated more securely into the formal education system, there is little doubt that it would enhance the profile of a youth and community profession that still finds itself struggling against public perceptions which trivialize the effects it has on the lives of the young people.

While the introduction of the Connexions programme has raised the profile of youth and community workers and the demand for their services, it has also tended to focus their activities on young people who are identified as having problems. While this is clearly a priority, social education must be made more generally available. It is simply too good not to share with all young people. Social educators working in partnership with schools and colleges have an exciting opportunity to do this.

Current problems in integrating education practice

Teachers' styles of practice are constrained by externally imposed curricula and compulsory attendance. In contrast, the kind of social education carried out by youth and community workers implies a more flexible, open-ended basis. Hardly surprising then, that where these two forms of education coincide, there are tensions over competing strategies, played out within the nature of the respective interventions that each make into the lives of young people.

Inevitably, there will be some schools in which partnerships may be hard to develop, most often because of resistance from the staff and consequently partnership initiatives would need to be encouraged by shifts in both education and youth policy. However, in recent years, the two professional areas have become much more closely associated within both schools and colleges. Mark Smith details some of the initiatives that are taking place, involving a growing army of personnel including classroom assistants, informal educators, youth workers, learning mentors and personal advisers.

Activities have included, for example:

- Working with students to set up study clubs and circles and homework clubs.
- Encouraging and supporting the development of groups around enthusiasms and interests such as music and sound systems, environmental issues and cross-community reconciliation.
- Developing alternative educational provision for young people experiencing difficulties in mainline classrooms.
- Working with individuals around personal difficulties they are experiencing with their lives. This could be to do with family relationships and friendships, schooling, health or around thinking about their future.
- Being around in hallways, canteens and recreation areas to help build an environment that is safe and convivial.
- Enhancing the quality of relationships and of college and school life generally through activities like residentials and 'fun days'.
- Opening up avenues for young people to engage with different political systems via school councils, student unions and youth forums.
- Assisting with the development of inclusive education. This may be through working with young people to accept others, and to make sense of the school environment.

(www.infed.org/schooling)

This present discussion explores the idea that the overall quality of the education delivered to young people would be improved by both formal and informal educators venturing across the 'Great Divide', which still separates the two areas of practice. A more holistic experience of education should be available to all young people, regardless of their academic ability. It is as unhelpful to overlook the personal and social needs of 'high achievers' as it is those who experience more difficulties succeeding in formal contexts, even though informal support is most urgently needed for those young people who have become disengaged from or disheartened by their experiences of formal education.

Changing the way we look at young people

Conceptions of young people have changed utterly over the past 150 years. Particularly in developed countries, young people now have a greater level of social legitimacy than ever before but perhaps we need still to consider the extent to which formal education practice retains a residual unwillingness to recognize the internal logic and rationality of the behaviour of young people. Here are two examples, one relating to a minority of students and one that applies to all young people. The purpose here is to illustrate the way that young people are not credited with the rationality of the choices they make, if those choices are in conflict with current educational discourse.

Truancy as a rational choice

Over the last ten years or more, there has been a pronounced change in the conceptualization of behavioural characteristics presented by young people in school. These include truancy and general disaffection and are seen as non-productive, dysfunctional and illegitimate by the DfEE and many teachers. In the past, a large number of studies have attempted to account for such conduct by using a pathological model, ascribing and reducing explanations to the personal inadequacies of the individual. However, this sort of model has been shown by subsequent research to be deficient.

Stoll and O'Keefe (1989/1993) have demonstrated that much truancy is based on a series of rational decisions taken by the young person. For example, students are most likely to absent themselves from classes that are seen by them as having the least relevance. Furthermore, a SCRE study (1996) has closely linked truancy to levels of educational achievement, suggesting that students are most likely not to attend when they recognize their inability to do well in that setting – predicting quite rightly, as far as they are concerned, that little learning will be achieved.

We would do well to consider the rationality of these decisions. Formal educators and those directing education policy have started to examine the 'intentionality' of those who truant or engage in disruptive behaviour, considering that this may be the result of structural problems within the school, a failure to accommodate the learning needs of such students. Where such an accommodation is made, the results are a significant reduction in truancy and an improvement in classroom behaviour. In schools where an inclusive kind of alternative curriculum has already been established, we can begin to see the kind of incremental benefits that more inclusive forms of education might engender.

A study by the National Foundation for Educational Research (NFER) has shown that different alternative curriculum programmes can be located at points along a continuum ranging from exclusion to inclusion of the pupil. At the exclusion end, the problem is located with the pupil whose behaviour is seen as unacceptable so that their needs have to be met by alternative provision outside the school, which effectively distances itself from the problem. At the other end of the continuum, schools accept that there is a need to revise their provision in order to meet pupil's different learning needs and in doing so tries to include them in a more appropriate form of education. Clearly such schools are engaged in promoting a critical reflection of educational practice and are operating as learning organizations, transforming themselves and showing an openness to new insights (www.nfer.ac.uk/research/papers/BERA.Cullen.doc).

Political protest as a rational decision

Article 12 of the UN Convention on the Rights of the Child (1990) asserts the right of young people to have a voice on issues that affect them. It is significant that the United States, a country that makes a virtue and a military reality of its obsession with individual freedoms, refused to ratify this article. However, young people have been slow to take advantage of this endorsement of their rights. Furlong and Cartmel refer to the fact that 'low levels of political participation among youth have been cause for concern in a number of industrialised countries' (1997: 96).

It is deeply ironic that when in April 2003, students were motivated to protest against what they saw as an unjust war, their actions were not seen as legitimate and they were met with the kind of condescension which might have made them doubt whether the calls for their political involvement were genuine. David Hart of the National Association of Head Teachers responded in a way that would be laughable, were it not so dismissive of the rights both of young people and of teachers:

> Heads should ban all protests during school. They should take disciplinary action against any members of staff who encourage the demonstrations and against any pupils who are absent when they should be in school . . . The right way to go about it is to give pupils the opportunity in school to debate the issues . . . They might benefit more from learning about the causes of war than by demonstrating against it.
>
> (Reported in BBC News, 21 March 2003)

Few comments could have illustrated any better the problematic discourse that still exists within parts of formal education and which is, at least in part, responsible for generating a negative reaction to schooling from both students and teachers! While schools must maintain a duty of care towards their students and events outside school need parents' permission, there remains an issue over how young people's opinions can be heard. First, there is a declaration that designated study time remain inaccessible to the wishes of students, regardless of the crucial nature of the issue. Second, there is a threat both to students and teachers which attempts to trivialize their ethical concerns. Third, there is a derisory attempt to offer an alternative to political action in the way of a debate and even this is degraded by the suggestion that young people need to learn more about the causes of war before they take to the streets. Again, as has been suggested in the Hutton inquiry, those young people had assessed the situation only too accurately and had come to the rational conclusion that there was no legitimate case for military action.

The comments of a student who was suspended because of taking part in a protest highlights the level of frustration felt by those who were disempowered by the experience:

> The majority of our school does not have democratic rights. They have no means to express themselves, and they don't have a voice in real terms. The only way we can, as minors, express ourselves is through demonstration.
>
> (Sachin Sharma reported on BBC News, 5 March 2003 and cited in
> www.infed.org)

We show a lack of respect for young people by ignoring such views. If we are as genuinely concerned about issues of citizenship as the government claims to be, we need to be prepared to listen with care and respond in a positive way. It can only be hoped that politicians who have long bemoaned young people's lack of political engagement have the good grace to squirm with embarrassment at the words of Neela

Dolezalova, an 18-year-old student who had walked out of school to join the demonstration:

> Everyone was determined to find a channel for the outrage they felt about the war. I realised that although this student peace movement is young and inexperienced, it is passionate, diverse and creative. Suddenly the politicisation of youth looks unattractive to those who have called us apathetic for too long.
>
> (*Guardian*, 22 March 2003)

The message seems to be that becoming a responsible citizen means accepting that your democratic rights are going to be compromised. Can active citizenship really be part of an educational discourse based on passive uncritical acceptance?

Enhancing the impact of formal education

As well as changes in national education policy, there is scope for re-evaluating the kind of relationships that exist between teachers and students, and whether developmental work could make these more productive. Teachers could be encouraged to engage in more critical self-reflective practice on this topic, highlighting good practice in dealing with problematic behaviour and responding to the perceptions of students.

Some consideration might, for example, be given to the role that some teachers play in generating flashpoints. In 2002, I conducted a series of informal interviews with youth workers operating in schools. Several of them mentioned the difficulty they found in persuading the teaching staff that badly managed interactions with students were sometimes creating and certainly exacerbating behavioural problems. Many of the explosive incidents that resulted in students being suspended or excluded took place in the classes of particular teachers. In discussions with youth workers, students repeatedly identified the same teachers, maybe four or five in each school. Many students talked of being provoked, of being goaded into an outburst.

Undoubtedly, youth workers are placed in a delicate position, trying to offer support to young people who feel aggrieved (perhaps with some justification) but being unable to challenge the nature of their relationship with teachers. There may be some scope for partnership working on topics like this. For example, workshops including both teachers and youth workers would provide a forum for an exchange of good practice and encourage both to develop a clearer understanding of each other's mode of practice and the problems they face. There is also scope for organizational learning to take place to help deal with unresolved classroom incidents like those identified above: 'not only an organisation in which learning opportunities for staff are encouraged and promoted, but one in which the whole organisation is open to new ideas, to learning from experience' (Coulshed and Mullender, 2001: 185).

First though, work needs to be done on changing the blame culture generated in part by the aggressive use of inspections. Teachers are more likely to fear failure rather than to see it as a learning opportunity; to care more about deflecting criticism than improving their practice. In *Educating the Reflective Practitioner* (1987) Schön has referred to professional practice often comprising a high ground overlooking a swamp:

On the high ground, manageable problems lend themselves to solutions through the application of research-based theory and technique. In the swampy lowland, messy, confusing problems defy technical solution.

(1987: 3)

Disruptive students are clearly a messy confusing problem and one that cannot be resolved without teachers being open to the opportunity to reflect on their practice and consider how improvements could be made. More suspensions, exclusions and referral units are technical solutions, which often merely deflect the problem elsewhere.

One solution to these problems involves joint training for teachers and youth workers as indicated in Box 13.1.

Box 13.1 Joint training workshops
Currently staff training for both teachers and youth workers is carried out separately. However, we might imagine scenarios where, based on an understanding of mutual interests in the same client group, teachers and youth workers might come together in workshop situations. These would enable each group to outline the difficulties they face and move on to developing joint strategies to confront those problems.

Discussion topics might include:

- The nature of the relationship between adults and young people in educational settings, considering the importance of mutual respect and potential areas of negotiation.
- The use of forum theatre or role play to deconstruct and analyse how conflict develops between adults and young people and how these might be resolved.
- Including young people as well as teachers and youth workers in a more general project to develop schools as learning organizations to address learning needs more directly.

As indicated above, education policy makers now seem to be reflecting on the way in which the curriculum could be revised to be less exclusive. This is much overdue in a situation where the implementation of the National Curriculum and Statutory Attainment Targets has forced teachers away from the process of education, towards more quantifiable goals. Blair and New Labour have invoked the mantra of the pursuit of excellence, with the inevitable corollary of a reduced emphasis being placed on the processual journey that less able students make to reach more moderate outcomes. Until recently, teachers have not been encouraged to place value on such 'soft' targets; they have seldom been praised for their ability to help students with less ability or poor motivation to experience the kind of positive unconditional regard offered them by social educators. Currently schools can be seen, while enhancing examination results for academically able, to be excluding the needs of those who do not fit into the demands of a formal educational curriculum. In this respect, the student who asks 'Why are we doing this?' or 'Why are we doing it in this way?' could be seen as asking a legitimate question that merits a considered response, rather than, as might be the case, being dismissed as impertinent and disruptive.

Young people might be inclined to ask why their learning does not include issues that will affect their futures far more than it will those who are responsible for delivering their education. Already young people have voiced their disapproval of military action in Iraq. They might also ask why they are not engaging in a critical examination of environmental issues, based on the evidence that older generations had left them with a dubious legacy of ecological problems.

Sustainable development, eco-literacy and the politics of interdependence

In the introduction, effective partnerships were seen as capable of generating a fertile space where new perspectives could take root. Globalization and particularly the freeing up of global markets, presents a challenge to formal and informal educators alike. How is it possible to help young people prepare for a life defined by patterns of consumption, in a world that pays scant regard to its resources and their equitable distribution? Neither group has a well-developed response to these questions but they are likely to become some of the most pressing concerns within the next half century. This is an area where partnerships start to define a potential strategy for survival based on mutual interdependence.

Fritjof Capra (1997, 2002) has spoken of the need for a 'Copernican shift' in our understanding of the world and a more general realization that the human race cannot go on treating the environment as if it were both separate from it and superior to it. He encourages us to adopt a sense of 'deep ecology', as opposed to the current shallow environmentalism that Andrew Dobson has described as: 'a managerial approach to environmental problems . . . without fundamental changes in the present values or patterns of production and consumption' (1995: 1). Capra proposes deep ecology as a holistic view of the world, seeing it as an integrated whole, where objects are viewed more as networks of relationships. The key concept is interdependence, a challenge to the aggressive individualism of the late twentieth century, which characterized formal education largely as a series of personal achievements.

The paradigm of deep ecology alongside a greater emphasis on young people becoming emotionally literate focuses on the importance of co-operation. This could become the basis for partnership work between teachers and social educators, integrating all aspects of the current formal curriculum with issue-based work on gender, equality and human rights. Such a partnership would provide a model that emphasizes the crucial nature of social action, developing in young people a realization that their learning directly informs their behaviour. If young people become more acutely aware that their actions can make a difference to the world they live in, their perspectives on learning will be transformed.

Conclusion

The educational partnerships proposed in this discussion are based on the need for more considered reflective practice within the education of young people. Policies need to be underpinned by an ongoing re-evaluation of their effectiveness in meeting the needs of successive generations of young people. What is argued here is that more holistic forms of education are required so that improvements in personal and social awareness can enhance more formal elements of the curriculum. Youth workers operating in schools are in a good position to drive forward such an initiative, yet to succeed it requires the active involvement of teachers. All those engaged in partnerships need to be committed to a reflective consideration of practice and display an openness to the potential learning that engagements with young people provide.

Questions for further discussion

1. Does the present National Curriculum offer young people only a partial preparation for their future lives? Are there identifiable gaps in current provision?
2. Does formal education lack coherence with its delivery of discrete subjects?
3. Can unifying concepts like deep ecology and emotional intelligence help create a more developed system of education?

References

Capra, F. (1997) *The Web of Life.* Flamingo, London.

Capra, F. (2002) *Hidden Connections.* Doubleday, New York.

Colley, H., Hodgkinson, P. and Malcolm, J. (2002) *Non-formal Learning: Mapping the Conceptual Terrain.* www.infed.org.uk.

Coulshed, V. and Mullender, A. (2001) *Management in Social Work.* Palgrave, Basingstoke.

Dobson, A. (1995) *Green Political Thought.* Routledge, London.

DfES (2002) *Green Paper on Extending Opportunities and Raising Standards for 14 to 19 Year Olds.*

DfES (2002) *Investment for Reform.*

Doyle, M. (2001) On Being an Educator, in L.D. Richardson (ed.) *Principles and Practice of Informal Education.* Routledge, London.

Eraut, M. (1994) *Developing Professional Knowledge and Competence.* London, Falmer Press.

Furlong, A. and Cartmel, F. (1997) *Young People and Social Change.* Open University Press, Buckingham.

Jeffs, T. and Smith, M. (1999) *Informal Education.* Education Now, Nottingham.

SCRE Study (1996) www.scre.ac.uk.

Schön, D.A. (1987) *Educating the Reflective Practitioner.* Jossey-Bass, San Francisco.

Stoll, P. and O'Keeffe, D. (1993) *Officially Present.* ILEA Education Unit, Warlingham.

Turner, B. (1999) McCitizens: Risk, Coolness and Irony in Contemporary Politics, in B. Smart (ed.) *Resisting McDonaldisation.* Sage, London.

Young, J. (1999) *The Exclusive Society.* Sage, London.

www.infed.org.uk

www.nfer.ac.uk/research/papers/BERA.Cullen.doc

Further reading

Kolb, D.A. (1984) *Experiential Learning – Experience as a Source of Learning and Development.* Prentice Hall, Englewood Cliffs/London.

Lorenz, W. (1999) *The Role of Training in Preparing Socio-educational Care Workers to Meet the Challenges of Social Change.* Address to 6th FESET European Congress.

Miller, T. (2002) Riding the Cusp/Courir deux lièvres à la fois, *European Journal of Social Education 2.*

O'Hagen, B. (ed.) (1991) *The Charnwood Papers.* Education Now, Ticknall.

Richardson, L. and Wolfe, M. (eds) (2001) *Principles and Practice of Informal Education.* Routledge/Falmer, London.

Smart, B. (ed.) (1999) *Resisting McDonaldisation.* Sage, London.

14

Effective partnerships to assist mentally-disordered offenders

Virginia Minogue

This chapter will:

- Examine why a partnership response is seen as appropriate in the provision of services for mentally-disordered offenders.
- Explore the development of partnership and multi-agency responses to mentally-disordered offenders, using case examples as illustrations.
- Discuss the benefits, difficulties and dilemmas arising from partnership working.
- Examine some of the issues of defining mentally-disordered offenders and the impact this may have on their access to appropriate care and treatment.

Introduction

In the course of an evaluation of an inter-agency mentally-disordered offender partnership group (Minogue 2000), agency managers were asked why partnership was the most appropriate approach to providing services to mentally-disordered offenders. One respondent simply replied, 'because it is the only way to do it'. This response may have been based on experience, a strongly held conviction, or could have been a reflection of local or national policy.

Interest in effective practice with mentally-disordered offenders, increased in the early nineteen nineties[1] and there were two probable elements to this, the first being the report colloquially known as the 'Reed Report' (Department of Health, Home Office 1992), which was the most far-reaching review of provision for mentally-disordered offenders that had, hitherto, been undertaken. The second key factor was the re-evaluation of the care and treatment afforded to mentally-disordered offenders brought about by the homicide committed by Christopher Clunis in 1992 (Reith 1998). However, although significant in marking a sea change in both professional and public interest, neither were remarkable in themselves as, some 16 years prior to the Reed Report, the Butler Committee (Home Office and Department of Health and Social Security 1975) had addressed very similar issues in relation to the care and treatment of 'offenders suffering from mental disorder or abnormality'. Furthermore, texts such as the Zito Trust (1995) and Reith (1998) reflect a long-standing concern about the care of the mentally disordered, instances of bad practice in the treatment of the mentally disordered, and the perceived risk posed by the mentally ill to others.

Early enquiries (Zito Trust 1995) into the care of the mentally disordered tended to focus on the quality of institutional care and their criticisms may have, in part, contributed to the move towards community-based care in the 1990s (Department of Health 1990). However, the complex nature of providing care and treatment in the community requires, for any seriously mentally-disordered person, a multidimensional package involving psychiatric and medical care, control and management, and possibly, public protection. Adding offending behaviour to this equation multiplies the factors to be considered in assessing risk and in the control and management of a case. This also underpins the unique nature of this minority group (mentally-disordered offenders) and the characteristics of mental disorder and crime. Clearly, not all mentally-disordered people offend and similarly, not all offenders are mentally disordered, but a subset of each group has both characteristics. Questions then arise, not only as to whether there is a relationship between the two conditions,[2] but also about the most appropriate method of care and treatment, i.e. from within health, social care or criminal justice systems. Mentally-disordered offenders cross service boundaries and, as such, become the responsibility of a range of professionals, each working from a differing set of values, policies and organizational structures.

The study of mentally-disordered offenders draws from a number of domains, criminology, sociology, mental health, psychiatry, to mention but a few. This, in turn, poses problems for multidisciplinary work as no one philosophy or professional discourse can, on its own, provide a satisfactory explanation or a framework. The study and management of mentally-disordered offenders illustrates how fine the dividing line can be between the perception and understanding of:

- sanity and insanity;
- acceptable and unacceptable behaviour;
- madness and crime.

It also illustrates how the boundaries between care and treatment can become similarly blurred and dependent on whether the offender/patient falls under the auspices of the criminal justice or health services. Robert Harris (1999) describes the mentally-disordered offender as a sort of borderline figure who occupies the space somewhere between mental disorder and criminality, between criminality and social problem, and between petty nuisance and social casualty.

This dichotomy presents the professional with several issues in determining the appropriate action:

- The general lack of any appropriate environment between hospital and prison.
- The need or otherwise to attribute a causal relationship between the mental disorder and the crime.

- The influence of subjective views on the clinical judgements of forensic practitioners.

The criminal law, in the context of this debate, is a relatively straightforward process when dealing with offenders free from mental disorders. However, dealing with a mentally-disordered offender is a far from straightforward process. The possibility of removing or 'diverting' the offender from the judicial process exists and can be utilized at several points in the process. Sections of the Mental Health Act 1983 (MHA 1983) can also be invoked as part of the sentencing process,[3] further illustrating how treating mental disorder challenges the boundaries between mental health and the law. The common factor in each instance is the assessment of the mental disorder and judgement of the offender's culpability in relation to their crime. These assessments contribute to determining their disposal.

Defining mentally-disordered offenders

Mentally-disordered offenders are one of the most difficult groups to categorize. Not only does the terminology used to describe them differ but also the definition of a mentally-disordered offender (Alberg *et al.* 1996; Department of Health, Home Office 1992; Home Office, Department of Health and Social Security 1975; Mental Health Foundation 1994; NACRO 1993). Although it may not be absolutely necessary to have a commonly agreed definition, lack of common understanding opens up the potential for ineffective or inappropriate responses to mentally-disordered offenders, or even the possibility of them falling through the net of services (Hagell 2002; Peay 1999; HM Government 1998). Mentally-disordered offenders are not a distinct group with clearly identifiable issues. Offending may range from comparatively minor offences such as petty theft or breaches of the peace, to serious offences of murder, while mental illness may range from a relatively mild depressive illness to paranoid schizophrenia. There may also be the additional impact of a substance misuse problem, behavioural disorder, personality disorder or sexual offending. The treatment needs of some patients categorized as mentally-disordered offenders may fall outside the boundaries of general psychiatric treatment, for example, sexual offending and violent behaviour. Some may also require a number of services working in co-operation to address a range of problems. However, this can raise issues of confidentiality.

As Clarke *et al.* (2002) point out, the relationship between mental disorder and crime is a complex one. The mental disorder may be a disinhibiting factor but there may be other criminogenic or associative factors of equal relevance. Attempts to define or establish categories become more complex if seen in the context of defining access to services. A serious incidence of offending is likely to increase the probability of intervention by the criminal justice system and lessen the possibility of accessing mental health care.

Even the most straightforward definitions can be problematic. The Reed Report (Department of Health, Home Office 1992), for example, referred to mentally-disordered offenders and others with similar needs as: 'a mentally disordered person who has broken the law'. This may intimate that a prosecution and contact with the courts is necessary, in order for an individual to be defined a mentally-disordered offender. This then excludes those who have not been prosecuted or convicted, although their behaviour may have posed significant risk to others. Furthermore, the shift in policy predicated by Home Office Circular 66/90 (Home Office 1990) and the Reed Report (Department of Health, Home Office 1992) saw the development of many diversion schemes. The majority of these worked on the principle of diverting the mentally disordered away from the criminal justice system at the earliest opportunity, i.e. pre-court. Many of these schemes, and other partnership arrangements, devised their own working definition of a mentally-disordered offender in order to clarify the target group (see Box 14.1).

Box 14.1 Definitions of a mentally-disordered offender

In 1996, in line with other definitions (NACRO 1993; Mental Health Foundation 1994), the Leeds Mentally Disordered Offenders Partnership Group (LMDOPG 1996) provided a broad and inclusive definition of a mentally-disordered offender as:

People who offend and who, without access to health and/or social care, have difficulty in maintaining independent and offending free lifestyles. This means:

- People with a mental disorder, as defined by the 1983 Mental Health Act;
- People with mental health problems linked to alcohol and substance misuse;
- People with significant behavioural and psychological problems associated with disordered personality development;
- Those offenders who commit sexual offences where mental health problems are evident, or disordered personality development;
- Offenders with problems of aggression associated with personality disorder who might benefit from complex psychological intervention and management.

(LMDOPG 1996: 1)

In 2001, LMDOPG opted for a simplified and less explicit definition of mentally disordered offender: 'All those with mental health problems who come into contact with the criminal justice system as a result of activities that may be considered criminal.'

Part III of the Mental Health Act 1983 is specifically concerned with patients involved in criminal proceedings. Despite this, it has limitations and does not deal adequately with those who require specific interventions, for example, those offenders who require psychological rather than psychiatric intervention, and substance misusers. Furthermore, it failed to clarify the nature and extent to which mental disorder should be seen as causing or impacting on offending behaviour and how this might affect any assessment of culpability or liability in prosecution procedures. As a result, the McNaughton Rules of 1843[4] remained the most significant determinant of a defendant's mental fitness in the legal arena. Evidence of the use of insanity as a defence for the commission of a crime stems from the sixteenth century (Gunn 1991), but it was the McNaughton trial in 1843 that led to the production of a set of rules on insanity. Critically, although this ruling placed the emphasis on the jury (comprising of lay people) making the decision about a defendant's sanity, it also introduced the concept of professional experts (i.e. psychiatrists) bringing medical evidence before the court.

By definition, mentally-disordered offenders fall within, or between, the remit of a number of different service providers across the health/social care or criminal justice sectors. This poses several challenges for those trying to determine an appropriate response:

1.   Should they see the mentally-disordered offender as a person with a mental disorder who also offends, or as an offender who also has a mental disorder? (For a further examination of these issues see Columbo 1997; Laing 1999; Fennell and Yeates 2002.)

2.   Should treatment of the illness or punishment of the offence be the primary concern?

3.   Where should the treatment or punishment be located – in the community, hospital or penal institution?

4.   How can two potentially disparate forms of state intervention, the criminal justice system and health care, offer treatment, care, punishment, restriction or rehabilitation, when operating from different ethical and philosophical standpoints?

Given the difficulties in categorizing mentally-disordered offenders, it is of little surprise that the main published statistics relate to those patients subject to a restriction order admitted to, detained in and discharged from hospitals. However, a systematic review of general population studies (University of York, NHS CRD 1999) demonstrated that the prevalence of mentally-disordered offenders in the population is relatively low. Up to the age of 26–30, prevalence was between 2.1 and 2.8 per cent for men and approximately half that number for women. All types of mental disorders were associated with all types of crime. Furthermore, it was apparent that the prevalence of mentally-disordered offenders in the general psychiatric population was also small. Those who were diagnosed with schizophrenia were not dangerous to others nor did they offend at any greater rate than the general population. Although the number of people being detained in high security and other hospitals has seen a steady increase over the last decade, there are still only approximately 100 patients per 3 million population.[5] They are four times more likely to be men than women (Home Office 2002).

However, examination of prison statistics demonstrates a somewhat different picture. A survey of psychiatric morbidity among prisoners in England (Singleton *et al.* 2000) found a prevalence of personality disorder in:

•   78 per cent of male remand prisoners
•   64 per cent male sentenced prisoners
•   50 per cent female prisoners

Psychosis was prevalent in:

- 7 per cent male sentenced prisoners
- 10 per cent male remand
- 14 per cent female prisoners

Further analysis revealed that nine out of ten detained young offenders showed evidence of mental disorder. Three-quarters of these had more than one disorder. Two-thirds of women prisoners in the survey were found to have a neurotic disorder, compared to women in the general population where only one fifth were assessed as having similar problems. Moreover, approximately 40 per cent female prisoners and 20 per cent of male prisoners had help or treatment for a mental or emotional problem in the 12 months before going into prison.

Developing inter-agency responses to mentally-disordered offenders

The 1959 Mental Health Act reflected a shift from institutional care to community care for the mentally ill. This gained momentum in the 1960s and 1970s (Jewesbury and McCulluch 2002) and was given further impetus in the 1980s and 1990s by the Tory government and its hospital closure programme. However, by the 1990s care in the community was heavily criticized (Zito Trust 1995; Howlett 1998; Reith 1998). This was in no small part due to the perceived failures in care indicated by the enquiries into serious incidents of harm involving mentally ill individuals (Ritchie *et al.* 1994; Woodley Team 1995; Royal College of Psychiatrists 1996). The government appeared to echo this view when the Secretary of State for Health made the following statement:

> The law on mental health is based on the needs and therapies of a bygone age. Its revision in 1983 merely tinkered with the problem. What I want now is a root and branch review to reflect the opportunities and limits of modern therapies and drugs.
>
> (Department of Health 1998a)

This presaged the publication of the government vision for the future of mental health services *Modernising Mental Health Services* (Department of Health 1998b), and subsequently the *National Framework for Mental Health* (National Health Service 1999), and the White Paper, *Reforming the Mental Health Act* (Department of Health 2000). The former introduced a raft of new or improved services such as outreach and crisis teams. However, both highlighted once again the tension between voluntary participation in health care and legally enforced compliance. These proposed reforms to the 1983 Mental Health Act will lead to the following:

- An extension of the powers to compel patients to undergo treatment both in hospital and the community.
- Decisions regarding the compulsory treatment of mentally-disordered offenders are likely to be made by the court rather than a Mental Health Review Tribunal (as per the 1983 Mental Health Act).

- Decisions about detention in hospital rather than care in the community would be taken after consideration of risk to public safety, and would obviously be informed by the nature of the offending behaviour.

Other policy changes are anticipated in relation to those with severe personality disorders (Home Office, Department of Health 1999). These arise out of concerns that those with a severe personality disorder, who present a high risk to the public, fall through the net of existing services. Under the proposed changes these individuals could be detained and not released until they are judged to be a low risk to the public, that is they would be subject to indeterminate detention.

There is no clear agreement about whether mentally-disordered offenders should be cared for by general psychiatric or forensic psychiatric services. There are advantages and disadvantages to both but those advocating specialist services argue that specific skills are required, as well as specific treatments and provision (Tighe *et al.* 2002). Some of this thinking underpinned the drive towards partnership responses to mentally-disordered offenders, which gained impetus in the 1990s following the publication of HO Circular 66/90 'Provision for Mentally Disordered Offenders'. This suggested that criminal justice agencies needed to increase their co-operation with health and social services (Home Office 1990). This circular was primarily aimed at the development of diversion schemes, the majority of which were based in police stations or courts. These schemes tended to involve a psychiatrist and/or community psychiatric nurse attending the police cells or court to undertake a psychiatric assessment of the defendant, as a result of a referral from the police, probation service, or other court-based service, and involved agencies co-operating by sharing information and discussing appropriate disposals. Other schemes were based on a 'panel assessment model', which involved a range of agencies forming a panel that met and formulated a management plan for each mentally-disordered individual referred to them (Hedderman 1993). Indications were that benefits were accrued in terms of provision of information, discontinuance of cases, increased understanding between agencies and, following initial pilots, other funding was made available to increase the number of diversion schemes nationally. However, an evaluation revealed that the panel assessment type schemes were not cost effective and recommended discontinuing them (Home Office 1995a).

By 1999, there were approximately 150 court diversion schemes in operation in England and Wales, plus a further 40 schemes operating in police stations (James *et al.* 2002). However, not all partnership schemes were based on a simple diversion model. Some took on a wider remit and attempted to bring together a broad range of agencies in the provision of a package of care, e.g. the Humberside scheme led by MIND (Staite *et al.* 1994), the Surrey Mentally Disordered Offender Project (Haynes and Henfrey 1995). The Humberside Project, in common with the Wessex Project (Swyer 1999), believed that to be successful in diverting the mentally disordered, the involvement of the prison service was crucial, offering the opportunity for more holistic provision across the social care and criminal justice systems, and also the possibility of involvement, by the prison service, in the joint commissioning of some health care services.[6] Crucial to this change in thinking (and willingness to work in co-operation) on the part of health, social care and criminal justice agencies, was the availability of funding from government departments through the Mental Illness Specific Grant, which contributed to the development of court assessment schemes, inter-agency projects and services.

Home Office Circular 66/90 (Home Office 1990) was followed by a further circular in 1995 (Home Office 1995b) reiterating the importance of inter-agency working, but also placing an emphasis on public safety considerations when making decisions regarding diversion. While still clearly supportive of diversion from the criminal justice system, this circular was a significant step away from wide-scale avoidance of prosecution for mentally-disordered suspects. Enquiries such as Clunis (Ritchie *et al.* 1994) had called into question the validity of diverting those who were suspected of committing serious harm, and some of those who had committed lesser crimes, from the courts. This was felt to ignore the victim perspective and also the need to challenge an offender's offending behaviour. Home Office Circular 12/95 was accompanied by an advisory booklet, prepared by the Home Office and Department of Health, which outlined action the relevant services *might* take and described a number of existing examples of 'good practice'. Perhaps inevitably, given the absence of clear research-based evidence at this stage, service development lacked clarity of purpose in its intended outcomes.

Joint working arrangements

The emphasis on 'inter-agency' working was reaffirmed and reinforced by the document *Building Bridges* (Department of Health 1995). This identified the agencies that should be involved in caring for mentally ill people, and outlined a number of key requirements for effective inter-agency working. For example, *Building Bridges* required a commitment to inter-agency working at all levels of the agency including senior management; a strategy which is jointly owned and agreed; agreed procedures; arrangements for exchanging information; consultation with, and commitment to, the involvement of service users and carers; joint commissioning in order to optimize resources; training within, and between, agencies which includes understanding of agency roles; review and evaluation.

Guidance was also published on the joint commissioning process advocated as an effective means of harnessing resources and coordinating services as well as overcoming some organizational boundaries. However, the Green Paper, *Developing Partnerships in Mental Health* (Department of Health 1997), stated that while in some areas health and local authorities were engaged in successful partnerships, this was not a consistent pattern across England and Wales. Further evidence of persistent inequalities in service provision is indicated, by a subsequent Secretary of State, in the publication of the *National Service Framework* intended to ensure national standards apply to all aspects of provision (NHS 1999).

Department of Health guidance had tended to focus on the joint working arrangements of health and local authority departments such as social services, which had become even more critical since the full implementation in 1994 of the Care Programme Approach (which was officially introduced in 1991). Clearly, collaboration between health, social care and housing services was integral to any successful implementation and throughput of services to the mentally ill. However, practically all the aforementioned literature had referred to the need to work with other public sector organizations. Indeed, a number of the schemes already developed had involved the police and/or probation service and it was generally acknowledged that those services should share their skills in risk assessment, and in working with offenders and particular groups, such as sex offenders (Audit Commission 1994; Department of Health 1997).

Although health and crime may not necessarily be linked in the perception of the general public, a document jointly produced by representatives of the Health and Probation Services was founded on the premise that crime had a definite impact on the nation's health (Home Office, Department of Health 1996). Apart from the impact of alcohol, drug, mental health problems and general health problems suffered by offenders, it was estimated that the effect on the health of victims of crime through their experience of being victimized was significant. Sex offenders, in particular, may have multiple victims. This advanced the view that benefits could be accrued by the two disciplines of health and criminal justice developing joint working and was recommended collaboration to implement the various aims of the 'Reed Review' (Department of Health, Home Office 1992), *Health of the Nation* (Department of Health 1992) and other documents. Principal amongst the reasons cited for collaborative working was improved risk assessment and management of mentally-disordered offenders. Addressing the needs of substance misusers and sex offenders would also offer the opportunity to reduce future offending and overall these factors would produce benefits for victims. Much of the guidance document *Building Bridges* (Department of Health 1995) focused on the development of joint policies and strategies, information sharing, offering joint training opportunities and maximizing access to effective services and offender programmes. Further suggestions included identifying liaison personnel in each agency, appointing managers from services to serve on boards or committees, and secondment of practitioner staff. An example of the development of joint working arrangements can be found in the following case study:

Case Study

In 1992, a multi-agency steering group was formed in the city of Leeds, West Yorkshire, to develop a diversion scheme at the Magistrates Court. In 1994, a partnership group was established to develop a strategic multi-agency approach to provide services for mentally-disordered offenders. This arose from a recognition that people with mental health problems who offend were not always dealt with appropriately, and a belief that a partnership response was the most effective way of addressing the issues. The partnership group, which comprised a range of agencies who were providers and purchasers of services, had a core membership comprising the health authority, the community (mental) health trust, social services, the probation service, magistrates court and police. The crown prosecution service and housing department also became members.

Terms of reference for the group were produced in February 1995 and followed by an 'action plan' in December 1996. The key objectives in the plan came under the headings:

1. Information awareness
2. Development of comprehensive services
3. Development of good practice

The partnership group effectively separated out the purchaser/provider functions by setting up a 'Provider Group' in 1996. The group produced its first strategy in May 1999 and listed its key strategic objectives and an action plan under three headings:

1. Policy
2. Practice
3. Information

A more comprehensive strategy document was produced in July 2001 (Leeds Mentally Disordered Offender Partnership Group 2001). The action plan contained four objectives with separate tasks identified under each one that were to be taken forward by a series of sub groups co-ordinated by a Mentally Disordered Offenders Development Officer.

An evaluation (Minogue 2000) found achievements could be categorized under the following headings:

• Relationship development and communication

1. Shared understanding
2. Agencies working together to achieve shared aims
3. Increased focus on mentally-disordered offenders and their needs
4. Liaison with and training of sentencers

• Mutual advantage and resource exchange:
1. Improved working relationships and inter-agency communication
2. Development of networks
3. Improved quality of work taking place in the courts through agencies allowing better access to their resources

• Specific outcomes:

1. Development of a city-wide strategy
2. Development of a court-based diversion scheme
3. Good practice protocols
4. Mapped the numbers of mentally-disordered offenders in the city
5. Production of a handbook for practitioners
6. Held inter-agency conferences and training
7. Development of care programme approach in a local prison
8. Undertook an audit of the use of acute beds by mentally-disordered offenders
9. Took part in an independent review of the partnership and held internal review

Apart from recognition that it was important to acknowledge the benefits of including criminal justice agencies on a consultative and cooperative level in determining services to the mentally-disordered offender, it is the relationship between the health and social services that is crucial in meeting the needs of the mentally ill. Community care legislation, and guidance on its provision, underlined this factor (NHS and Community Care Act 1990; Department of Health, Home Office 1992; Department of Health 1995). The points at which mentally-disordered offenders link the health and criminal justice systems have already been outlined, but the mentally-disordered cross the boundaries of health and social care even more frequently. It is hard to visualize cases (other than long-stay hospital patients where rehabilitation is not envisaged), where all needs are met by one service (see Figure 14.1).

Inpatient care may be predominantly the domain of health care workers but community care and rehabilitative services will be delivered by a range of practitioners from health and social services, for example, approved social workers, residential social workers, occupational therapists, community psychiatric nurses. Unlike 'physical' diseases, mental disorder rarely presents as a single episode and hence patients move from the care of one or more services to others over varying periods of time. Service models, therefore, have to ensure that they are built on systems that incorporate effective care management and public protection and that there are strong interfaces between health, criminal justice and other agencies, across the different levels of health care (see Figure 14.2).

Holistic partnership provision?

For holistic partnership provision, encompassing community care, to become a reality (thus avoiding the critical conclusions of the enquiries mentioned several times previously), effective targeting and delivery of services is incumbent on health and social services. Community care reforms implicitly assumed that the required improvements would result but perhaps did not pay sufficient regard to the fundamental differences in models of mental disorder employed by health and social services, i.e. bio-medical and social care models.

The casual observer might conclude that community care has failed the majority of mentally-disordered patients (Blom-Cooper 1999; Reith 1998). However, Taylor and Gunn (1999) point out that fewer homicides are committed by the mentally disordered than there were 30 to 40 years previously, and research into the rehabilitation of former hospital patients by Leff (1997) suggested that, generally, care was satisfactory. Undoubtedly, there were difficulties in operationalizing community care initiatives, particularly the Care Programme Approach, which carried no additional funding to assist in implementation and administration. Consequently, differences in the scale of implementation, planning and procedures, existed between health authorities (Association of Metropolitan Authorities 1994) in the first few years following its inception.

Also crucial to successful implementation was the level of co-operation between health and social services and, to a certain extent, the voluntary and independent sector. Although research, such as Henwood (1995), pointed to the improvements brought about by community care – for example, improved joint working and

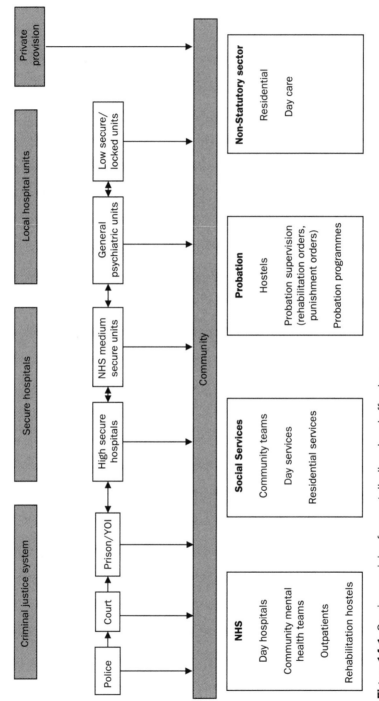

Figure 14.1 Service provision for mentally-disordered offenders

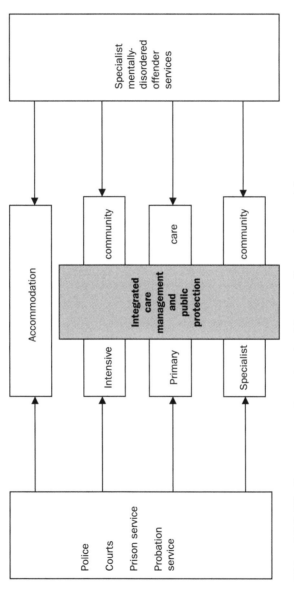

Figure 14.2 Effective care management and public protection service model

relationships between services – recognition of the necessity for specialist skills, plus issues such as resourcing the provision of services remain critical.

Conclusion

Mentally-disordered offenders pose particular issues for the agencies providing care and treatment but the basic needs of the individuals receiving the care, and the basic principles of partnership working, are similar. Undoubtedly, there have been significant steps forward in inter-agency working in this area and strategic agreements exist between many of the main agencies. However, partnership cannot simply exist at a strategic level. Front-line staff need to understand the nature of partnership and be given adequate training in order for them to jointly manage care and public protection. Service users and carers are best placed to be able to identify their needs and to inform service development. Changes in general health and mental health services (NHS 1999; NHS 2000; Department of Health 2000, 2001a, 2001b, 2001c) that have placed the patient much more centrally in the planning and delivery of services have gone some way to addressing the need to involve the service user. However, the mentally-disordered offender is not always included, particularly where there are specific issues surrounding risk or public protection.

As Figures 14.1 and 14.2 illustrate, the provision of care for mentally-disordered offenders is complex as it may cross different service tiers. The pattern of service delivery may be more complex still if the individual spends time in prison and is not identified through the in-reach or liaison systems linking the prison with community provision (in some establishments these may not yet be available). The most effective responses are those that are part of a co-ordinated partnership approach. However, setting up a partnership is only one element of what is needed. Operational policies and protocols are vital to a successful partnership but will require monitoring and evaluation to ensure they work in practice. Moreover, an agreement between agencies to work in partnership does not in itself ensure quality services or equal access to services. Unless different professional groups and organizations are prepared to remove some of the boundaries that prevent good communication, information sharing and cross-fertilization of skills, and work towards developing shared philosophies, it is unlikely that partnership working will be sustained in the longer term. A further fundamental aspect to a successful operational partnership is an effective communications network. Communication is fundamental on two levels: communication between strategic planners, managers and operational staff; information sharing between agencies to ensure effective care management and public protection. Partnership involves all stakeholders and this includes service users. Service user involvement in service planning and delivery, and in the monitoring and evaluation of services is key to ensuring that provision is effective and relevant.

Finally, forward steps in any future attempts to develop and improve 'effective partnerships to assist mentally-disordered offenders' should, I would propose, include two further radical developments. One stakeholder group rarely given prominence in discussions about partnership working and mentally-disordered offenders is their victims or the relatives of victims (where the offence is against the person). Is it time to include this stakeholder group as a key player in any partnership approach to service planning, co-ordination and delivery? Secondly, Wolff (2002) had highlighted the policy implementation failures in the attempts to develop more integrated partnership services for mentally-disordered offenders. Has the time not arrived for the traditional key players in this arena – health, social services and criminal justice agencies – to turn to new wave management and business improvement theory, in order to iron out the process and communication failures which have frequently marked much of the partnership approaches to mentally-disordered offenders? Approaches to quality improvement such as the European Excellence Model (Nabitz *et al.* 2000; Stahr *et al.* 2000) might very well assist all partnership players to break down the individualistic agency philosophies and processes which have hampered partnership working in the past by using such models as the building blocks of a truly *partnership* response to the needs of the mentally-disordered offender. Such an approach could turn partnership working on its head by beginning with the required outcome – care for the mentally-disordered offender – rather than with the individual contribution of each agency.

The way forward

Agencies involved in the care of mentally-disordered offenders need to build on the information sharing protocols that exist between them for dealing with risk management and public protection issues. Improved information sharing between agencies would address many of the criticisms relating to the failures in inter-agency communication that have led to serious incidents of harm. All stakeholders, including service users, carers and victims, should also be involved in the planning and delivery of services, if services are to be effective and relevant.

There are a high number of detained young offenders who show evidence of mental disorder, addressing their needs prior to them entering the criminal justice system should help to reduce the numbers of mentally-disordered offenders in the prison system. The needs of those with a psychopathic disorder need to be similarly addressed, to avoid extended periods in secure conditions under proposed legislation.

A critical evaluation of the range of inter-agency partnerships that have been developed in response to mentally-disordered offenders is needed. Although there have been evaluations of court diversion schemes and of local partnerships, there has been no meta-analysis to determine which models are most effective.

Questions for further discussion

1. Are services for mentally-disordered offenders best provided by general psychiatric services, forensic psychiatric services, or specialist multidisciplinary teams?
2. How can service users be involved in service planning and delivery, alongside other stakeholders, in a meaningful way?
3. To what extent does the Department of Health and Home Office provide a clear lead on dealing with mentally-disordered offenders?

Notes

1　Buchanan (Buchanan 2002) identifies 19 circulars containing guidance on mentally-disordered offenders issued between 1990 and 1999.
2　Opinion on the relationship between crime and mental disorder differs. A great deal of the research has concentrated on the link between violence and mental health. For an overview of the research in this area see: The NHS Centre for Reviews and Dissemination (2000) 'CRD Report 16 – Scoping Review of Literature on the Health and Care of Mentally Disordered Offenders'. University of York.
3　Section 37 of the MHA 83 allows the Court to make a Hospital Order, or an Interim Hospital Order can be made under Section 38, detaining a convicted patient in hospital for treatment. Section 41 adds a restriction to a Hospital Order requiring authority from the Secretary of State for leave of absence or discharge from hospital. Section 37 also allows the making of a Guardianship Order placing a person under the guardianship of the local authority. Sections 35 and 36 allow the courts to remand a defendant to hospital for the preparation of reports or for treatment.
4　McNaughton committed an offence of murder (the victim was the Prime Minister's secretary) but was found not guilty by reason of insanity. This provoked a public outcry forcing the Law Lords to outline the criteria for the decision, thereby producing the rules of insanity known as the 'McNaughton Rules'.
5　In 2001, 3,002 were detained in hospital under restriction with 614 having been admitted during that particular year.
6　Prison health care remained outside the remit of the NHS and governors were required to devolve part of their budget to the purchase of health care services.

References

Alberg, C., Hatfield, B. and Huxley, P. (eds) (1996) *Learning Materials on Mental Health – Risk Assessment*. University of Manchester, Manchester.

Association of Metropolitan Authorities (1994) *Review of Mental Health Services: Issues for Local Government*. Association of Metropolitan Authorities, London.

Audit Commission (1994) *Finding a Place: A Review of Mental Health Services for Adults*. HMSO, London.

Blom-Cooper, L. (1999) Public inquiries in mental health (with particular reference to the Blackwood case at Broadmoor and the patient complaints of Ashworth Hospital), in D. Webb and R. Harris (eds) *Mentally Disordered Offenders. Managing people nobody owns*. Routledge, London.

Buchanan, A. (2002) Who does what? The relationships between generic and forensic psychiatric services, in A. Buchanan (ed.) *Care of the Mentally Disordered Offender*. Oxford University Press, Oxford.

Clark, T., Kenney-Herbert, J. and Humphreys, M.S. (2002) Community rehabilitation orders with additional requirements of psychiatric treatment, *Advances in Psychiatric Treatment*, 8: 281–8. The Royal College of Psychiatrists.

Columbo, A. (1997) *Understanding Mentally Disordered Offenders – A Multi-Agency Perspective*. Ashgate Publishing Ltd, London.

Department of Health (1990) *NHS and Community Care Act 1990*.

Department of Health (1992) *Health of the Nation.* Department of Health, London.

Department of Health (1995) *Building Bridges: Arrangements for Inter-Agency Working for the Care and Protection of Severely Mentally Ill People.* HMSO, London.

Department of Health (1997) *Developing Partnerships in Mental Health.* The Stationery Office, London.

Department of Health (1998a) Frank Dobson Outlines Third Way for Mental Health. Available from http://www.coi.gov.uk/coi/depts/GDH/co14465e.ok.

Department of Health (1998b) *Modernising Mental Health Services: Safe, Sound, Supportive.* The Stationery Office, London.

Department of Health (2000) *Reforming the Mental Health Act.* Department of Health, London.

Department of Health (2001a) *Health and Social Care Act 2001.* Department of Health, London.

Department of Health (2001b) *Involving Patients and the Public in Health Care.* Department of Health, London.

Department of Health (2001c) *Research Governance Framework.* Department of Health, London.

Department of Health, Home Office (1992) *Review of Health and Social Services for Mentally Disordered Offenders and Others Requiring Similar Services.* Final Summary Report Cm. 2088. HMSO, London.

Fennell, P. and Yeates, V. (2002) To serve which master? – criminal justice policy, community care and the mentally disordered offender, in A. Buchanan (ed.) *Care of the Mentally Disordered Offender.* Oxford University Press, Oxford.

Gunn, J. (1991) The trials of psychiatry: insanity in the twentieth century, in K. Herbst and J. Gunn, (eds) *The Mentally Disordered Offender.* Butterworth Heinemann Ltd, Oxford.

Hagell, A. (2002) *The Mental Health of Young Offenders. Bright Futures: Working with Vulnerable Young People.* Mental Health Foundation.

Harris, R. (1999) Mental disorder and social disorder. Underlying themes in crime management, in D. Webb and R. Harris, (eds) *Mentally Disordered Offenders. Managing People Nobody Owns.* Routledge, London.

Haynes, P. and Henfrey, D. (1995) *Progress in Partnership and Collaboration: An Evaluation of Multi–agency Working for Mentally Disordered Offenders in Surrey.* Brighton, Health and Social Policy Research Centre, University of Brighton.

Hedderman, C. (1993) *Panel Assessment Schemes for Mentally Disordered Offenders.* Home Office Research and Policy Unit, London.

Henwood, M. (1995) *Making a Difference: Implementation of the Community Care Reforms Two Years On.* Nuffield Institute for Health, King's Fund, London.

HM Government Cabinet Office (1998) *Bringing Britain Together: A National Strategy for Neighbourhood Renewal.* The Stationery Office, London.

Home Office (1990) Probation Circular 66/1990 *Provision for Mentally Disordered Offenders.* Home Office, London.

Home Office (1995a) Probation Circular 21/1995: Home Office Research Study 138 *Public Interest Case Assessment Schemes.* Home office, London.

Home Office (1995b) Probation Circular 12/1995 *Mentally Disordered Offenders: Inter-agency Working.* Home Office, London.

Home Office (2002) *Statistics of Mentally Disordered Offenders 2001.* Home Office Research Development and Statistics Directorate, London.

Home Office and Department of Health and Social Security (1975) *Report of the Committee on Mentally Abnormal Offenders* (The Butler Committee). Cmnd 6244. Department of Health and Social Security, London.

Home Office, Department of Health (1996) *A Guidance Document Aimed at Promoting Effective Working Between the Health and Probation Services.* HMSO, London.

Home Office, Department of Health (1999) *Managing Dangerous People with Severe Personality Disorders.* The Stationery Office, London.

Howlett, M. (1998) *Medication, Non-Compliance and Mentally Disordered Offenders. A study of Independent Inquiry Reports.* The Zito Trust.

James, E., Farnham, F., Moorey, H., Lloyd, H., Hill, K., Blizard, R. and Barnes, T. (2002) Outcome of Psychiatric Admission Through the Courts. RDS Occasional Paper Number 79. Home Office Research Development and Statistics Directorate, London.

Jewsebury, I. and McCulluch, A. (2002) Public Policy and Mentally Disordered Offenders in the UK in A. Buchanan (ed.) *Care of the Mentally Disordered Offender.* Oxford University Press, Oxford.

Laing, J. (1999) *Mentally Disordered Offenders in the Criminal Justice System.* Oxford University Press, Oxford.

Leeds Mentally Disordered Offender Partnership Group (1996) *Action Plan 1996/7.* Leeds Mentally Disordered Offender Partnership Group, Leeds.

Leeds Mentally Disordered Offender Partnership Group (1999) *Mentally Disordered Offender Strategy 1999–2001. Breaking Down Barriers – Building Bridges.* Leeds Mentally Disordered Offender Partnership Group, Leeds.

Leeds Mentally Disordered Offender Partnership Group (2001) *Leeds Strategy for Mentally Disordered Offenders.* Leeds Mentally Disordered Offender Partnership Group, Leeds.

Leff, J. (1997) *Community Care – Illusion or Reality.* John Wiley, Chichester.

Mental Health Act 1983. London, HMSO.

Mental Health Foundation (1994) *Promoting Care and Justice.* Mental Health Foundation, London.

Minogue, V. (2000) Effective Partnership Working: Developing a Collaborative Response to Mentally Disordered Offenders. PhD thesis, unpublished.

Nabitz, U., Klazinga, N. and Walburg, J. (2000) The EFQM Excellence Model: European and Dutch Experiences with the EFQM Approach in Health Care, *International Journal of Health care Quality Assurance,* 12(3): 191–201.

National Association for the Care and Resettlement of Offenders (1993) *Diverting Mentally Disturbed Offenders from Prosecution.* NACRO, London.

National Health Service (1999) *Modern Standards and Service Models. Mental Health National Service Frameworks.* Department of Health, London.

National Health Service (2000) *The NHS Plan.* Department of Health, London.

Peay, J. (1999) Thinking horses, not zebras, in D. Webb and R. Harris (eds). *Mentally Disordered Offenders. Managing People Nobody Owns.* Routledge, London.

Reith, M. (1998) *Community Care Tragedies: A Practice Guide to Mental Health Inquiries.* Venture Press, Birmingham.

Ritchie, J.H., Dick, D., Lingham, R. (1994) *Report of the Inquiry into the Care and Treatment of Christopher Clunis.* HMSO, London.

Royal College of Psychiatrists (1996) *Report of the Confidential Enquiry into Homicides and Suicides by Mentally Ill People.* Royal College of Psychiatrists, London.

Singleton, N., Meltzer, H. and Gatward, R. (2000) *Psychiatric morbidity among prisoners.* Office for National Statistics, London.

Stahr, H., Bulman, B. and Stead, M. (2000) *The Excellence Model in the Health Service: Sharing Good Practice.* Kingsham, Chichester.

Staite, C., Martin, N., Bingham, M. and Daly, R. (1994) *Diversion from Custody for Mentally Disordered Offenders.* Longman, Harlow.

Swyer, B. (1999) The Wessex Project – resettlement of prisoners with mental disorder in Hampshire, *Criminal Justice Matters*, 37: 51.

Taylor, P.J. and Gunn, J. (1999) Homicides by people with mental illness: myth and reality, *The British Journal of Psychiatry*, 174: 1–14.

Tighe, J., Henderson C. and Thornicroft, G. (2002) Mentally Disordered Offenders and models of community care, in A. Buchanan (ed.) *Care of the Mentally Disordered Offender*. Oxford University Press, Oxford.

University of York, The NHS Centre for Reviews and Dissemination (1999) *CRD Report 16 – Scoping Review of Literature on the Health and Care of Mentally Disordered Offenders*. The University of York.

Wolff, N. (2002) (New) Public management of mentally disordered offenders Part II: A vision with promise, *International Journal of Law and Psychiatry*, 25: 427–44.

Woodley Team (1995) *The Woodley Team Report*. East London and the City Health Authority, London.

Zito Trust (1995) *Learning the Lessons*. The Zito Trust.

15

Working across the interface of formal and informal care of older people

Pat Chambers and Judith Phillips

This chapter will:

- Explore the extent to which carers of older people are able to work in meaningful partnerships with the private, voluntary and independent sectors of health and social care.
- Discuss the social policy and legal context of 'caring' in defining 'who' carers are and 'what' we know about the way in which they receive services.
- Explore the diversity of the caring experience.
- Analyse 'models' that have been developed to explain the relationship between carers and service providers and explore their potential for understanding carers' relationships with a multiplicity of service providers.

Introduction

In this chapter we draw on the general literature on informal care and, more specifically, on recent research that one of us undertook with 'working' carers of older adults, that is, those carers who are in full-or part-time paid employment as well as undertaking unpaid, so-called informal care of an older relative (Phillips *et al.* 2002). We suggest a way of working that acknowledges the complexities of the experience of being a carer of an older person and identify some key issues for good practice in 'working together'. We conclude with a note of caution.

Social and legal context of caring

During the 1970s the idea of care being undertaken by the community instead of just care in the community (Bayley 1973) came to underlie much of the thinking about community care. Increasing public and governmental disquiet about the spiralling welfare costs of a rising elderly population further fuelled the debate about 'who' was going to provide the bulk of care, and with the advent of the 1979 Conservative government committed to the reduction of the overall costs of welfare and the development of a mixed economy of care (Bernard and Phillips 1998), 'informal care' (that is, care provided by family and friends), became an explicit component of social care provision enshrined in *The NHS and Community Care Act* (Department of Health 1990). The care provided by 'informal carers' was acknowledged as a vital resource which, depending on the outcome of a 'needs led' assessment of the person being cared for, would be partnered by the 'formal' sector of care: local authority social services departments; private agencies; and the voluntary sector. Indeed, throughout the last decade of the twentieth century, the increasing reference to carers in public policy documents has been striking. *The Carers (Recognition and Services) Act* (Department of Health 1995) gave carers access to a 'carer's assessment subsequent on an assessment having been carried out on the person being cared for' and was hailed as a further acknowledgement of the government's commitment to partnership.

A significant milestone in the recognition of carers as potential 'partners in care' was the publication, in 1999, of *The National Strategy for Carers* (Department of Health 1999a) that for the first time identified the need for a legislative framework for practical support to be provided directly to carers. More importantly, this was followed, in 2000, by *The Carers and Disabled Children Act* (Department of Health 2000), which gives carers a right to ask for an assessment in their own right, and the inclusion in the National Service Framework for Mental Health of a standard specifically relating to carers: Standard 6 – Caring about Carers (Department of Health 1999b). Carers' needs were also acknowledged in the *National Service Framework for Older People* (Department of Health 2001). We will argue later in this chapter that these recent initiatives have important implications for partnership working.

The government's commitment to partnership, however, is a recent development, with carers often being invisible in policy and taken for granted for many years. It was only when feminist writers in the 1980s (Finch and Groves 1983; Ungerson 1987; Lewis and Meredith 1988) challenged the gendered and unequal nature of caring that their voice became heard. Furthermore the explosion of research on caring in the 1990s (see, for example, Parker 1990; Twigg 1992; Twigg and Aitken 1994; Phillips 1994), alongside the activities of the carer lobby led by the Carers National Association (now Carers UK) and the work of the King's Fund Informal Carers Unit, demonstrated that the reality of 'partnership' was often different. 'Informal' care often superseded the 'formal' contribution, carers' assessments were patchy, limited to those carers providing a substantial amount of care on a regular basis, and there was no guarantee of services. The Social Services Inspectorate (SSI) carried out an inspection of local authority support for carers in 1996 and produced a highly critical report: *A Matter of Chance for Carers* (SSI 1996). The inspectors found that support for carers was dependent on where carers lived and who they were in contact with, rather than on what they needed. They praised carers' groups and acknowledged that support for carers of older people was better developed than support for other groups, particularly those carers who supported people with mental ill-health.

Since the SSI report a number of policy and research initiatives have sought to grapple with the place of 'informal care' or 'family care' (Nolan *et al.* 1996) within overall social care provision and to extend the way in which partnerships between formal and informal care might be forged. In particular, there have been a number of detailed explorations of what informal care is about, the nature of caring relationships, who undertakes care and what are the problems encountered in the delivery of care (see, for example, Brechin *et al.* 1998; Nolan *et al.* 1996, 2001) and, more recently, the experience of 'juggling' work and care (Phillips *et al.* 2002). However, Banks (1999) urged caution suggesting that despite the prominence of carers in policy and research, carers' concerns were still not embedded in mainstream thinking; partnership was far from being a reality. One reason for this, we argue, is that 'partnership' implies a level of equality between the partners, which may not be the case if people or organizations are merely 'working together'. While the impact of carers (and service users) has grown significantly over the last 15 years, carers are still relatively powerless when compared to service providers. Reasons for this have included:

- Stereotyping of carers as a homogenous group.
- The myriad of health and social care services provision within the statutory, voluntary and private sectors.
- Paternalism of health and social care professions.
- Resource constraints and eligibility criteria.
- The costs of caring.
- Multiplicity of potential partnerships.
                    (Twigg and Aitken 1994; Nolan *et al.* 1996; Brown *et al.* 2001)

However, let us turn briefly to current demographic data in order to ascertain 'who' carers are and 'what' we know about them. Then, drawing on the findings of *The National Strategy for Carers* (Department of Health 1999a), we will summarize what carers themselves say they require in order for partnership to be successful.

According to the 2001 census (Office of National Statistics) there are 5.2 million carers in England and Wales, a million of whom provide care for more than 50 hours a week. Over 225,000 people providing more than 50 hours unpaid care per week state that they are 'not in good health' themselves and more than half of the people providing this much care are over the age of 55; it is at these ages that the 'not good health' is highest. The age group where the largest proportion provides care is in the fifties: more than one in five of people aged 50–59 are providing some unpaid care. This confirms the findings from *The National Strategy for Carers* (Department of Heath 1999a) that the likelihood of becoming a carer increases with age, with the peak age being 45–64. Many carers in this age group are working either full or part time. For example, in 1999 2.7 million people combined work with informal care for another adult (Department of Health 1999a). *The National Strategy for Carers* also notes that nine out of ten carers care for a relative, of whom two out of ten care for a partner or spouse and four out of ten care for parents. One half of all carers look after someone over 75.

Once we move away from the numbers of carers, and start to identify and describe both 'who' does care and 'what' is their experience, our task becomes difficult. As we noted earlier in this chapter, the 1980s saw a burgeoning of feminist literature which highlighted the gendered nature of caring (Finch and Groves 1983; Ungerson 1987; Lewis and Meredith 1988). However, most commentators now acknowledge that while it is true that more women than men are carers, the picture is much more complex. Carers are a diverse group of people in terms of age, marital status, gender, ethnicity, sexuality, disability, education, health, household composition, family, income, employment status and, of course, in terms of willingness, capacity and expertise to care. Some are more politicized than others and feel able to claim both the title and identity of 'carer', whereas others reject it in favour of their status or relationship as relative: daughter, wife, husband, etc. (see, for example, Henderson 2001). Indeed some carers share care with other family members, while others are sole carers. The relationship that they have with the person they care for will be individual and located in their own biography and life course (Nolan *et al.* 1996; Brechin *et al.* 1998) and will inevitably be influenced by the views and expectations of others, including other family members. That caring relationship will, in turn, develop its own history, of which a relationship with formal services may be an increasingly substantial component. Furthermore, carers differ in both the quantity and the type of care that they offer. Some carers undertake the regular physical labour of personal care and supporting domestic tasks, either living with or near to the person they care for, whereas others may 'care at a distance', offering emotional support, organizing and overseeing care services. Indeed, carers differ in the amount of support they want and receive from formal services and perhaps more importantly, in the relationships they develop with a variety of service providers, for example, local volunteer support groups.

While it is impossible to do justice in a chapter such as this to the multiplicity of caring experiences, the examples in Boxes 15.1, 15.2 and 15.3, of women caring for their mothers, serve to illustrate the diversity of the caring experience.

Box 15.1

When my mother left mental hospital I was told to accept what she had become. She just sat staring at the wall. I have worked hard to rehabilitate her and though this has cost me a great deal both mentally and physically, I have a great deal of satisfaction seeing that my efforts have been worthwhile and have proved the medical profession wrong (cited in Nolan *et al.* 1996: 93).

Box 15.2

There was this terrific pressure because the (paid) carer would leave at say 4 p.m. and I needed to be there shortly afterwards. If I was late . . . then I had to telephone my mum's neighbours and let them know I would be late. I would stay with mum, give her tea, chat, help with continence, shower, undress and help her to bed and read to her etc., then go home and start studying or spend some time with my partner. We had a bizarre existence and it was extremely stressful and pressurised . . . the possibility of giving up work was very much on my mind as I didn't know how I could continue to cope with no end in sight, and also my family, especially my grandfather, was very critical of me trying to continue with my career . . . At times, I was accused of neglecting mum and did feel that I was not doing a good job. Others were critical of a 'stranger' looking after her when it should have been me . . . (Mia, cited in Phillips 2000: 47–50).

Indeed, it would be fair to say that the differences between carers may well outweigh their commonalities and any attempts by service providers to develop partnerships have to recognize and work with both uniqueness and diversity.

There are clearly both costs and benefits to being a carer. Early feminist literature, in an attempt to emphasize the physical labour of caring and demonstrate that the 'personal is political' (Ungerson 1987), tended emphasize the 'burden' of caring for women. Carers UK, in its literature, has emphasized the physical, emotional and financial costs of caring for all carers. The following case study (Box 15.3), taken from recent research with working carers, exemplifies some of these costs.

Box 15.3

The constant juggling put stresses and strains on them all (Ursula, two sisters and brother, all of whom had multiple demands with their own jobs and families). Despite the support of the team Ursula worked with, and of her manager who was very good, Ursula became ill herself. She had to have a few weeks off work but still kept going to her mother's. One of her sisters also lost her job due to the inflexibility and demands of the children's home where she worked . . . Towards the end, Ursula says, 'We were all so stressed. We were tired and there was friction in the family. That sounds petty but that's how it gets. But we managed to keep it together . . . there was no sort of fighting in front of her or anything [but] there was tension'. Looking back, Ursula feels angry about the responsibilities she had to take on, the travelling she had to do, the work and social things she missed out on.

('Ursula Vine – the reluctant worker' cited in Phillips *et al.* 2002: 35)

Ursula's description of a family under stress is not uncommon and we would argue that the costs of caring can be major barriers to partnership working. It is difficult for a carer to consider herself to be an equal partner with formal services when she is constantly juggling many roles and trying to maintain some control over her whole life, not just the care-giving component. This is not to suggest that carers are passive 'victims'. To the contrary, as Nolan *et al.* (1996: 79) remind us: 'Far from being a passive and largely reactive group, carers are characterised by being pro-active and purposeful in bringing a range of methods to bear on the difficulties they face.' Carers, they argue have to learn, if they did not know already, how to be resourceful in relation to finding relevant information, seeking help from formal services and seeking out a confidante. For some carers, this is an empowering experience which enables them to work side by side with formal services but for others these coping responses result in stress and exhaustion that contribute instead to an increasing sense of powerlessness and isolation.

Nonetheless, there is increasing evidence that some carers find care-giving to be a satisfying and rewarding experience. Nolan *et al.* (1996), for example, while noting the embryonic nature of literature on the rewards of care-giving compared to the burgeoning literature on burden and stress, highlight the reciprocal nature of care-giving, the potential to develop relationships and the subjective meaning of care for both the care-giver and the cared-for person. The continuation of ongoing loving relationships, the capacity to 'give back', doing a good job and gaining satisfaction, are some of the benefits cited by daughters who cared for their mothers, in research carried out by Lewis and Meredith (1988). More recently, Karen, a 46-year-old part-time district nurse has looked after her 72-year-old mother since her father died of cancer some five years ago. She says:

> What goes round comes round. You're cared for, you care and you're cared for. That's how it is . . . Only do it if you want to. If it's not something that you want to do – not everybody can do it – then don't do it. Find another way round it. There are good care homes and because someone is in a care home, it doesn't mean that the family doesn't care – it means they can't care.
>
> (Cited in Phillips *et al.* 2002: 23)

Karen is a working carer who is supported by a range of informal and formal networks and services. She clearly feels that she has some control over her decision to care, and has a sense of empowerment and satisfaction that is derived from that control. As we have demonstrated in previous examples, not all carers are in such position.

The National Strategy for Carers (Department of Health 1999a) sought, through consultation with a multiplicity of stakeholders, to document these diverse experiences of caring and put forward a realistic strategy for carers that would make working in partnership a reality rather than a pipedream for ALL carers. The document identified that in order to care effectively, carers need a partnership with service providers, which is based on respect and recognition of carers' expertise. This must be accompanied by: accessible, relevant and comprehensible information; recognition both as individuals and as a collective; a multi-agency approach which incorporated health, housing and employment as well as social care; and transparency in relation to policy and practice. So often, by focusing on the negative burden of caring, 'partnership' with statutory service places carers in a deficit role. Instead, *The National Strategy for Carers* (Department of Health 1999a) recognized that carers are service users, service providers and above all, citizens.

As such, carers have the right to expect:

- Freedom to live a life of their own, including spending time with family and friends outside of caring responsibilities or remaining in work.
- Maintenance of their own health and well-being.
- Confidence in the standard and reliability of services.
- To share caring responsibilities with service providers and feel that the person they care for is respected; this includes practical and emotional support that contributes to their well being and knowing that assistance will be available in a crisis.

(Department of Health 1999a: 24)

In addition, those carers who work or care at a distance may need the following: time off from work in a crisis; the use of a telephone to arrange care/check arrangements; help from the local carers' centre; particular support from statutory services in their relative's area. In summary, in order to achieve partnership:

> Carers need caring for. Most of them need high quality, reliable and responsive support from statutory or voluntary services. Many need help from their employer. Carers have many of the same needs as the rest of the population . . . carers have less opportunity to get what they need.
>
> (Department of Health 1999a: 83)

The National Strategy for Carers (Department of Health 1999a) stressed the importance of involving carers in discussions about care delivery, in planning care and in providing feedback on services and initiatives and significantly, highlighted the urgency for legislation to enable local councils with social services responsibilities to provide services direct to carers. Along with the Government's previous initiatives to support carers in their caring role (Health Improvement Programmes; requirement for consultation in Joint Investment Plans, NHS surveys of patients and carers; Patient Partnership Strategy; consultations with carers' organizations and the active development of carers' support groups), it provided impetus for *The Carers and Disabled Children Act* (Department of Health 2000). The Act, which came into force on 1 April 2001, gives local councils the power to supply certain services to carers following assessment. There is also, as indicated earlier in this chapter, a new right to a carer's assessment, even where the person cared for has refused an assessment for, or the provision of, community care services. The extension of direct payments has enabled some carers to purchase services they are assessed as needing. It is still early days, and the potential of this Act for empowering carers, and thus enabling them to become partners in care, has yet to be fully evaluated. Nonetheless, it is clearly a significant milestone in recognizing carers in their own right.

Furthermore, resultant good practice guidelines issued by the Department of Health have highlighted the need for carers' employment to be a main factor in assessment. This is clearly significant, given the increasing numbers of carers of older people who are also in paid employment. The needs of working carers have also been addressed by other government departments. For example, the 1999 Employment Relations Act gave employees the right to unpaid 'reasonable' time off to deal with unexpected or sudden situations relating to those that they care for. The Department for Education and Employment subsequently launched the Employers for Work-Life Balance Initiative, encouraging organizations to make a commitment to support carers in the workforce and the *Work-Life Balance Campaign*, which sought to encourage employers to develop more flexible working practices (Department of Trade and Industry 2002). However, according to Phillips *et al.* (2002: 2) existing family-friendly schemes are still primarily designed for working parents of young children and most current schemes rarely address the needs of employees who care for older or disabled adults. Yet again, it would appear that there is a wide gulf between policy and practice.

Understanding the experience of carers

Recent initiatives, therefore, have sought to raise the profile of carers, and develop partnerships between carers and those who provide formal services at both macro-level and micro-level. Firstly, at the macro-level of 'community' or 'workplace', there is the potential for partnerships to develop in relation to planning and provision of services. A carer, either as an individual or as a member of a carers' organization may, for example, be invited onto a working party to develop new initiatives or may be consulted about the development of an ongoing service. At this level, the carer is a representative, the 'voice' of carers. Given the diversity of carers and experiences identified earlier, this, of course, can be problematic, and the potential and effectiveness of such partnerships weakened if that diversity is neither acknowledged nor incorporated into service delivery. What is missing from a lot of the discussion surrounding these initiatives, however, is not just a lack of recognition of the reality of that diversity but also a lack of clarity concerning the differential power imbalance between the formal and the informal sectors of care: carers do not have access to the power and resources available to the formal sectors, and as such may find themselves at a constant disadvantage. There may, however, be unanticipated consequences of recent policy and practice, according to Leece (2003: 27). She suggests that the increasing 'commodification' of care inherent in health and social care policy in recent years and, we would argue, especially in relation to caring relationships, may cause a shift in this balance of power, with informal carers reassessing their position and demanding payment, better support or indeed refusing to continue providing care for their relatives.

At a micro-level, carers are personally at the interface of formal and informal service provision but in an ambiguous position. As service users, there is potential for partnership development with formal service providers in their own right, through community care processes of carer assessment and care delivery. For those carers who are also in paid employment there is, in addition, a need to develop collaborative working arrangements with their employers. As service providers that potential development will be via the person they are caring for, who will also be subject to community care processes. It is well documented, however, that community care processes have the potential to either empower or further disempower carers and service users, who find themselves dependent on the skills, values and practice of individual workers and local systems and resources (see, for example, Hughes 1997; Oliver and Sapey 1999). Within that caring relationship, a carer may be working in partnership with the person they care for, may be acting as advocate for that person or may even find that they are in conflict with that person. What emerges is a very complex web of relationships, which itself may be a barrier to developing partnership with formal service providers.

So, given the barriers to partnership working identified so far, to what extent does the social and legal context that is being developed enable carers to develop real partnerships with service providers? A number of 'models' have been put forward that have attempted to conceptualize the differential relationships that carers have with the health and social care sector. These models have sought to both better understand and inform practice and, for the purposes of the current discussion, enable us to analyse the potential for partnership and collaboration. We will focus here on two.

Just over ten years ago, Twigg and Aitken (1994) suggested a framework that sought to explore the way in which service providers respond to carers. They contended that service agencies and professionals, generally lacking an explicit rationale for work with carers, tended to adopt instead one of four implicit models (see Table 15.1).

Each of the 'models' reflects a different relationship that formal service providers adopt, often unwittingly, with carers. According to Twigg and Aitken (1994: 12), 'carers as resource' reflects the predominant reality of social care, embodied in the *NHS and Community Care Act* (Department of Health 1990). Care provided by carers is a 'given' against which agencies operate: it is 'freely available' with no 'cost' attached to it; and there seems to be an assumption by both service providers and the wider public that informal care is preferable with the social care system only needing to step in when informal care support is unavailable. The 'cared for' person is the focus of intervention and the concern with carer welfare is marginal. The primary focus of agency intervention is that of maintenance. Alternatively, 'carers as co-workers' are jointly involved in the enterprise of care. Ideally, the divisions of formal and informal care are transcended in this joint enterprise and partnership is achieved. The reality of the differing worlds of formal and informal care, with potentially diverse values and expectations, means that this rarely happens (Twigg and Aitken 1994: 14). The primary aim of the formal care system is to assist 'carers as co-workers' to carry on caring. In the model of 'carers as co-clients' the aim of the

Table 15.1 Four models of carers (Twigg and Aitken 1994: 13)

	Carers as resources	*Carers as co-workers*	*Carers as co-clients*	*Superseded carer*
Definition of carer	Very wide	Wide	Narrow	'Relatives'
Focus of interest	Disabled person	Disabled person with some recognition of the carer	Carer	Recognized but in relation to both carer and disabled person
Conflict of interest	Ignored	Partially recognized	Recognized fully but only one way	Recognized but in relation to both carer and disabled person
Aim	Care maximization and minimization of substitution	Highest quality of care for the disabled person. Well-being of carer as a means to this	Well-being of the carer	Well-being of carer and independence for the disabled person but seen as separate

service system is primarily to support those carers who are most stressed and heavily burdened. Carers are regarded as clients and the focus of attention is on the carer and their needs, sometimes at the expense of the cared-for person.

Finally, 'the superseded carer': here the aim is to replace current informal care relationships either in the interests of the person being cared for or, in some cases, to enable a person to give up caring. This model is often employed with parent carers of disabled adults, as a way of developing independence for the 'cared for' person. Twigg and Aitken (1994) argue that these models are ideal types of response and that no one agency draws exclusively on one model. However, they go on to suggest that there is evidence that different models are stressed at different levels of organizations. For example, those workers with social work training tend to be more comfortable with the 'co-worker' model, whereas managerial staff find more favour with 'carers as resources'. There would also appear to be differences in emphasis between socially and medically oriented practitioners, with a tendency by medical staff to view carers as: 'an unquestioned background resource' (Twigg and Aitken 1994: 15). It would seem then that the potential for partnership is heavily dependent not only on the model of carer that is adopted, but also on 'who' in an organization is involved in assessment, including the professional orientation of that person. Increasing multiplicity of service providers, drawn from the voluntary and private sectors whose workers have varying degrees of training, as well as an increasing variety of health and social service providers, adds even greater complexity and possibility of variation in practice.

While acknowledging that these models might be appropriate in describing given circumstances, Nolan et al. (1996) suggest that none of the models is adequate as a basis for intervention across the interface of formal and informal care because they fail to really reflect ideals of empowerment, partnership and choice. Moreover, they contend that underpinning Twigg and Aitken's framework is the principle that all parties (formal and informal care providers) bring something of value to an encounter and share views in moving towards a common goal (Nolan et al. 1996; Brown et al. 2001:30). The literature, they go on to argue, suggests that this is often not the case, and that professionals and family carers frequently have differing and not necessarily complementary goals and sources of knowledge. Furthermore, what is needed is a working model that reflects more adequately the goals of partnership and empowerment inherent in policy and practice guidelines and recognizes the power differentials of formal service provision and family care.

This critique has led them to develop such a model, 'carers as experts', that can be used as a basis for assessment and intervention (Nolan et al. 1996). The model incorporates a number of basic assumptions. Firstly, important though the problems of caring are, a full understanding of carers' needs will not solely be achieved via assessment of the 'difficulties' of caring but instead must be grounded in knowledge of the expertise that is derived from a 'caring career'. This might include, for example, past and present relationships, rewards of caring, coping skills and resources. Secondly, assessment must incorporate the subjective experience of the carer, and the carer's willingness and/or capacity to care. Thirdly, a life course approach to 'caring' is adopted, which acknowledges temporality, that is 'the changing demands of care and the way in which skills and expertise change over time' (Brown et al. 2001: 31).

And finally, if carers are conceptualized as 'experts', then it becomes possible to help them attain further competence, skills, resources, etc., enabling them to provide quality care without detriment to their own health.

The National Strategy for Carers (Department of Health 1999a) also recognized the importance of carers' expertise and recommended the following strategies to support partnership:

- Active monitoring and provision of information by GPs and Primary Health Care Teams who are in touch with carers.
- Training to 'care' course to be developed in consultation with carers: practical skills such as lifting and handling; stress management; 'taking care of yourself'.
- Carers' breaks.
- Carers' support services and carers' centres, which incorporate information and advice, emotional support and befriending schemes.

We would concur with the basic assumptions of this model of 'carers as experts'. Indeed, without recognition of such expertise, partnership may well be impossible.

Developing good practice

At this point it is useful to summarize our discussion so far. We have charted the policy context of partnership in relation to carers and sought to develop an understanding of the diversity and complexity of the caring experience. We then examined two models that seek to explain the relationship between carers and service providers, and the usefulness of these models as bases for developing partnership. Our final task then, arising from this discussion, is to identify key issues for practice in order to maximize meaningful partnerships across the interface of formal and informal care.

At a micro-level, it is clearly crucial for service providers to acknowledge both power differentials and temporality. Not all carers will experience the same sense of powerlessness and not all carers will be at the same stage in their 'caring career'. As we have previously acknowledged, many carers will also be differentially engaged in full- or part-time paid work. Carers' assessments must be routinely offered and carers must be encouraged to participate. In order to promote collaboration, a life course perspective, which is grounded in an understanding of the diversity of carers and the multiplicity of caring experiences, must be adopted during assessment and the provision of support must be appropriate to the stage of 'caring career' that the carer has reached. The subjective experience of the carer must be accounted for alongside the more objective criteria such as 'hours spent caring', and the 'burden' of caring must not be assumed. Indeed, an exploration of the positive aspects of caring and the recognition of carer expertise will be more conducive to developing a partnership, and less likely to pathologize either the carer or the cared-for person. Such an approach is advocated by Askham (1998), who suggests a broad definition of support for carers which includes any action that helps carers to: take up or decide not to take up a care-giving role; continue in the care-giving role; or end the care-giving role. She stresses a variety of possible interventions: training and preparation for caring; information; emotional support; instrumental help. We would argue that this requires a framework for assessment, grounded in the recommendations of *The National Strategy for Carers* (Department of Health 1999a) and the rights outlined in *The Carers and Disabled Children Act* (Department of Health 2000), that takes account of differences, acknowledges power, is sensitive to dynamics of care and is able to collect relevant information. In addition, the person carrying out the assessment must have understanding and knowledge of the diversity of caring experiences and must be able to adopt a person-centred, life-course approach to understanding caring relationships.

For interventions to be successful, then, the carer must be valued as a whole person, a citizen with a multiplicity of roles and responsibilities. This will require of service providers both flexibility and an understanding of what is or is not acceptable or appropriate at a particular time. Ongoing recognition of the temporal nature of caring, and the way in which needs and support will inevitably change, is essential. A 'one-off' assessment will clearly not suffice. Instead, service providers must be prepared to build evaluation and reassessment into partnership arrangements. The entire collaborative enterprise must be underpinned by anti-discriminatory practice (Burke and Harrison 2002) and information must be shared with all those involved in the delivery of a care package.

At a macro-level, it is recognized that support for carers in the area where they live works best when a range of local organizations work in partnership to maintain and develop a community service to carers. This might include a range of organizations: social services; housing; transport; education; health trusts; general practitioners; employers; volunteer bureaux; benefits; carers' groups (Department of Health 1999a: 68). It must also include private and voluntary agencies that are at the forefront of service delivery. These must be more than 'talking shops' and the commitment to partnership needs to be developed and regularly reviewed, perhaps through the development of shared policy and practice guidelines. One example of a local partnership is 'Partnerships for Carers in Suffolk'. This comprises Suffolk Carers, a number of local authorities' social services and education departments, the health authority, voluntary organizations, NHS trusts and Primary Care Groups. Each partner has 'signed up' for the Charter for Carers in Suffolk, which emphasizes the following: carers' right to recognition; choice, information; appropriate practical help; assistance towards the financial costs of caring; and co-ordinated services. Furthermore, each of the partners is committed to implementing an action plan.

Communication, information and recognition are crucial to developing and maintaining partnership. Formal care services must work together with individual carers and their organizations, to develop appropriate and accessible systems that recognize carers' needs. There are a number of examples of good practice of innovative systems in different parts of the United Kingdom. For example, Newcastle City NHS Trust has appointed a nurse specialist in carer support to work with carers and educate professionals. A GP Carers' Project in York and Selby has developed a range of initiatives to provide carers with information and support; these include, carer messages on prescriptions, the use of notices to identify carers and carer-designated notice boards. Other initiatives have included: handbooks for carers (Cambridgeshire), a free-phone, designated carers' line and carers' packs (Rhondda Cynon Taff Social Services Department (Department of Health 1999a).

Partnership arrangements with employers are an effective way of supporting working carers of older people and can benefit both carer support services and employers themselves (Department of Health 1999a: 69). In the organizations they studied, an NHS Trust and a social services department (Phillips et al. 2002), they were able to identify a number of 'family friendly' policies. These included: extended leave; short-term leave; time off in lieu; shorter week and reduced hours; flexitime; job share; eldercare information; dependent leave; special leave; and counselling. However, the authors were critical that the way in which these policies were translated into practice was heavily dependent on managerial discretion and support, knowledge of staff and the sub-cultures of the organization. There are interesting parallels here with the way in which carers in general report their experience of formal services: so often, despite policies for partnership being in place, their experience is dependent on the way in which they interact with a particular health or social worker, and the way in which organizational systems and constraints help or hinder (Twigg and Aitken 1994; Department of Health 1999a; Carers Association Southern Staffordshire 2003). It is vital that training for those who work with carers is provided, both in the workplace and the community, in order that policy is translated into practice. Disappointingly, Phillips et al. (2002) also found that partnership arrangements between public, private and voluntary agencies to support working carers of older people were virtually non-existent. We endorse their advocacy for such developments at a local level and argue for a pooling of knowledge about working carers and joint initiatives between employers from public, voluntary and private sectors, in order to develop effective partnership arrangements.

Conclusion

In this chapter our focus has been to explore the extent to which carers of older people are able to work in meaningful partnership with formal care services. We have demonstrated that carers are characterized by their diversity, differential access to resources and power, and expertise. We have argued that an understanding of diversity, power and expertise is crucial in working across the interface of formal and informal care. We have acknowledged that for such partnerships to be effective, a range of organizations may need to be involved. We have drawn attention to the different levels of partnership that carers may find themselves engaging in, both willingly and unwillingly, and have raised a discussion of models which seek to describe those relationships. We have sought to identify key issues for practice in working across the interface of formal and informal care, and have provided some specific examples of good practice. Inevitably, then, in a chapter of this size we have been unable to pay much attention to the 'cared-for' person and what has been described as the politics of care (Brechin et al. 1998; Priestley 1998, 1999). We wish, therefore, to end with a note of caution. Any attempt to develop partnerships with carers must not be at the expense of further disempowering the cared-for person. Partnerships with carers must, therefore, encompass relationships of care that seek to enable and empower the cared-for person. This will inevitably add further complexity to an already complex web of relationships between the formal and the informal sectors of care. Cooperation, understanding and a commitment to working together must, therefore, be the starting point to any relationship between formal care services, carers and the cared-for person, with partnership as the goal to strive for.

Questions for further discussion

1. How might you begin to develop a partnership with a carer during a carer's assessment? What would this depend on?
2. Highlight the dilemmas for carers in caring at long distances.
3. How would you reconcile the needs of carers with the needs of the 'cared-for' person in developing a partnership across the interface of formal and informal care?

References

Askham, J. (1998) Supporting caregivers of older people: an overview of problems and priorities, *Australian Journal of Ageing*, 17(1): 5–7.

Banks, P. (1999) *Carer Support: Time for a Change of Direction*. King's Fund, London.

Bayley, M. (1973) *Mental Handicap and Community Care*. Routledge and Kegan Paul, London.

Bernard, M. and Phillips, J. (1998) *The Social Policy of Old Age: Moving into the 21st Century*. Centre for Policy on Ageing, London.

Brechin, A., Walmsley, J., Katz, J. and Peace, S. (eds) (1998) *Care Matters: Concepts, Practice and Research in Health and Social Care*. Sage, London.

Brown, J., Nolan, M. and Grant, G. (2001) Who's the expert? Redefining lay and professional relationships, in M. Nolan, S. Davies and G. Grant, *Working with Older People and their Families: Key Issues in Policy and Practice*. Open University Press, Buckingham.

Burke, B. and Harrison, P. (2002) Anti-oppressive practice in R. Adams, L. Dominelli and M. Payne, *Social Work: Themes, Issues and Critical Debates* (2nd edn). Palgrave, Basingstoke.

Carers' Association Southern Staffordshire (2003) Discussion with one of authors.

Department of Health (1990) *The NHS and Community Care Act*. HMSO, London.

Department of Health (1995) *The Carers (Recognition and Services) Act*. HMSO, London.

Department of Health (1999a) *The National Strategy for Carers*. HMSO, London.

Department of Health (1999b) *National Service Framework for Mental Health*. HMSO, London.

Department of Health (2000) *The Carers and Disabled Children Act*. HMSO, London.

Department of Health (2001) *National Service Framework for Older People*. HMSO, London.

Department of Trade and Industry (1999) *Employment Relations Act*. The Stationery Office, London.

Department of Trade and Industry (2002) *Work-Life Balance Campaign*. www.dti.gov.uk

Finch, J. and Groves, D. (1983) *A Labour of Love: Women, Work and Caring*. Routledge and Kegan Paul, London.

Henderson, J. (2001) He's not my carer – he's my husband: personal and policy constructions of care in mental health, *Journal of Social Work Practice*, 15: 149–60.

Hughes, B. (1997) *Older People and Community Care*. Open University Press, Buckingham.

Leece, J. (2003) The Development of Domiciliary Care: What does the future hold? *Practice*, 15(3): 17–30.

Lewis, J and Meredith, B. (1988) *Daughters who Care: Daughters Caring for Mothers at Home*, Routledge and Kegan Paul, London.

Nolan, M., Grant, G. and Keady, J. (1996) *Understanding Family Care: A Multidimensional Model of Caring and Coping*. Open University Press, Buckingham.

Nolan, M., Davies, S. and Grant, G. (2001) *Working with Older People and their Families: Key Issues in Policy and Practice*. Open University Press, Buckingham.

Office of National Statistics (2001) *Census 2001*. www.statistics.gov.uk

Oliver, M. and Sapey, B. (1999) *Social Work with Disabled People* (2nd edn). Macmillan, Basingstoke.

Parker, G. (1990) *With Due Care and Attention: A Review of the Research on Informal Care* (2nd edn). Family Policy Studies Centre, London.

Phillips, J. (1994) The Employment Consequences of Caring for Older People, *Health and Social Care in the Community*, 2: 143–52.

Phillips, J. (2000) Working carers: caring workers, in M. Bernard, J. Phillips, L. Machin and V. Harding-Davies, *Women Ageing: Changing Identities, Challenging Myths*. Routledge, London.

Phillips, J., Bernard, M. and Chittenden, M. (2002) *Juggling Work and Care: The Experiences of Working Carers of Older Adults*. The Policy Press, Bristol.

Priestley, M. (1998) Discourse and resistance in care assessment: Integrated living and Community Care, *British Journal of Social Work*, 28: 659–73.

Priestley, M. (1999) *Disability Politics and Community Care*. Jessica Kingsley, London.

Social Services Inspectorate (1996) *A Matter of Chance for Carers*. HMSO, London.

Twigg, J. (ed.) (1992) *Carers: Research and Practice*. HMSO, London.

Twigg, J. and Aitken, K. (1994) *Carers Perceived: Policy and Practice in Informal Care*. Open University Press, Buckingham.

Ungerson, C. (1987) *Policy is Personal: Sex, Gender and Informal Care*. Tavistock, London.

16

Partnerships and capacity building for African-Caribbean and Asian elders with dementia

Neil Moreland, David Jolley, Kate Read and Michael Clark

This chapter will:

- Utilize the findings of two research projects (Moreland 2001, 2003) into ethnic minority community experiences of health and social services for older people with dementia and their carers to examine current issues and developments in provision.
- Examine the meaning(s) of partnership and community capacity building in the context of the defined needs of the African-Caribbean and Asian carers and the older people with dementia for whom they care.
- Consider the implications of the research findings for service development within the overall framework of the 'New Public Management' of health and social services.

Part one: the Wolverhampton context

> Happy families are all alike; every unhappy family is unhappy in its own way.

Leo Tolstoy provides the starting line of this chapter for, in the context of older people with dementia and their carers, the opening line of the novel *Anna Karenina* is a pertinent example of the literary imagination encapsulating a sociological truth (Routh and Woolf 1977). The various illnesses and degenerative cognitive conditions that constitute dementia cause the people who suffer dementia and their carers to be constituted within an ontology of complexity (Wojan and Rupasingha 2001). That is, dementia affects sufferers in different ways, and with differing rates of deterioration and manifestations, the result of which is to create a wide range of situations and support needs. Time after time, research and first-hand accounts of the experience of dementia by individuals, both alone and within families, points to the trauma and disruptive effects of the disease upon 'normal' family relations and life in general, both for the sufferers (e.g. Friedel 2002; Aggerwal *et al.* 2003) and their families (e.g. Menne, Kinney and Morhardt 2002). This complexity of living arrangements and support needs is the main rationale behind the implementation guidance of the

National Service Framework for Older People (Department of Health 2001) and some of the social service framework standards such as D39, which benchmarks the 'Percentage of people receiving a statement of their needs and how they will be met' (Department of Health 2002).

In meeting the support needs of older people with dementia, it is clear that a great deal of the caring is carried out informally. Hirst (2001), who carried out a meta-analysis of the trends in informal care in Great Britain during the 1990s, found that the overall numbers of the population involved in informal care was decreasing, but that the proportion of carers as a percentage of the whole was increasing. At the same time, Hirst suggests that the provision of informal care by friends and neighbours decreased in the 1990s resulting in an overall decline in care-giving between households. Moreover, Hirst suggests that the trend is for parents increasingly to be looked after in their own homes by non-resident daughters and daughters-in-law.

Having said that, large numbers of men as well as women provided informal care for a spouse or partner by the end of the 1990s (Hirst 2001). As many of these carers are themselves becoming old and frail, it has become even more important to provide support for carers, including time for them away from their caring duties. Nocon and Pearson (2000: 345), for instance, support the implementation of the Carers Act and standards, as such developments are helping to reverse previous assumptions that 'the availability of informal care (has been) a reason for *not* providing services' (brackets added, emphasis in original).

As can be seen in other chapters in this book, there are a number of developments occurring in care and carer support needs that are underpinned by Acts of Parliament. It is not intended here to describe such developments, for the focus of this chapter is the consideration of a triumvirate of related concepts and issues, those of empowerment, partnership and community capacity building. Each of these three concepts and issues was explicit to varying degrees in the two projects that now collectively go under the names of 'Twice a Child I' and 'Twice a Child II'. Those projects will be described briefly before the substantive issues arising from them with regard to empowerment, partnership and community capacity building are considered.

The 'Twice a Child' research projects

The original Twice a Child I project was initiated in December, 2000, and jointly funded by Wolverhampton Social Services and the Department of Health. The project was based within Dementia Plus West Midlands, and was designed to take further two earlier pieces of work. The first small project was carried out in 1996, and researched the characteristics and support needs of white older people with dementia and their carers in Wolverhampton (Jolley *et al.* 1996). It became obvious at that stage that it was desirable to carry out similar research with the African-Caribbean and Asian communities in Wolverhampton. It was not until 2000, however, that further impetus was given and funds provided, as a result of the second project concerned with ethnic elderly dementia in Wolverhampton (Dementia Plus West Midlands 2000). As a result of the ensuing conference, the Department of Health agreed to provide some funding and support for the small-scale research project that became Twice a Child II.

A major difficulty experienced in Wolverhampton was the availability of up-to-date statistics about the ethnic minority communities in Wolverhampton, for the best available figures were from the 1991 census, which were already nearly ten years out of date. The statistics did suggest that both the African-Caribbean and Asian communities had age profiles that were younger than that of the white population. At the 1991 census, 18.6 per cent of the borough's population were from 'black and minority ethnic groups', with those from the Asian sub-continent being the largest group (59 per cent of the 18.6 per cent) (Phillipson 2001: 46). At the same time, while close to one-fifth of the population of Wolverhampton as a whole were of retirement age in 1991, the African-Caribbean and Asian elderly constituted only 5.3 per cent of those over retirement age. A resulting concern was the numbers of older people with dementia from the two communities, for if the proportions were similar to the white population, the number of known older people with dementia from the two communities should have been greater than the numbers actually known to health and social services. In the event, the research was able to confirm that there were only a very small number of hidden older people with dementia in the two communities, disproving at least locally the assumption that 'they look after their own, don't they?' (SSI 1998). Okuyiga (1998) supports this when he wrote that:

> Changing family patterns and lifestyles within ethnic minority communities mean that it is no longer the case that there are always relatives to provide support and care when it is needed. There is evidence that there are lonely, vulnerable people in these communities who need to know where they can go to access information, advice and help.
>
> (Okuyiga 1998: 4)

To check out such assumptions, the research samples in TACI (Twice a Child I) consisted of interviews with the representatives of 11 different organizations from each of the two communities in Wolverhampton (African-Caribbean and Asian Communities), followed by interviews with ten carers of older people with dementia from each of the two communities (N = 20). In both sets of interviews there was a concern to elicit their knowledge and understanding of dementia. The community representatives were asked also about the capacity of their organizations to provide support and assistance for older people with dementia. The carers were asked about their experiences of dementia and the effects upon the person with dementia for whom they have a responsibility, as well as their experiences of, and perspectives upon, health, social services and voluntary organizations in Wolverhampton.

Current community capacity in Wolverhampton to support older people with dementia and their carers

The representatives from the churches, temples, voluntary groups and agencies were quizzed as to their understanding of dementia – what it is; the current situation of dementia in the community; and the extent to which they were willing or able to commit their organizations to participate in community-based initiatives in dementia care. The eventual title of the research – 'Twice a Child' – was chosen, as it was the commonsense way in which the African-Caribbean community in particular described dementia in a shorthand but easily understandable way. For the research, what was initially important about the perspectives of the community representatives was the confirmation that there were only a very small number of people potentially with dementia that were known to them, but not to the health and social services (less than five people in total in the two communities). On that basis, the health services in Wolverhampton can be considered to be effective in identifying and assessing older people with dementia from the African-Caribbean and Asian communities. It also strikes back, yet again, at the assumption commonly held of the ethnic minority communities that they 'look after their own, don't they?' (SSI 1998).

Secondly, the representatives and their organizations had a desire to help, but their facilities and capabilities were considered insufficient to provide such assistance without a great deal of capacity building, both in terms of building and skills/ capabilities. The commitment to be involved more fully in the caring and support process for older people with dementia was there, but the capacity of the community organizations to do so manifestly was not. There was one obvious exception to this incapacity in the African-Caribbean community, for the African-Caribbean Community Initiative (ACCI) had gained beacon status as a voluntary organization dedicated to providing advice, help and assistance to members of their community over the whole range of needs, including those associated with older people with dementia. ACCI runs a general carers' group that includes older people with dementia, and provides some voluntary support to carers for respite, shopping and other duties. While there are voluntary agencies in the Asian community also, the existence of over 100 organizations within the Asian community in Wolverhampton is obviously a factor affecting the development of services and support. Overall, there-fore, the capacity of the two communities to provide services and support was in need of development. We return to the issue of community capacity building below.

The TACI carer experiences and perspectives of services

The average ages of the Asian older people with dementia was 70 for the men, and 82 for the women, while the similar ages for the African-Caribbean older people were 65 and 69 years respectively, reflecting the younger age profile overall of the African-Caribbean community in Wolverhampton. At the same time, the average age of the carers was higher for the African-Caribbean community than the Asian community. The average age of the African-Caribbean carers was 58 for the three men carers, and 47 for the seven female carers. The respective ages for the Asian community was a single Asian man carer aged 75, and an average age of 48 years for the nine Asian female carers. Besides the emotional and practical difficulties experienced by the carers in their caring role, many of the carers themselves also had medical conditions that affected their capacity to care for the older person with dementia for whom they had responsibility.

In asking the carers about their experiences of the services provided by GPs, specialist health services and the social and voluntary sectors, the concern of the research was to elicit the views of the carers with regard to:

- the promptness of the services provided;
- the relevance of the services provided;
- the helpfulness of the services provided;
- levels of overall satisfaction, as well as services desired but not provided.

In their evaluation of the services by the carers, only the specialist psychiatric doctors and community mental health nurses (CMHN) received substantial approval for the promptness and relevance of the services they provided. The carer experiences of GPs (for many the first line of call) was very mixed, and emphasized that the GPs have critical positions as first line informants about dementia, but also as gatekeepers to further specialist assessment and services. GPs who were rated highly by both sets of community carers were likely to quickly supply an initial concern of dementia, ensure rapid throughput to specialist services, and provide information, support and understanding. Additionally, the Asian carers in particular gained from a common heritage, culture and identity with their GPs.

Social services provision was not rated very highly by either set of carers, despite the majority of older people with dementia having some social service care plan and support, primarily in terms of day and respite care, though other services were accessed. Difficulties experienced by the carers centred upon the paucity of information about available services and eligibility criteria, the slowness in developing and implementing a care plan, and the varying degrees of cultural insensitivity experienced by the carers and the older people with dementia. That is, apart from a specialist Asian day centre that is not set up to cater for dementia sufferers, the day and respite services are staffed and run as 'white' services. Lest social services be unjustly accused of racism, it is important to recognize that developments have occurred to reduce such cultural insensitivity, including the development of culturally relevant surroundings, activities, languages and food in day and respite centres, but that such developments take time within overall council policies and practices that (for instance) abhor rapid action alternatives such as compulsory redundancies. The issues of service responsiveness were taken up in the second research project – Twice a Child II (TACII). It should also be noted that some of the dissatisfaction with social services was a matter of poor communication in that some assessments and services had been delivered but clients were not aware of this.

The TACII project

TACI ended in July 2001, when a conference took place to disseminate the findings, and to ensure that all the relevant service providers were aware of the desirable developments identified as a result of TACI, especially in the areas of community involvement, capacity building and culturally sensitive provision. TACII, which focused upon new carer experiences of the services and the experiences and perspectives of service managers (especially social services) was completed in 2003, and reported upon at a number of conferences (see Moreland 2003; Read et al. 2003).

In TACII, a number of carers who had been involved in TACI (five per community, N = 10) and new carers (five per community, N = 10) were interviewed to ascertain their views and perspectives upon the health, social and voluntary services received. For the TACI carers, there was obviously the necessity to bring the caring situation up to date, and to review their subsequent experiences of the different service sectors. Indeed, many of the older people with dementia from TACI had become even more incapacitated, and many were now in sheltered accommodation, with the carers taking a more pastoral caring role than before. In addition, many of the issues from TACI were the same, with the result that the research was able to identify a number of 'lessons' that should be recognized and acted upon in order to improve the experiences and thus lives of the older people with dementia and their carers. That is, the importance of GPs as the initial access point for services was confirmed, as was the approval of the specialist health services. Social services were still criticized for the slowness of assessment, and time lags in getting care packages agreed and established. Other major issues were still ones of knowledge about dementia itself amongst the communities, but also about the range of services available and eligibility criteria. In addition, social services were perceived to be much more geared up to the needs of the Asian community than the African-Caribbean community in Wolverhampton. It was strongly suggested, for instance, that there should be a specialist community mental health nurse for the African-Caribbean community so that the very well-received services provided by the Asian CMHN could be replicated for the other community.

The research process in TACII also involved interviews with managers in various organizations, in particular with senior social services personnel, as their services received the most criticism. In all, eight interviews with service providers were carried out, including one with the service manager of ACCI, and one with the chairperson of Wolverhampton Alzheimer's Society. Throughout, the commitment of all the interviewees to their clients was exemplary, as was their desire to improve service provision, though within tight budget and activity constraints. Consequently, there had been a number of developments since TACI. Examples of developments since TACI are:

- The creation of a Asian Carers' Support Group, now numbering over 100 carers.
- The creation of informational leaflets and tapes in different Asian languages on understanding dementia and carer issues.
- Wide-ranging informational talks about dementia carried out in and across the two communities, and the Asian community in particular.
- The building of a secure housing facility for Asian women suffering from dementia and allied illnesses.
- Specialist talks to all GPs about dementia and cultural manifestations and issues thereof.
- Social services staff voluntarily receiving Asian language tuition, and taking up the opportunity to visit and learn about specialist Asian facilities and cultural aspects.

These are important developments, though both staff and carers were aware of the necessity for further developments. To assist this process, the TACII Report identified a number of 'lessons' to be learned and implemented. The main lessons were as follows:

1. Recognize and relate to the variety of circumstances of the older people with dementia and their carers.

2. Respond to the continuous desire for information about dementia and its manifestations.

3. Recognize the continuing importance of GP responses to carer and patient needs and satisfaction.

4. The desirability of single, integrated care package assessments.

5. Regular care package reviews to recognize changing circumstances.

6. The desirability of culturally sensitive services.

7. Provide for a role for community and voluntary organizations in partnerships.

Unlike other social services such as Bradford (Read *et al.* 2003), Wolverhampton social services to date has not sought to develop community capacity to directly provide services to any great extent, so there are few service level agreements with voluntary agencies or charities. This is changing, however, as the communities themselves find their voice, but also as a result of central government emphasis upon a greater private and charitable involvement in service provision. Lesson seven above, for instance, is an indicator of central government pressures for change, such as the personalization of services through participation (Leadbetter 2004). In considering participation, community capacity building and empowerment, therefore, we have to recognize the national context of developments as well as subject these concepts to further analysis in the light of the two Twice a Child research projects and reports.

Part two: partnerships and community capacity building: the drive for a 'new public management' and service provision

Since the 1980s, there has been a more or less continuous central government driven interest in change in public sector service provision towards what has been character-ized as a 'new public management' that is counterpoised against an 'old' public management model. In effect, the old model of public management was essentially a post World War Two creation, at least in the developed world, though the model was actually a long time in the making. The post-1945 'Keynesian economic consensus' led to the expansion of the state into areas of social provision that became known as the Welfare State. Perhaps the most important assumption underlying the Welfare State was the necessity for the state to alleviate or make good the deficiencies of the capitalist markets, giving rise to a 'provider or supply side-led' command model of welfare provision.

The rise of the 'new right' in the 1980s, including neo-liberal economic theory (Baiman 2001; Hutton 1995), contested such statist models (Jessup 2002), proclaim-ing that the inefficiency of public bureaucracies meant that individual personal needs were not being met sufficiently well or effectively. Consequently, the defining characteristics of the new public management model of the welfare state were:

Its entrepreneurial dynamic, its reinstatement of the market as a potentially more efficient provider of public services than the state, and its proclaimed intention to transform managerial behaviour in the public sector. The practical realisation of the model usually produced the following public sector reforms:

- Restructuring through privatisation.
- The restructuring and reduction of central social services.
- The introduction of competition, especially by contracting public services to the private sector.
- The improvement of public services by means of service charters and the conducting of performance audits and assessment.

(Minogue 2002: 134)

Such dynamics and activities are now commonplace, and demonstrate the extent to which the new public sector management approach has become the dominant ideology of health and social services. Allied developments that have assisted this development have been the rise of the quality movement (Wilkinson and Wilmott 1995) and concepts of service quality (Rust and Oliver 1994), which emphasize user empowerment (Dooher and Byrt 2003) and definitions of quality – covering service encounters (initial and subsequent interactions with service providers); overall service satisfaction; and communally defined concepts of service quality (Bitner and Hubbert 1994). To speak of a 'dominant ideology', however, is not to say that such views have percolated and permeated the local providers of services equally well, for that manifestly is not so. Instead, local institutional adaptations of the ideology have occurred to fit local circumstances, priorities and perceptions of need.

Local adaptation in the health and social services

Despite suggesting that all health and social services in England and Wales have been subjected to the ideology and practices associated with 'new public management', we are aware that we have to be careful of assuming that the internal institutional arrangements and behaviours of health and social service departments in councils and health trusts simply and straightforwardly reflect and embody the wider ideological situation. This is not so, for there are other countervailing factors that exist inside organizations besides the central government 'regulatory pillar' (Scott 1995: 35), which establish the 'rule-setting, monitoring and sanctioning activities of institutions'. In our view, at least two other 'pillars' have existed locally to alter or downgrade the significance of the central regulatory pillar. These 'pillars' or buttresses are the cognitive and normative pillars (see Figure 16.1).

The cognitive pillar refers to the symbols and meanings assigned to external stimuli by staff within an institution. These are the socially constructed meanings and understandings common to staff, and which constitute the prism through which external factors are viewed and assigned weight and significance. An example of a cognitive pillar might be the use (and non-use) of direct payments to carers, a way of promoting carer decision making in service provision. Direct payments are social care monies provided directly to carers so that they may purchase a service to suit their

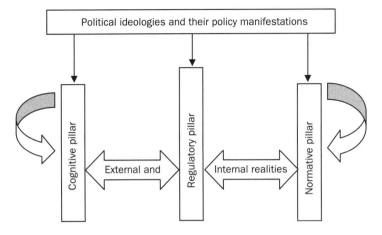

Figure 16.1 Pillars that influence organizations

needs as defined by them. In Wolverhampton social services, while the possibility of direct payments has been available for a number of years, take-up has been low, for the direct payments service has not been publicized. When asked why, a senior commissioning manager indicated that the authority has not deemed direct payments to be a particularly helpful way of ensuring the services are provided and used. It is important to realize that this stance is not illegal or underhand, but a perspective based upon a clear history and tradition of providing services in certain ways that are, for the members, considered superior ways of doing so. Without compulsion or a change of priorities, this situation is likely to remain the same in the near future.

This brings us to the third and related pillar that buttresses social action and behaviour – the 'normative pillar'. This pillar is closely allied to the cognitive pillar, but refers specifically to the shared values and norms – the pervasive culture – that guides the actions of institutional members. Actions here are thus associated not only with a perspective upon external realities, but also with a moral rightness – a belief by the group of key personnel (e.g. officers) that what is being done, and how it is being done, is right and proper and the best way of meeting defined needs. Diffused across all these pillars, of course, are sets of external and internal realities, e.g. the number of day care places, the numbers of social and health care staff with permanent contracts, and so on, which establish parameters for action and inaction by health and social services personnel, even though those self-same realities have, in all probability, been created because of the differential impact in the past of the different pillars. Overlying such pillars, in addition, are political ideologies and their policy manifestations, for it is no coincidence that the City of Wolverhampton which has a long-held Labour local government, has found it hard to adjust and accept the strictures of the regulatory pillars sustained by alternative political ideologies, such as those of neo-liberal doctrines (Baiman 2001).

At the same time, the continual drip feed of central government statements and actions, and their embodiment in agencies such as the NHS Modernisation Agency, means that some movement does occur, and alternative perceptions come into being and bring about effects. Indeed, it has been observed that one of the major impetuses for the Twice a Child research projects was the desire by the local health and social services to be seen to be leaders in service development for their local ethnic minority populations. At the same time, the failure of social services to overtly carry out some key actions arising from TACI, such as the publication and dissemination of eligibility criteria for services, suggests that the commitment to partnership, community involvement and capacity building is uneven amongst the senior staff of the services concerned.

Partnerships in theory

It is important in any analysis of partnerships for there to be a clear definition of partnerships, and to distinguish partnerships from participation and/or consultation, for in using the former, many commentators and professionals actually mean one or other or both of the latter. To begin with, the least involved relationship – consultation – is the process of seeking information, advice, opinions or perspectives from individuals, social groups and institutions who have an interest in an issue, and whose views are considered worthy of collection and consideration (Pendleton 2003). In consultative processes, the consulted usually have no formal role or right of participation in decision making, except perhaps a weak claim to have their views heard and taken account of (which is not the same necessarily as being listened to).

Participation is a stronger type of relationship involving some form of incorporation into the fact-finding and executive processes. Participation, however, does not have to be based upon equality of status, and indeed often is not. Participation is usually considered to be a means of involving and co-opting sections of the community into policy and decision making. Guijt and Shah (1998), for instance, state that:

> The aim of participatory development is to increase the involvement of socially and economically marginalized people in decision-making over their own lives. The assumption is that participatory approaches empower local people with the skills and confidence to analyse their situation, reach consensus, make decisions and take action, so as to improve their circumstances. The ultimate goal is a more equitable and sustainable development.
>
> (Guijt and Shah 1998: 1)

These are laudable aims, though the realities are often different and less satisfactory from the perspective of the marginalized groups. That is, participation can be a form of co-option into decision-making processes where the actual act of involvement is considered to be sufficient to warrant and expect the subordinate groups to accept the actual decisions made, even where the decisions manifestly are not attuned to the interests or needs of the group. After all, if you have had the opportunity to comment and participate, you ought to accept the outcomes!

Additionally, participation, particularly where it is spasmodic and temporary, does not by itself enhance the capacity of social groups to participate fully in decision making, for that requires skills of involvement and persuasion as well as the capacity to articulate and present persuasively an account of the needs of the group.

Consequently, participatory activities and techniques such as focus groups and small scale research projects can just lead to 'consultation fatigue' (see Rowntree Trust web site: www.jrf.org.uk/knowledge/forums/forum.asp?forumID=1), and a perception that such activities do not alter the core experiences or advance the needs of a group or defined community, such as an ethnic minority, within an area or region. As Tett, Crowther and O'Hara (2003: 39) suggest, 'rather than create more opportunities for democratic engagement, partnerships may simply serve to incorporate communities and professionals more deeply into arrangements that they have little genuine control over that do not really serve their best interests'. To guard against this, and for fatigue not to happen, there has to be sufficient development, which is acceptable to a community group, for that group to continue to participate.

This then takes us on to the definition and meaning of partnerships themselves. Following Tett, Crowther and O'Hara (2003: 39), we can say that partnerships occur 'when a change in process, product or output takes place that requires contributions from all the organizations involved'. It follows from this that there are degrees of formality in partnerships (the extent to which they are formally constituted through memoranda of co-operation), but also that the organizations concerned do not necessarily contribute equally. Partnerships appear to be facilitated when the collaborators recognize areas of interdependence and mutual action. That is, there is an accepted basis for collaboration and joint action; when the partnerships are fit for their intended purpose; and when the collaborating organizations are stable.

The Ontario development pack for aboriginal partnerships (see www.aboriginalbusiness.on.ca/resource_kit/ch3/ch3_1.html) suggests that there are four common attributes that collectively set partnerships apart from other types of relationships (Figure 16.2).

For partnerships to work, there has to be mutual benefits. That is, the partnership arrangements must deliver something of value to each party. There normally is shared responsibility, where both parties contribute resources and share the risks.

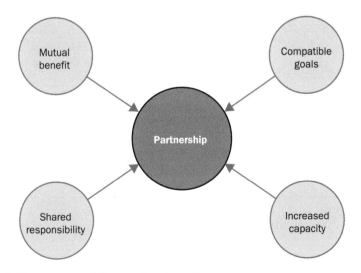

Figure 16.2 The common attributes of partnerships

Ideally, there should also be a strategic fit and compatibility between the goals of the partners, and recognition that the partnership enables the parties to do more together than any one organization could do alone. In all of this, it must be borne in mind that partnership are a means to an end, not an end in themselves – for a good partnership opens new opportunities, helps to mobilize resources and develop capabilities that would otherwise have been difficult for either partner to do alone.

The Ontario project suggests that there is a number of critical success factors in partnerships. In their view, these factors are:

- Relationship building on principles of honesty, sharing and kindness
- Mutual respect
- Mutual knowledge and understanding
- Mutual trust
- Explicit goals
- Clear roles and responsibilities
- Open dialogue and communications
- Creativity
- Flexibility
- Sustained commitment

Additionally, there are three main types of partnerships: joint ventures, strategic alliances or comprehensive partnerships. Joint ventures are a form of partnership where a new organization is specifically created by the partners to achieve a defined purpose, or set of purposes, through jointly sponsored action. Strategic alliances – the second form of partnership – usually have a more narrowly focused set of purposes. In strategic alliances, the partners remain legally separate entities but agree to collaborate in a principal area, such as (in our case) service developments to meet the needs of ethnic minority older people with dementia and their carers in the City of Wolverhampton. Finally, comprehensive partnerships occur when the partners remain legally separate entities but make a commitment to collaborate across a number of inter-related areas on a long-term basis, often involving community development activities. Service level agreements, and the sharing of tasks and responsibilities, are the hallmarks of comprehensive partnerships. But what happened in the Twice a Child projects?

Partnership in practice in the Twice a Child projects

It is clear that that the main form of partnership utilized in the two Twice a Child projects was that of a strategic partnership. A steering group that had representatives from the following organizations managed the two projects:

- Dementia Plus West Midlands
- African-Caribbean Community Initiative

- Alzheimer's Society, Wolverhampton
- Asian Women's Adhikar Association
- BME Housing Consortium
- Department of Health
- Wolverhampton Health Authority
- Wolverhampton Health Care NHS Trust
- Wolverhampton Race Equality Council
- Wolverhampton Social Services

This is an impressive list, and indicates a great deal of community involvement, though a selective one also, for there are many organizations representing the African-Caribbean and Asian communities in Wolverhampton that were not present. This was a major reason behind the TACI survey of what were considered to be the most important community organizations outside the steering group. In effect, however, because of the predominance of public health and social service provision in Wolverhampton, the real power rested with the health and social service managers who were involved in the two projects. That is, the proposals for development that came out of TACI, and which formed the focus of TACII concerning the extent of their achievement, were predominantly pressure group suggestions for change. Though a number of the proposals were taken up, a number were not, suggesting differences in priorities between the statutory agencies and the strategic alliance that constituted the Twice a Child steering groups.

There was one example, however, of a joint venture in practice if not in law. The BME Housing Association, in collaboration with the Asian Women's Adhikar Association, developed plans and built a small complex of sheltered housing for Asian women with dementia in Wolverhampton. Improvements for the African-Caribbean community, however, are less well developed, and may in part be due to a perception that existing organizations, such as ACCI, are already sufficiently able to represent and meet the needs of their community. At the same time, some community capacity building has been carried out, but mainly at the levels of knowledge and community representation of needs. It has already been suggested that this limited development of community capacity is due to local political and ideological realities, allied to real issues over current authority policies and practices on service planning, staffing, redundancy and redeployment.

Community capacity building

The phrase Community Capacity Building describes precisely what it is. Undertaken either by the communities alone or in concert with other agencies such as health and social services, community capacity building focuses upon the development of the capacities of a community (e.g. the African-Caribbean or Asian communities in Wolverhampton) so that they are able to raise their profile in the 'quest for social justice, particularly around the right to receive equal treatment in all aspects of public sector health and social care activity' (Read *et al.* 2003: 32). Capacity building is all about developing grass roots community support for organizations and individuals who are able and willing to further the interests of that community by:

- Collecting and disseminating information about services to the community (e.g. outreach work to the communities about dementia by the health and social services, as well as by the local community organizations themselves such as ACCI).
- Developing the structures by which the community can come together and voice their concerns individually and collectively (e.g. through health and social service sponsored focus groups).
- Developing members of the communities themselves so that they are able, willing and confident enough to collate and represent the views of the community to the health and social services, as well as pursue individual cases of need.
- Assistance in developing community organizations themselves so that they are able to provide voluntary support to complement health and social service provision (e.g. Wolverhampton ACCI Carer's Group).
- Development of the capacity of community-based organizations to provide services to their community under formal service level agreements (e.g. culturally sensitive day care provision).

Carrying out such developmental tasks is not just the responsibility of either the community or the health and social services. Rather, the responsibility is a joint responsibility of community and services. There is the necessity to manage such developments, both by reaching out to the community, but also by in-reach activities within health and social services – activities such as ethnic minority recruitment and training initiatives by health and social services to ensure that culturally relevant staffing and services are available to those community members that need and want them. In-reach can involve:

- the re-orientation and refocusing of existing services;
- extending service through alternative modes of provision;
- innovating in-service provision to provide locally novel solutions.

In the experience of the Twice a Child projects, the achievement of such developments requires the active support and interventions of a senior change champion as well as building upon developments being pushed through the national 'regulatory pillar' that was considered earlier. That is, changes which are in tune with wider developments are more likely to be implemented than those that are not. Doing this requires the capacity of managers to anticipate and address staff worries about themselves and their futures, for it is important to take staff along with the changes, and to allow for small steps as well as giant leaps.

Conclusion

The Twice a Child projects have demonstrated both achievements and some shortcomings in community partnerships and involvement in the development of health and social services. In many ways, the projects were just steps on the road to greater community empowerment and involvement in service provision for older people with dementia and their carers. There are still many worthwhile developments that need to happen but with will, foresight and patience on all sides, there is a great deal of hope for the future provision of such services, either by the statutory agencies or the communities themselves. Developments need to be in the form of partnerships, and involve the development of the capacity of communities themselves to pursue their interests and needs. In Wolverhampton, the African-Caribbean and Asian communities have both sought to carry out such developments, but it is clear that there is yet still more to come. On that basis, watch this space!

Questions for further discussion

1. To what extent have the seven lessons described in this chapter been realized in your own experience?
2. What three key activities would you need to engage in, in order to build community capacity in your area of practice?
3. How closely to the findings of the two Twice a Child projects resemble care of people with dementia in your own experience?

References

Aggarwal, N., Vass, A.A., Minardi, H. A., Ward, R., Garfield, C. and Cybyk, B. (2003) People with dementia and their relatives: personal experiences of Alzheimer's and of the provision of care, *Journal of Psychiatric and Mental Health Nursing*, 10: 187–97.

Baiman, R.P. (2001) *Political Economy and Contemporary Capitalism: Radical Perspectives on Economic Theory and Policy*. M. E. Sharpe, London.

Bitner, M. J. and Hubbert, A. R. (1994) Encounter Satisfaction Versus Overall Satisfaction Versus Quality, Chapter 3 pp. 72–94, in R.T. Rust and R.L. Oliver (eds) *Service Quality: New Direction in Theory and Practice*. Sage, Thousand Oaks, CA.

Dementia Plus West Midlands (2000) *Beginning to Explore Ethnic Elderly Dementia In-depth (BEEDI)*. Wolverhampton: Dementia Plus West Midlands (mimeo)

Department of Health (2001) *National Service Framework for Older People*. Department of Health, London.

Department Of Health (2002) *Social Service Performance Assessment Framework Indicators, 2001–2002*. Department of Health, London.

Dooher, J. and Byrt, R. (eds) (2003) *Empowerment and the Health Service User* (Volume Two). Mark Allen Publishing, Dinton.

Friedel, M. (2002) Awareness: A personal memoir on the declining quality of life in Alzheimer's, *Dementia*, 1(2): 359–66.

Guijt, I. and Shah, M. (1998) *The Myth of Community: Gender Issues in Participatory Development*. Intermediate Technology Publications, London.

Hirst, M. (2001) Trends in informal care in Great Britain during the 1990s, *Health and Social Care in the Community*, 9(6): 348–57.

Hutton, W. (1995) *The State We're In*. Cape, London.

Jessup, B. (2002) *The Future of the Capitalist State*. Polity Press, Cambridge.

Jolley, D., Read, K., Swindlehurst, L. Werrett, J., Clifford, C. and Chung, M.C. (1996) *An Analysis of the Characteristics and Needs of Known Dementia Sufferers and their Carers in Wolverhampton*. University of Wolverhampton CHPRD, Wolverhampton.

Leadbetter, C. (2004) *Personalisation Through Participation*. Demos, London (see www.demos.co.uk).

Menne, H.L., Kinney, J, M. and Morhardt, D.J. (2002) Trying to continue to do as much as they can do, *Dementia*, 1(2): 367–82.

Minogue, M. (2002) Power to the people? Good governance and the reshaping of the state (Chapter 7, pp. 117–35), in U. Kothari and M. Minogue (eds) *Development Theory and Practice*. Palgrave, London.

Moreland, N. (2001) *Twice a Child I: Dementia Care for African-Caribbean and Asian Older People in Wolverhampton*. Dementia Plus West Midlands, Wolverhampton.

Moreland, N. (2003) *Twice a Child II: Service Development for Dementia Care for African-Caribbean and Asian Older People in Wolverhampton*. Dementia Plus West Midlands, Wolverhampton.

Nocon, A. and Pearson, M. (2000) The roles of friends and neighbours in providing support for older people, *Ageing and Society*, 20: 341–67.

Okuyiga, A. (1998) Reaching Ethnic Minorities, *Journal of Dementia Care*, 6(3): 1–10.

Ontario Native Affairs Secretariat (1998) *The Power of Partnerships: New Opportunities for Aboriginal Peoples and Ontario Business: The Partnership Development Kit*. Ontario, Canada: ProvincialGovernment(accessedatwww.aboriginalbusiness.on.ca/resource_kit/index.html. Last accessed 4 April 2004).

Pendleton, D. (2003) *The New Consultation: Developing Doctor Patient Communication*. Oxford University Press, Oxford.

Phillipson, C. (2001) *The Family and Community Life of Older People: Social Networks and Social Support in Three Urban Areas*. Routledge, London.

Read, K., Rouf, A., Jolley, D. and Henderson, J. (2003) *Double Take: A Tale of Two Cities: Improving Services for Older People from Black and Minority Ethnic Communities in Bradford and Wolverhampton*. Bradford Social Services and Dementia Plus West Midlands, Bradford.

Routh, J. and Wolff, J. (eds) (1977) *The Sociology of Literature: Theoretical Approaches* Sociological Review Monograph 25. University of Keele, Keele.

Rust, R.T. and Oliver, R.L. (eds) (1994) *Service Quality*. Sage, London.

Scott, W.R. (1995) *Institutions and Organizations: Theory and Research*. Sage, London.

Social Services Inspectorate (SSI)(1998) *They Look after their Own, Don't They? The Inspection of Community Care Services for Black and Ethnic Minority Older People*. Department of Health, London.

Tett, L., Crowther, J. and O'Hara, P. (2003) Collaborative partnerships in community education, *Journal of Education Policy*, 18(1): 37–51.

Wilkinson, A. and Willmott, H. (eds) (1995) *Making Quality Critical*. Routledge, London.

Wojan, T.R. and Rupasingha, A. (2001) Crisis as opportunity: local context, adaptive agents and the possibilities of rural development, *Regional Studies*, 35(2): 141–52.

PART 3

Developing and improving partnerships

17

Learning from partnerships: themes and issues

Ros Carnwell and Julian Buchanan

This chapter will reflect on the different examples of partnership working this book in order to:

- Examine the different meanings and interpretations given to the notion of partnership.
- Discuss the political imperatives for working in partnership.
- Explore the challenges of working in partnership.
- Highlight examples of good practice.

The meaning of partnership

In Chapter 1, Carnwell and Carson explore the meaning of partnership and collaboration. Following a review of literature, they highlight the main attributes associated with these two concepts, and referring to case studies within this book, they assess the utility value of them. In distinguishing between the two concepts (see Table 17.1), they argue that collaboration (the verb) is *what* partners (the noun) *do* when they *work together*. However, in addition to these main attributes, the different case examples of working together explored in this text have also illustrated a wider range of possible attributes as indicated in the third column.

Carnwell and Carson argue that 'respect' is a main attribute of successful collaboration. This is illustrated in Chambers and Phillips's reference to *The National Strategy for Carers* (DoH 1999), in Chapter 15, which is based on 'respect' and recognition of carers' expertise. The importance of 'teamwork' is highlighted by Corby in Chapter 12, in order to encourage interprofessional teams to work together to protect children. Interestingly, Corby's suggestions for working together mirror closely the attributes listed for both partnership and collaboration. He recommends:

- the establishment of a common purpose;
- a sympathetic evaluation and understanding of each other's roles;

Table 17.1 Attributes of partnership and collaboration

Main attributes of partnership	Main attributes of collaboration	Additional possible attributes
Trust in partners	Trust and respect in collaborators	Communication
Respect for partners	Joint venture	Mutual benefits
Joint working	Teamworking	Shared responsibility
Teamwork	Intellectual and cooperative endeavour	Strategic fit and compatibility between the goals of the partners
Eliminating boundaries	Knowledge and expertise more important than role or title	Recognition that partnerships enable parties to do more together than any one organization could do alone
Being an ally	Participation in planning and decision making	Joint training
	Non-hierarchical relationship	Involvement of service users in decisions about their care
	Sharing of expertise	
	Willingness to work together towards an agreed purpose	
	Highly connected network	
	Low expectation of reciprocation	

- positive ongoing contact between professionals;
- secondments between agencies to facilitate better communication and under-standing of respective roles, developing respect for the roles of others, and counteracting stereotyping.

Other attributes referred to are those of 'trust', 'joint working' and the importance of knowledge and expertise in comparison to role or title. As Wyner (Chapter 9) points out, it is easier to successfully negotiate with a person from a different agency if some basic trust and understanding has been built up through meeting individually or as a group. While individuals within different agencies may appreciate the importance of joint working and develop trust with other professionals, it is helpful to have formal policy/practice support to validate and affirm this use of time and energy. Wyner provides a useful example of how the Rough Sleepers' Unit produced a local strategy on rough sleeping for their area, which actively encouraged improved joint working between agencies.

Joint working is an attribute that Carnwell and Carson note in current health and social policy, see for example, *Building Bridges* (DoH 1995), which makes reference to joint commissioning, in order to optimize resources. The wider possible attributes listed in column three of Table 17.1 seem more reminiscent of *Building Bridges'* reference to training within, and between, agencies, which includes understanding of agency roles. Other examples highlighted by different authors include: the need for mutual benefits (which could resemble a willingness to work together towards an agreed purpose); shared responsibility, where both parties contribute and share resources; a strategic fit and compatibility between the goals of the partners; and recognition that the partnerships enable the parties to do more together than any one organization could do alone (Moreland *et al.*, Chapter 16). Joint training is also frequently referred to, for example, by Buchanan and Corby (Chapter 11) in relation to agencies developing a shared understanding of different agency roles and function, Corby (Chapter 12) in relation to child protection and by Wyner (Chapter 9) with reference to homelessness and the need to develop an understanding of each other's services, and the roles and restrictions that agencies are bound by.

In relation to the importance of knowledge and expertise, Buchanan and Corby (Chapter 11) provide some interesting evidence of how drug dependency workers were much better prepared for dealing with drug users than other professional groups, and in fact considered that other professions tended to overreact as a result of their lack of knowledge. They also point out, however, that other professional groups that specialized in other areas, such as child protection, provided a broader generic service. It is quite possible that such differences in expertise and professional orientation might affect the relationship between professional groups and hence their ability to work together.

It is also interesting that none of the attributes of either partnership or collaboration include 'communication', yet it is frequently mentioned by authors of this book. Chambers, for example, mentions in Chapter 15 the need to communicate with carers in order to work successfully in partnership and Corby (Chapter 12), when stressing the need for more joint training in order to protect children, states that this should focus specifically on communication and barriers to it, such as stereotyping and ignorance of the roles and duties of others. Wilson (Chapter 10) also refers to the need for the establishment of clear lines of communication between the different centres in order to provide efficient and safe management of patients and accurate dissemination of information regarding treatments for children who are found to be HIV positive, when they are referred to tertiary centres some distance from the District General Hospital. Wyner (Chapter 9) discusses how communication in the homelessness sector revolves around establishing good relations with individuals and having meetings that are effective and satisfactory for all concerned. Another important example of communication is illustrated in Minhas's personal account of being a recipient of human services during the 1950s and 1960s. Minhas (Chapter 5) portrays a failure of health, social and educational professionals to communicate to him significant decisions affecting his health and social welfare. As he so eloquently states:

> Most crucially . . . perhaps clear explanations (reasons for the decisions) given in a sensitive and supportive way may have ameliorated some of the sense of absolute powerlessness I felt when, for example, I was told whether I was to stay with strangers in Farnham or with Kathleen in Fulham, or whether I was going to

the children's home in Winchester during the summer holidays or to stay with my 'uncle's' family in Liverpool.

What is so important about Minhas's experience, of course, is that it also illustrates the point that not a single attribute listed in the first two columns of Table 17.1 refer to involvement of service users in decisions about their care; most literature on partnerships focuses instead on partnerships between different agencies.

Policy imperatives for partnership working

Such is the importance of 'joined-up' thinking within current health and social policy that almost all of the authors have referred to policy drivers and explained how these policies have influenced and shaped the development of services for specific client groups. Indeed, Allison (Chapter 3) cites McLaughlin (2004) who argues that partnership provides a 'core theme' within social policy, which can consistently be observed in a range of diverse areas including health and social care, urban regeneration, education, crime and biotechnology. In Chapter 2, Parrott explores the key policies that have influenced the development of joint working. He explains how the election of a Labour government in 1997 seems to have been a landmark in the implementation of partnership strategies for developing public services, despite the fact that most local authorities had been pursuing partnership arrangements for many years. Examples he provides of how this was exemplified in practice include social service representation on the boards of Primary Care Groups and Trusts, and partnership focused approaches to allow the creation of pooled budgets. Such initiatives were also encapsulated within the terminology of 'joined-up government' and the drive towards the creation of 'seamless services', which reflected the importance that New Labour attached to working across what had previously been considered unhelpful professional and organizational divides. As Parrott points out, New Labour's partnership philosophy is embedded within its 'Third Way' approach to delivering services. It promotes closer relationships at all levels of the organization, and encourages contractual developments between statutory, voluntary and the growing independent sector. This is a much stronger vision of partnership than previously promoted concepts, such as inter-agency working. Parrott suggests that the previous emphasis on joint planning, commissioning and provision of services has now given way to integration, with agencies working more collaboratively formally and informally.

Within other chapters of this book, it becomes evident how government policy plays out in service developments. Some developments foster partnerships between different agencies, while others encourage partnerships between professionals and service users. Wilson provides an example of the latter in Chapter 10, in which the Department of Health has identified the need for patients to become 'experts' about their own health, so that they can become key decision makers in the treatment process. By ensuring that knowledge of their condition is developed to a point where they are empowered to take some responsibility for its management and work in partnership with their health and social care providers, patients can be given greater control over their lives (DoH 2001). This emphasis on partnership with service users is also reflected in Article 12 of the 1990 UN Convention on the Rights of the Child, which asserts the right of young people to have a voice on issues that affect them (see Miller, Chapter 13). The principle of incorporating and empowering service users so they can be properly represented within partnerships poses a real challenge, and from the examples in this book, service users are not always given a voice.

Minogue (Chapter 14) makes reference to the prominence given to partnership working in the Green Paper, *Developing Partnerships in Mental Health* (DoH 1997), to inter-agency working by the document *Building Bridges* (DoH 1995) and collaborative working in *The National Service Framework for Mental Health* (NHS 1999). While the Green Paper highlights a lack of consistency in the development of successful partnerships across England and Wales, *Building Bridges* states that agencies should be involved in caring for mentally ill people, and outlines a number of key requirements for effective inter-agency working. These requirements include: commitment to inter-agency working at all levels of the agency; a jointly owned and agreed strategy and procedures; and involvement of service users and carers. Key to *The National Service Framework for Mental Health* is the need to ensure that national standards apply to all aspects of provision and to improve risk assessment and management of mentally-disordered offenders by collaborative working. Herein lies a tension, the development of partnerships across the UK will inevitably result in different groupings of agencies and individuals, together with a diverse array of working relationships and practices – making consistency and national standards more difficult to maintain.

The government's interest in partnership has also extended as far as rural communities and Pugh (Chapter 6) draws attention to the *Care in the Country* report (SSI 1999) and the rural White Paper, *Our Countryside, The Future* (MAFF 2000). In the latter, a Rural Services Standard was established, in which polices were 'rural proofed', meaning that they had been considered and developed not solely from an urban perspective. However, the different partnerships that emerge in this text are not so easily replicated in the rural context given the differences in opportunities, resources, population density, public transport and road access – a point which Pugh argues has financial and resource implications that are rarely taken into account by UK-wide policy directives.

Challenges of working in partnership

Most of the challenges of working in partnership arise as a result of moral and philosophical issues, structural/political issues and more practical concerns. In Chapter 3, Allison points out some of the ethical and moral tensions that might arise when working together. For example, she refers to the need to recognize the limits to one's expertise and competence regardless of how long one may have been doing the job, while also highlighting that in interprofessional settings, it is uncomfortable to feel ill at ease or unskilled. There is a tendency to want to demonstrate competence and make a good representation on behalf of the agency in such settings.

More general problems are helpfully highlighted by Pugh in Chapter 6, when he cites Hague's (1999) review of multi-agency initiatives. Some problems of partnership are listed in Box 17.1.

Box 17.1 Potential problems in partnership working

- Tendency of some agencies to 'defend their own turf'.
- Confusion and lack of clarity about roles and responsibilities.
- Tendency to marginalize equality issues, such as gender and ethnicity.
- Wastage of scarce resources, especially of smaller agencies, in unproductive discussion.
- Futile attempts to co-ordinate systems that are already inadequate or disorganized.
- Difficulties in resolving differences of power, resources and philosophy between agencies.
- A tendency for larger agencies to take over the work and marginalize the smaller agencies.
- Larger agencies may leave too much of the work to smaller ones.
- Tendency to marginalize service users and prospective clients.

Many of the problems listed above are evident in this book. Resolving these differences in power, resources and philosophy between agencies is illustrated in Minogue's concern (Chapter 14) with how two potentially disparate forms of state intervention – the criminal justice system and health care – offer treatment, care, punishment, restriction or rehabilitation, given their different ethical and philosophical standpoints. Tensions arising from different philosophical positions can also be seen in Miller's description (Chapter 13) of the philosophical differences between how teachers intervene in the lives of young people compared to the interventions of youth and community workers. While teachers' styles of practice are constrained by externally imposed curricula and compulsory attendance, in contrast youth and community workers are able to draw on a more flexible, open-ended approach to provide wider social education. These differences in philosophy, Miller argues, result in tensions over competing strategies, played out within the nature of the respective interventions that each profession makes into the lives of young people.

The tendency to marginalize service users and prospective clients, also highlighted by Hague, can be seen in Wilson's chapter (Chapter 10), Buchanan and Corby (Chapter 11) and in Minhas's chapter (Chapter 5). Wilson states that an important barrier to working in partnership is fears, misconceptions and negative attitudes to certain groups of service users, such as those who are HIV positive, while Minhas recounts his own personal experience of marginalization by not being involved in decisions about his care. Roberts, in Chapter 7, also emphasizes issues of marginalization in relation to Gypsy Travellers, particularly in relation to how they have been rejected by many societies for several hundred years and continue to be so. Marginalization is further illustrated by Bates (Chapter 4) when he cites Hague *et al.*'s (1996) findings that many survivors of domestic abuse felt reluctant to offer their services to local initiatives because of the power imbalance between the 'professionals' and survivors; some even felt that they might be used by the project primarily to give it legitimacy. Similar concerns are succinctly expressed by Moreland *et al.* in Chapter 16, when they describe 'participation as a form of co-option into decision-making processes where the actual act of involvement is considered to be sufficient to warrant and expect the subordinate groups to accept the decisions made, even where those decisions manifestly are not attuned to the interests or needs of the group. After all, if you have had the opportunity to comment and participate, you ought to accept the outcomes!' At a more practical level, Chambers and Phillips (Chapter 15) argue that it is difficult for carers to consider themselves to be equal partners while attempting to juggle many roles and maintaining some control over their whole life, not just the care-giving component.

In Chapter 4, Bates elaborates further on some of these issues at a more structural level, arguing that professionals working together will inevitably find themselves in conflict as their different disciplines rely on different discourses. It is his contention that power and meaning operate differently within and between groups and that this is translated into how service users are treated and processed. Some service users may historically have been used to a fairly disempowering and patronizing relationship from particular agencies and will need to be empowered before they can fully partici-pate and play a meaningful role in collaborative provision. As empowering users requires statutory bodies to relinquish some of their power, this is likely to remain contentious – though some professionals may be more willing than others to devolve power to marginalized groups. This is exemplified in Minhas' personal experience (Chapter 5) in that he spent years attempting to access services individually, with no 'key worker' to ease this process. As he gained entry to educational systems he seems to have become more empowered and through that process was more able to access the services he needed.

Evidence of successful partnerships

What we have highlighted thus far in this chapter is that, despite the government rhetoric to improve partnership working and the vast amount of literature that engages in some level of debate about the nature or partnership, collaboration and working together, there are many challenges and barriers that beset public service agencies when making partnership working happen. However, what this book has illustrated is the extent to which partnership working has been successful in enabling professionals and service users to work together. As a consequence, it can be seen from many of the case studies that partnership work has enabled some agencies to deliver a more effective service. The remaining section of this chapter outlines some of the successful partnerships and summarizes their key features.

Successful partnerships seem to be operating at one or more of three levels: a macroscopic (strategic) level, a medioscopic (operational) level, and a microscopic (practice) level. There are examples within this book of strategic (macroscopic) partnerships. For example, Moreland *et al.* (Chapter 16) explain how 'Twice a Child' projects relied upon joint responsibility between community health and social ser-vices, which required in-reach, as well as out-reach activities within health and social services. These included reorientation and refocusing of existing services; extending services through alternative modes of provision; and innovating in-service provision to provide locally novel solutions. Another example is evident in Minogue's chapter (Chapter 14), when she explains how a multi-agency steering group was formed in the city of Leeds, West Yorkshire, to develop a diversion scheme at the magistrates court for mentally-disordered offenders. This arose from a recognition that people with mental health problems who offend were not always dealt with appropriately, and a belief that a partnership response was the most effective way of addressing the issues. The strategic nature of this group is reflected in the agencies involved (health authority, the Community [Mental] Health Trust, social services, the probation service, magistrates court and police, the crown prosecution service and housing department), as well as in the development of terms of reference, key strategic objectives, an action plan and comprehensive strategy document. Minogue explains how this strategic approach led to a number of operational (medioscopic) achievements. These achievements included: the development of a court-based diversion scheme, good practice protocols, and liaison with and training of, sentencers. Interestingly, she explains how the main deficiencies are linked to knowledge and information awareness such as: confidentiality protocols, and involvement of service users and carers. Involvement of service users and carers as a weakness is hardly surprising, given that they did not appear to be included in the membership of agencies involved at a strategic level. Chambers and Phillips (Chapter 15) provide a third example of a macro-level partnership, 'Partnerships for Carers in Suffolk'. The partnership comprises Suffolk Carers, a number of local authorities' social services and education departments, the health authority, the Association of Voluntary Organizations, NHS trusts, and primary care groups. Each partner has 'signed up' for the Charter for Carers in Suffolk, which emphasizes carers' right to recognition; choice; information; practical help; financial assistance towards the costs of caring; and co-ordinated services. Each partner is also committed to implementing an action plan.

At the medioscopic (operational) level, a key feature of a successful partnership seems to be the nature of the agencies involved. In Chapter 8, for example, Blyth describes a successful partnership combining public and community services – the Coventry Partnership – which provides services to victims of domestic violence. Blyth argues that the balance of power between the voluntary and statutory sectors was one of the reasons for the partnership's success. This is because, while structural power was provided by statutory organizations, the voluntary sector women's organizations were able to better represent the voices of survivors of domestic violence and ensured the partnership remained properly focused on work that made a real difference to their lives. Blyth also points out the critical role of the co-ordinator in successful partnership, who requires the skills to operate across agency boundaries, build bridges between different interest groups, broker difference and build consensus (Webb 1991). In this situation, the different expertise and experience of the statutory and voluntary agencies seems to have been complementary and kept the agencies focused and working together more effectively.

This balance achieved by different agencies working together is also illustrated in Wyner's description of Hamden's weekly agency meeting in Chapter 9. These meetings arose out of an agreement that better partnership working would develop if colleagues from different agencies met together regularly to discuss issues. She describes this as an 'information-sharing forum with an objective of improving liaison between organizations so that they could each offer an informed and unencumbered response to the clients, where overlaps were less likely to happen, and where staff didn't work at cross purposes. There was particular concern to minimize the potential for homeless people to split and manipulate agencies, particularly for those whose lives were desperate and chaotic and who had borderline or other personality disorders, which was not uncommon. She recounts how a GP explained that talking to drug and alcohol workers in multi-agency meetings had enabled a more complete picture of patients' needs and was, therefore, less likely to undo the good work that had been achieved.

At the microscopic (practice) level of partnership working Roberts describes (Chapter 7) the Multi-agency Traveller Forum for Gypsy Travellers in Wrexham in North Wales. She explains how during the early stages of the development of the team the emphasis was on 'how best can we work together', developing terms of reference for the group, and identifying the skills, knowledge and expertise held within this diverse gathering of professionals and lay interested parties. The forum subsequently provided a mobile caravan for the delivery of health and social welfare information and advice. In effect, this has become a private space, within which Gypsy Travellers can discuss culturally difficult issues including: sexual health topics; pregnancy; informal counselling; domestic violence; and mental health worries. In some respects, this example crosses the boundary between the operational level and practice level as the members of the team struggle with operational issues, such as team membership and working together, which they then translate into more practical issues of identifying skills and knowledge within their members. Another example of practice-level partnership can be seen in Chapter 13, in which Miller explains how the professions of education and youth and community work have recently become much more closely associated within both schools and colleges. He cites the work of Smith who details some of the initiatives that are taking place, involving '. . . a growing army of personnel including classroom assistants, informal educators, youth workers, learning mentors and personal advisors . . .' (Smith 2002: 1). Some of the activities in which they are engaged include: working with students to set up study clubs; supporting development of interest groups; developing alternative education for young people experiencing difficulties in mainline classrooms; and organizing residentials and fun-days.

Conclusion

This chapter has explored the nature of partnership and collaboration as it is illustrated within case studies and examples throughout this book. The attributes of partnership and collaboration have been discussed and policy drivers have been explained. What has emerged from the chapters herein is that partnership working will by its very nature be fluid, but this can enable the agencies involved to respond better to the rapidly changing communities and needs that they serve. By comparison, agencies that work alone have a tendency to develop parochial interests and drift towards serving the needs of the employees and employers rather than responding to service user needs. Working in partnership is not easy, however, due to a number of reasons. Partnerships have to be sustained over a long period of time and this requires energy and commitment of all partners. This vulnerable lifespan is appropriate given that organizations can, over time, go stale and struggle to respond to changing demands. Expending time and effort sometimes means that partners may become involved in activities that are arguably not cost effective. Furthermore, partnerships can sometimes rely too heavily upon the enthusiasm of a particular agency or individual and this may result in tensions between agencies. Their fluid nature can also make partnerships susceptible to being dominated by powerful individuals or agencies. Nevertheless, it is possible that long-term partnerships could erode the diverse identities of different agencies as they blend and converge.

Perhaps the future of partnerships lies primarily in a shared vision for service delivery. This shared vision should then be translated into three levels: strategic, operational and practice. Within the strategic level there should be a synergy between voluntary and statutory agencies and recognition of the need to understand and promote differences between agencies rather than to compete for resources. At the operational level, while policy directives will help drive resources, listening to service users and developing partnerships with voluntary groups will help keep service relevant and meaningful. At the practice level, greater understanding between personnel would be achieved by secondments between agencies, perhaps for six-month periods. The need to involve service users is also key to the development of partnerships, but this concept is under-developed both philosophically and practically. More equal representation of service users would be achieved if service providers employed them, even if only on a consultancy or part-time basis.

References

Department of Health (1995) *Building Bridges: Arrangements for Inter-Agency Working for the Care and Protection of Severely Mentally Ill People*. HMSO, London.

Department of Health (1997) *Developing Partnerships in Mental Health*. The Stationery Office, London.

Department of Health (1999) *The National Strategy for Carers*. HMSO, London.

Department of Health (2001) *The Expert Patient: A New Approach to Chronic Disease Management for the 21st Century*. Department of Health, London. Crown Copyright.

Hague, G., Malos, E. and Dear, W. (1996) *Multi Agency Work and Domestic Violence: A National Study of Inter Agency Initiatives*. Polity Press, Bristol.

Hague, G. (1999) Smoke screen or leap forward: inter-agency initiatives as a response to domestic violence, *Critical Social Policy*, 53: 93–109.

McLaughlin, H. (2004) Partnerships: panacea or pretence? *Journal of Interprofessional Care*, 18(2): 103–13.

Ministry of Agriculture Fisheries and Food (2000) *Our Countryside: The Future a Fair Deal for Rural Communities*. DETR, Wetherby.

National Health Service (1999) *Modern Standards and Service Models. Mental Health National Service Frameworks*. Department of Health, London.

Social Services Inspectorate (1999) *Care in the Country – Inspection of Community Care Services in Rural Areas*. Department of Health, London.

Smith, M.K. (2002) Informal Education in schools and colleges in *The Encyclopaedia of Informal Education*, http://www.infed.org/schooling/inf-sch.htm. Last update: 14 February 2004.

Webb, A. (1991) Co-ordination: A Problem in Public Sector Management, *Policy and Politics*, 19(4).

18

Developing best practice in partnership

Julian Buchanan and Ros Carnwell

Introduction

For many decades health and social agencies have worked separately and independently with multi-agency practice an exception, rather than a rule, but over recent years partnerships have become a dominant model for tackling difficult health and social problems. Key factors that have brought about the shift towards partnership practice include:

- An increasingly complex society leading to multifaceted needs that can no longer be met by a sole agency.
- Changes in the structures, roles and function of statutory agencies, which made them more fluid, adaptable and able to work alongside other agencies.
- The political drive from government policy for 'joined-up' thinking, which has resulted in a range of legislation and policy directives requiring agencies to work collaboratively in partnerships to deliver seamless services.

In the past, the focus was more often upon the client seeking help from an individual agency. The response to client need tended to be a specific intervention strategy or therapy delivered exclusively from within the agency. While not mutually exclusive, the focus today draws upon enabling the individual to access a range of services and facilities available from different agencies – statutory, voluntary and private. These agencies often work in collaboration with each other, sometimes informally, sometimes within formalized partnerships, to provide packages of care. A partnership may include various statutory, voluntary and independent/private organizations, and sometimes, though not often enough, service user involvement. This approach reflects the more diverse and fluid nature of society, the changing nature of the welfare state, the multifaceted nature of individual needs, and the shift away from exclusive statutory provision to the expansion of 'contracted out' services provided by the voluntary and independent sector. This approach is at the heart of New Labour's 'Third Way'. The concept of partnership is now embedded within mainstream health and social care provision.

This shift of focus has significant implications for professionals in the health and social care sector (including criminal justice workers), many of whom have been used to working exclusively within their own organization and responding to need through their own in-house therapies, treatments or interventions. A particular challenge is ensuring staff possess the appropriate knowledge, skills and values to be able to work flexibly to develop, establish and maintain effective partnerships. Training and professional courses tend to lack interdisciplinary opportunities for learning together with students from related disciples (such as nursing, social work, community work, youth work, medicine, probation work), though there are now a growing number of modules appearing on courses that are concerned to equip students to understand inter-agency and partnership practice.

Relatively little has been written about partnerships, and what literature there is tends to concentrate upon the concept of partnership, or ideological basis of partnership. What is particularly lacking is literature concerned with the development of theory/practice knowledge in relation to partnership work that would inform and enable workers at the 'front line' to be better equipped. There are a proliferation of partnerships, yet a dearth of knowledge, and a lack of training and education opportunities to inform practice wisdom to work effectively in partnership.

Key principles for effective practice when working in partnership

This final chapter will attempt to draw out some of the main messages from the text by identifying key principles for effective practice when working in partnership. We offer 14 key principles of effective practice:

1. Devote time to creating, nurturing and maintaining partnerships

Effective partnerships seem more successful when partners relate well and understand each other's roles. A good partnership cannot be rushed into existence. It is likely to require an initial heavy investment of time and even when established it will need ongoing attention. This is often best achieved by face-to-face contact that encourages informal, open dialogue between all partners exploring philosophy, vision, strategy and practice, while at all times clarifying difference and sameness, strengths and weaknesses. This may be supplemented by new electronic forms of communication including email, dedicated mail databases, discussion boards, electronic communities etc. Once partnerships are formed, agencies may find it useful to maintain dialogue and understanding through regular meetings, electronic communication and by involving staff from different agency partners in shared training events and role shadowing.

2. Develop a mutual understanding and respect between agency partners

A lot of misunderstanding occurs when agencies fail to appreciate the different roles and functions of the other agencies with whom they are seeking to work closely. Stereotypes and agency sub-cultures can hinder good working relationships with other agencies and fuel parochial attitudes and rivalry. Staff from all agencies need to be informed about each other's roles, and feel comfortable in embracing and respecting agency differences even though at times they may be philosophically at odds with their own. This level of mature understanding, agreement and respect is not easily achieved and will often require considerable dialogue and investment of time to properly appreciate how other agencies 'see', and what they do.

3. Allow time for partnerships to develop

In a climate of standardization and 'top down' policy-driven practice, an attempt may be made to force partnerships into existence by legislation. This can happen but they will need time to develop as they are more fluid and organic by nature and are not easily created by bureaucratic mandates. This flexibility is, of course, a major strength of a partnership in that it is able to cater and respond to diverse local needs. This may sit uncomfortably with a centralist agenda, which promotes the creation of national standards, consistency and the roll out of fixed models of partnership across the UK. Although easily created by statute or policy directives, regional and local differences will result in different partnership arrangements. Models of practice are, therefore, best created at local levels to reflect the unique circumstances, such as rurality or cultural diversity. Otherwise, there is a risk of 'false partnerships' being created where agencies come together to fulfil a legal, political or policy requirement to be 'seen' as a working in partnership, though in practice not operating as one. This can benefit the agency but doesn't benefit the service user.

4. Guard against multi-agency inertia

Meeting together and discussing agendas, roles, philosophies as well as what the partnership could achieve is a relevant and important part of partnership development, but there is a risk that partnerships may become talk shops. Places where good intentions and ideas are explored but never implemented. Personal agendas (sometimes hidden) and status arising from participating in partnerships can for some individuals be their sole purpose in participating, these individuals can be quite destructive to the progress of any partnership.

5. Shared interest in service delivery

As bidding for new tenders, contracts and monies becomes an integral part of the 'modernized' welfare state, it is easy for agencies to seek partnerships to attract funding, without giving proper consideration as to whether the partnership will, in practice, improve service delivery – chasing power and status, and losing sight of the needs of service users. Agencies and partnerships can sometimes end up focusing upon the needs of their staff rather than the needs of clients. Effective partnership requires agencies to be focused on a shared commitment and interest to the needs of the client, and a belief that much more can be achieved for the benefit of the client by working together rather than working separately.

6. Develop strategic and operational commitment

Partnerships have a better chance of success when ownership and support exists both amongst grassroots staff at operational and practice level, as well as from staff at a managerial and strategic level. Support from legislative and policy directives can validate and sanction such moves. Without backing at this level, resources can be more difficult to acquire and the authority of the partnership can be undermined. Partnerships that are driven by enthusiastic individuals may be valid and effective, but if they lack strategic support, they can soon be left floundering once key personnel leave.

7. Establish the basis and boundaries of the partnership

This is a difficult issue to explore and may seem inappropriate, but the 'what if' questions need exploring in order to be clear about the basis and boundaries of the partnership. The range of issues that may occur are wide ranging, but common issues may include:

- Can agencies withdraw from the partnership at any stage without notice?
- Are agencies able to compete independently to bid for contracts that the partnership may be also bidding for?
- Should agreements concerning service delivery be signed to form a legally binding contract?
- If legal or financial problems occur for the partnership, do all agencies share the burden equally?

8. Maintain identity and difference

Agencies form partnerships to work closely together and gain benefit from what the other partner agencies can offer. There is a risk, however, that agencies who form a partnership could lose their focus and identity to a new corporate identity. A shared identity does help integration, so partners no longer see their separate identities as so significant. This does, however, present a constant tension within partnerships as the creation of a new single corporate agency could risk losing the benefits afforded by the many different agencies working together. This may be a particular issue for partnerships that unite together in shared premises, such as Drug Teams or Youth Offending Teams. While partnerships should not be discouraged on account of this, the risk of agencies losing their identity needs to be acknowledged.

9. Promote corporate identity

Agencies working collaboratively together in partnership may rigorously defend their own distinct identity, which arguably strengthens the partnership, but there needs to be a corporate identity too, which is widely understood and promoted. If agencies are so busy promoting their own identity who is promoting the partnership? One agency could take on this role but that may lead to a power imbalance. All could share the role but that would necessitate a considerable depth of understanding by all agency partners to avoid mixed messages. One solution to this problem is the appointment of an independent Chair who has no allegiance to any single agency, can steer meetings, and is able to act as a consultant promoting the partnership to outside bodies.

10. Concentrate on process not just practice

In a climate of centralized bureaucracy and managerialism that is preoccupied by objectives, targets, deliverables and outcomes, there is a danger of losing sight of the needs of the client. Practice with clients driven by procedures can sometimes lead to 'empty' relationships in which staff go through all the right motions but fail to meet the client's real need. The evidence in this book suggests clients do not want to receive a service that leaves them feeling like they had just been processed along a conveyor belt in the health and social care factory. It is clear that clients are concerned about the way in which they are treated and not just about what services they receive. Clients want 'human-friendly' services that are delivered by agency staff who have a genuine empathy and understanding of their situation and who are able to communicate clearly, honestly and respectfully.

11. Involve and listen to service users

There are few partnerships who properly involve service users in the running of them. It is easy for agencies to lose sight of the needs of clients while building the partnership. Service-user involvement can help to address this problem and hold agencies to account by reminding them of why they exist. Service users can also provide valuable insights into their needs, which are not always fairly or comprehensively understood by agency representatives. It is easy for agencies to make erroneous assumptions about the needs of clients, or develop unfair stereotypes or prejudices. This is less likely to occur if service users are able to participate actively in the partnership. In order to enable service users to participate on an equal basis, partnerships may consider employing service users to work in the partnership, perhaps on a part-time basis. This also addresses the problem of service users being unfairly expected to give up a lot of time on a voluntary basis.

12. Guard against exploitation and power imbalance

Partnerships bring together a wide range of agencies; some may have considerable resources, a high percentage of qualified staff, and excellent administrative support, while other partner agencies may be largely dependent upon unqualified staff and volunteer administrative support. It is easy in these circumstances for the larger agencies to dominate the partnership and stifle the contribution of smaller agencies. Whenever possible, partners should be equal, when they are not, the basis and rationale for inequality needs to be openly established and agreed. Equality in partnership does, however, raise structural conflicts related to historical and largely fixed differences between partners concerning terms and conditions of service, leading to wide variations in the partnership in relation to qualifications, salaries, pay, pensions and annual leave.

13. Clarify the boundaries of confidentiality

This is a perennial issue that should not be avoided as it will eventually emerge when a serious issue arises. To what extent can agencies share information across the partnership, and precisely what information can be shared? Guidelines need to be established regarding sharing of information across boundaries and data protection. Signed consent from clients should also be obtained.

14. Evaluate the success of partnerships

It cannot be assumed that because partnerships are formed, they are working effectively. Factors such as different identities, different educational qualifications, different working conditions, as well as differences in vision, mission and cultures in organizations can all play a part in limiting effectiveness. Mechanisms are needed, therefore, at all levels of each organization within the partnership to ascertain effectiveness. Questions that could be asked within the evaluation include:

- Does each partner have equal commitment to the partnership and, if so, how is this demonstrated?
- Does the partnership promote ethical standards within its working practices?
- How is effective practice promoted and maintained throughout the partnership?
- How are professional conflicts between partners managed?
- Does the partnership have a corporate identity that is shared across agencies inside and outside the partnership?
- Does the partnership adequately take into account the need for comparable working conditions for comparable grades of staff?
- Is joint training in operation where needed?
- What are the service users' views and experiences of the partnership?
- What gaps in service delivery can be identified?
- What are the training needs of partner members?

Conclusion

This book seeks to help fill the current knowledge gap concerning the nature, context and form of partnerships. Part 1 explored the context within which partnerships operate. Part 2 looked at a partnership approach to tackling some of the most pressing and difficult health and social issues in the UK. We have been able to highlight many examples of partnership currently in existence responding to complex needs, such as homelessness, domestic violence, travellers, and so on. The benefits and challenges involved in working in partnership have been carefully explored throughout. Our key concern is to develop 'effective practice', which actually makes a difference to the lives of vulnerable people in need. In many situations, this is best achieved by agencies working collaboratively together in partnership. We hope that the key principles we have presented in this final chapter offer a way forward for developing successful partnerships.

Index

Page numbers in *italics* refer to boxes, *n* indicates chapter note.

KEY CONCEPTS AND DEBATES IN HEALTH AND SOCIAL POLICY

Nigel Malin, Stephen Wilmot and Jill Manthorpe

This book identifies key social policy concepts and explores their relevance for health and welfare policy, and for the practice of professionals such as nurses and social workers who are involved in the delivery of services and provision. The text adopts ideologies of welfare approach using examples of recent policy shifts to illustrate theoretical and political tensions. This shift in emphasis away from the traditional approach of documenting policy areas is an important feature of the book. The concepts are organized in terms of doctrinal contests. This allows the authors to explore the tension between different approaches and ways of defining social policy. The aim is to help professionals identify these tensions, to be aware of the strategic choices which have been made in national and agency policy, and to locate their own practice in relationship to these choices. It draws upon the continuing debate around the Third Way and New Labour policies as they apply to health and social welfare; and identifies tensions within a non-ideological, pragmatic set of practices.

Key Concepts and Debates in Health and Social Policy has been written with students and practitioners in mind. It is a valuable resource for a wide range of health and welfare professionals, especially in nursing, social work and occupational therapy. It is also suitable for use on professional training courses, and with students of social policy and health studies.

Contents
Introduction – The Third Way: a distinct approach? – Identifying the Health Problem: need or risk? – Responsibility and Solidarity – Consumerism or Empowerment? – Central Planning and Market Competition – Controlling Service Delivery: professionalism versus managerialism – Community Care and Family Policy – Evaluating Services: quality assurance and the quality debate – Prioritizing and Rationing – Conclusion – Index.

176pp   0 335 19905 4 (Paperback)   0 335 19906 2 (Hardback)

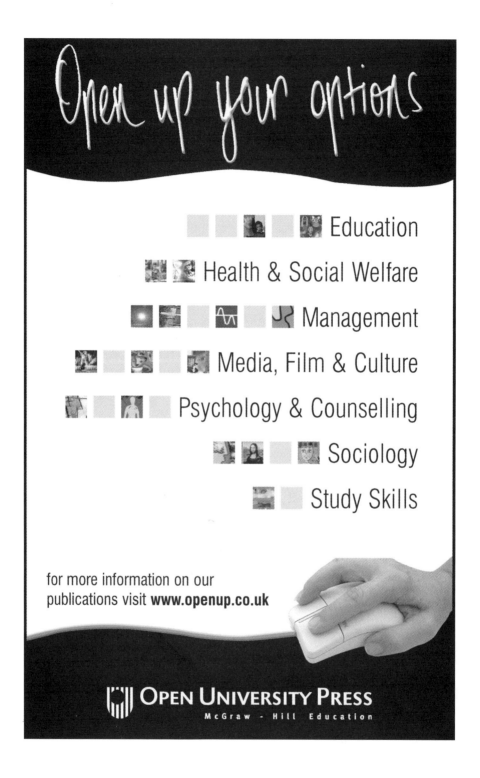